BALANCING
EMPATHY
AND
INTERPRETATION

BALANCING EMPATHY AND INTERPRETATION

Relational Character Analysis

by Lawrence Josephs, Ph.D.

JASON ARONSON INC.
Northvale, New Jersey
London

The author gratefully acknowledges permission to reprint the following:

Selected excerpts from *The Collected Papers, Volume 2* by Sigmund Freud. Authorized translation under the supervision of Joan Riviere. Published by Basic Books, Inc. by arrangement with Hogarth Press and the Institute of Psycho-Analysis, London. Reprinted by permission of Basic Books, a division of HarperCollins Publishers, Inc.

Selected excerpts from *The Standard Edition of The Complete Psychological Works of Sigmund Freud*, translated and edited by James Strachey. Reprinted by permission of Sigmund Freud Copyrights, the Institute of Psycho-Analysis, and Hogarth Press.

Production Editor: Elaine Lindenblatt

This book was set in 10 point Palacio by TechType of Upper Saddle River, New Jersey, and printed and bound by Haddon Craftsmen of Scranton, Pennsylvania.

Library of Congress Cataloging-in-Publication Data

Josephs, Lawrence.
   Balancing empathy and interpretation: relational character analysis / by Lawrence Josephs.
      p. cm.
   Includes bibliographical references and index.
   ISBN 1-56821-447-2
   1. Typology (Psychology) 2. Psychoanalytic interpretation.
   3. Empathy. 4. Personality assessment. 5. Intersubjectivity.
   I. Title.
   RC489.T95J67   1995
   616.89–dc20   94-46147

Manufactured in the United States of America. Jason Aronson Inc. offers books and cassettes. For information and catalog write to Jason Aronson Inc., 230 Livingston Street, Northvale, New Jersey 07647.

To Aaron and Matthew

CONTENTS

Acknowledgments ix

Introduction xi

Part I: Psychoanalytic Technique 1

  1: Working from Surface to Depth 3

  2: Reichian Character Analysis 25

  3: Defense Analysis and the Therapeutic Alliance 43

  4: The Principle of Multiple Function and the Structural Model 77

  5: From Ego-syntonicity to Self-syntonicity 105

  6: The Analysis of Transference 143

  7: The Analysis of Countertransference 169

Part II: Relational Character Analysis 195

  8: Impression Management and the Need to Be Seen as Normal 197

  9: Strategic Thought in the Analysis of Defense 233

  10: Personal Idiom and the Principle of Identity Maintenance 275

  11: Sadomasochism, Perversity, and the Unconscious Sense of Self 305

12: Role Reversibility and the Bipolarity of Self
      and Object Experience   329

13: Ambience and Interpretation   375

Conclusion   397

References   417

Index   423

ACKNOWLEDGMENTS

I wish to thank Ona Nierenberg, M.A., for her deconstructionist reading of my book. She questioned my unquestioned assumptions, forcing me to clarify and sharpen my arguments. I owe Dr. Joel Weinberger a special debt of gratitude for enabling me to see where and how my thinking was more original and dialectical than I had consciously realized. As always, my greatest support has been Dr. Laura Josephs, who has unfailingly encouraged me through innumerable revisions and self-doubts. And Aaron and Matthew Josephs have been an incredible delight throughout the entire process.

INTRODUCTION

To speak of *empathic character analysis* could seem like an oxymoron to those who associate the term *character analysis* with the approach of Wilhelm Reich (1933). Reich advocated a confrontational method of resistance analysis that was seen by contemporaries such as Fenichel (1953) and Sterba (1953) as unduly adversarial, provocative of negative transference, and injurious to the patient's narcissism. Ego psychologists went on to refine the technique of character analysis in emphasizing such ideas as developing a working alliance and analyzing resistance to the awareness of resistance by carefully working from surface to depth. These refinements were thought to add the essential elements of tact, timing, and dosage that seemed to be lacking in Reich's approach. Nevertheless, Kohut (1984) criticized what he labeled the "penetration-to-the-unconscious-via-the-overcoming-of-resistances model" (p. 113), which he believed characterized the classical approach to treatment even with its ego-psychological emendations, the tradition in which Kohut was originally trained.

Kohut (1984) contrasted the traditional approach to defense/resistance/character analysis with his own approach in which he conceived "so-called defense-resistances" as "valuable moves to safeguard the self, however weak and defensive it may be, against destruction and invasion" (p. 141). If resistance is to be understood as a developmental necessity to be tolerated and appreciated, then any approach that questions, challenges, or confronts the patient's resistance—no matter how tactful, well timed, or carefully dosed—is likely to be experienced as lacking in empathy. Kohut's approach was to maintain an empathic stance, a stance in which the analyst attempts to consistently interpret from within the patient's subjective frame of reference or point of view.

The basic technique of character analysis, making the ego-syntonic ego-dystonic, would seem to be incompatible with the self psychological approach as Kohut developed it, as it requires questioning, challenging, and confronting the patient's point of view. By remaining committed to the empathic stance, the self psychological analyst attempts to studiously avoid invalidating the patient's subjective reality or imposing the analyst's external frame of reference on the patient as though the analyst's viewpoint constituted an authoritative objective reality in contrast to the patient's unrealistic perceptions. Lichtenberg and colleagues (1992) stated, "An inherent contradiction exists between the empathic mode of perception and the traditional treatment of defenses by confrontation and interpretation. . . . [D]efenses and defense mechanisms tend to be dealt with from the perspective of the outside observer . . . the inherently oppositional stance (regardless of tone) of the penetrator of deceptions and the searcher for hidden secrets" (pp. 153-155).

Self psychologists imply that traditional approaches to defense, resistance, and character analysis are the antithesis of a genuinely empathic analytic attitude. Classical analysts imply that self psychologists, in being overly sensitive to the patient's narcissistic vulnerabilities, work in a manner antithetical to the rigorous analysis of patients' unconscious character resistances and unconscious conflicts. Yet this controversy is not simply between self psychology and classical analysis, for it also informs the well-known debate between Kohut and Kernberg. In treating more severe character pathologies, to what extent should analysts actively confront and analyze primitive defenses such as splitting, projective identification, idealization, and devaluation versus empathize with the emergence of archaic selfobject needs?

This controversy also emerges in the tension between certain relational perspectives and self psychology. To what extent should analysis be a dynamic encounter between two clearly separate subjectivities whose different and conflicting perspectives and personalities are mutually analyzed versus a relationship in which the analyst's individuality is submerged as he or she becomes empathically immersed in the subjective world of the patient and is experienced as an attuned selfobject? If the patient treats the analyst as a narcissistic extension of the self, should it be analyzed as a resistance to acknowledging anxiety-laden unconscious perceptions of the analyst's individuality and countertransference, or should it be tolerated and empathically appreciated as a necessary developmental need? Contemporary Freudians and self psychologists also clash in regard to the dynamic tension between empathy and analysis. To what extent is self-experience rigorously analyzed as a compromise formation that serves multiple and conflicting functions versus empathically appreciated in terms of a superordinate function such as the need to affirm an essential sense of selfhood? The dynamic tension between empathy and analysis seems to inform a wide variety of contemporary controversies in regard to psychoanalytic technique. Given these conflicting perspectives on the nature of the therapeutic process, how do we know what genuinely constitutes empathic analysis?

I believe that the attempt to empathically interpret from the patient's point of view is always an ideal endeavor, an aspiration that one may attempt to approximate but could never fully achieve, for the analyst cannot help but interpret the patient's point of view through the lens of the analyst's own subjective point of view. This insight seems to be the basis for Atwood and Stolorow's (1984) development of an intersubjective approach. The analyst inevitably interprets the patient's point of view in the light of the analyst's own preconceptions. Mitchell (1993) discussed the limitation of the phenomenological approach in psychoanalysis that attempts to capture and portray the patient's subjective experience without the imposition of the analyst's own theoretical assumptions. According to Mitchell, "The phenomenological solution, while decrying objectivism in any form, ironically represents the return of a naive realism. . . . Although the analyst as scientific observer has no privileged vantage point from which to discover the truth, it is assumed that the patient does, and the analyst has the power to know what the patient knows, even if the patient is not aware of it herself" (p. 54). As Schafer (1983) noted, analysts create as well as discover their facts.

Kohut's (1959) definition of empathy as "vicarious introspection" does not seem to take full account for the fact that introspection, be it vicarious or otherwise, is not simply an act of scientific discovery but is also an act of interpretation that reflects the implicit organizing principles of the person doing the introspection. Kohut (1984) defined empathy as a "value-neutral tool of observation which can lead to correct or incorrect results" and "as 'vicarious introspection' . . . one person's attempt to experience the inner life of another while simultaneously retaining the stance of an objective observer" (p. 175). I would question whether it is possible to empathically understand another in a value-neutral way that does not express the observer's subjective biases. I would also question whether it is possible to so clearly judge the correctness or incorrectness of one's empathic observations as though standards for assessing the validity of an observation were not open to debate.

Even self psychologists who think of themselves as "constructionists," such as Lichtenberg and colleagues (1992), seem to believe that they can mitigate the effect of their preconceptions on the analytic process. In their discussions of "empathic perception," they highlight the element of discovery rather than of creativity. To speak of empathic *perception* rather than of empathic *understanding* seems to imply something that approximates direct access to the patient's subjective experience although we know that even the act of perception is an act of construction. According to Lichtenberg and colleagues (1992), "We attempt to understand from within the perspective of the analysand and thereby mitigate (clearly not eliminate) the imposition of our perception of reality onto the analysand" (p. 118). They seem to imply that this situation is something over which the analyst has some degree of control rather than consider the possibility that the analyst's perception of reality saturates the clinical encounter. Perhaps there is no understanding of the patient that is not achieved through the imposition of the analyst's preconceptions.

I would suggest that the patient at some level, consciously or unconsciously, is always cognizant of the fact that the analyst's attempts at empathy consistently embody the organizing influence of the analyst's preconceptions. The patient cannot help but recognize that the analyst's mind applies different principles of organization than the patient's mind. As a consequence, the patient is at some level consistently reacting to that difference, curious yet fearful of the nature of the analyst's preconceptions to which the patient's subjective universe will be assimilated. It usually does not take too long for a patient in analysis to reliably predict in advance how the analyst is likely to interpret the patient's material. Despite the analyst's attempt to empathize with the patient's subjective point of view without imposing preconceived notions, the patient nevertheless plausibly experiences the analyst as assimilating the patient's material according to some preconceived story lines and narrative traditions.

Case reports in the clinical literature illustrate the analyst's deployment of preferred story lines. Case reports as a literary genre tend to be fairly predictable from the theoretical orientation of the writer in terms of the way the story is likely to end, for there is rarely a surprise ending. Spence (1987) likened the psychoanalytic case history to a Sherlock Holmes novel in which the mystery is always solved in the end. In looking at psychoanalysis as a narrative endeavor, Schafer (1983) suggested that there are Freudian story lines, Kohutian story lines, Kleinian story lines, and so on. Each analyst possesses a preferred set of story lines, each with its own understanding of the nature of the patient's subjectivity. From a narrative perspective, it becomes difficult to argue that one story line is more objective, empathic, or experience-near than another. Comparisons reflect aesthetic sensibilities more than anything else.

The analyst's application of a preconceived narrative tradition exerts an interactional pressure on the patient in analysis that tends to evoke certain subjective states in the patient while leaving dormant other potential subjective states. The analyst's witting or unwitting application of his or her own theoretical preconceptions evokes the very material that those theoretical preconceptions seek to explain. The analyst's attempts to function as a person who consistently interprets the world from the patient's subjective point of view without imposing preconceptions tend to evoke in the patient the experience of the analyst as an extension of the self. The empathic approach of Kohut diminishes experiences of the analyst as a separate person with a mind of his or her own. The patient may react to that lack of separateness positively as a benign, nonintrusive presence or negatively as a distressing lack of personal presence. In contrast, a character-analytic approach exerts a virtually opposite inter-actional pressure. It evokes in the patient the experience of the analyst as a separate person with a view of reality quite distinct from the patient's point of view. The patient may perceive the analyst's separateness positively as a thought-provoking encounter that facilitates envisioning the self from novel and multiple perspectives or negatively as a persecu-tory imposition of an invalidating and alien reality. Different patients will respond to different interpretive frameworks/ interactive styles differently. Yet each interpretive framework/ interactive style pushes the patient to respond in a general direction in keeping with the analyst's expectations.

Often the idea of clinical technique is understood as a set of hard-and-fast rules concerning the proper or right way to conduct a psychoanalysis. For this reason many clinicians eschew the idea that the conduct of a psychoanalysis can be boiled down to a technique, for it seems to imply treating all patients identically. In treating patients in some rigidly pre-scribed manner, the analyst denies the individuality of the patient and the uniqueness of the particular analytic dyad. Yet if it is acknowledged that all analysts cannot help but work with patients in the light of their theoretical preconcep-tions, then one crucial aspect of their preconceptions is their implicit theory of technique. Technique, in this sense, is not so much a prescribed set of rules as it as an implicit strategy of engaging the patient in an analytic process, a strategy that derives from one's theoretical beliefs. When Freud likened the technique of psychoanalysis to a game of chess, he was implying that the analyst as well as the patient were strate-gists engaged in a game of move and countermove. To discuss principles of technique is to discuss clinical strategies that will determine the analyst's moves. To deny that the analyst possesses and implements such clinical strategies in the treatment situation is to portray the analyst as only a passive, receptive processor of the patient's material with no intentional agenda of his or her own. Since the analyst's implicit clinical strategy or agenda is an important aspect of the analyst's personal participation, exerting a powerful interactional pressure on the patient, it is important for the analyst to recognize its presence and assess its impact.

Each interpretive framework and the clinical technique derived from that framework tends to evoke and highlight certain dimensions of subjective experience while concurrently diminishing others. Though interpretive frameworks are often conceived as all-encompassing explanatory systems that leave no aspect of human subjectivity unexplained, each interpretive framework is more like a spotlight sharply focusing attention on a particular phenomenon while simultaneously leaving in the dark all that exists outside the perimeter of the spotlight. Each interpretive framework results in a kind of tunnel vision. For example, character analysis tends to highlight the patient's existence as a character but downplays the patient's existence as a self. In contrast, self psychology tends to highlight the patient's existence as a self but downplays the patient's existence as a character. I believe that people exist as both characters and selves. Character and self are both holistic concepts that refer to the person's existence as an integrated unit, but each concept looks at the whole person from contrasting frames of reference. To look at a person as a character is to conceive the person from an external frame of reference as an object in the eyes of others, whereas to look at the person as a self is to conceive the person from a subjective frame of reference as a subject from the person's own point of view. Character analysis objectifies the patient, whereas self psychology subjectifies the patient. To the extent we all exist and relate to each other as subjects as well as objects, each approach could be said to encapsulate a limited vision of the potentials of the clinical encounter.

The issue tends to become polarized because of certain anxieties that the clinical encounter evokes in the practitioner. When the clinical emphasis is on empathizing with the patient's point of view, there is a tendency to worry about the dangers of objectifying the patient. An effort is made to minimize the possibility that an authoritarian dogmatic analyst could impose a false reality to which the patient would be forced to submit. The clinical emphasis on empathic understanding serves to avoid that dreaded possibility. In contrast, when the emphasis is on addressing unconscious defensive activity, there is a tendency to worry about the dangers of subjectifying the patient. The prospect of a naive analyst taking everything the patient says at face value is alarming. In unconsciously colluding with the patient's unconscious character resistances, the analysis remains stuck at a superficial level. A clinical emphasis on character analysis attempts to avoid that dreaded possibility by consistently interpreting the patient's ego-syntonic and ego-dystonic character resistances.

Clinical technique need not become so polarized an issue. A dialectical approach that allows the analyst to move freely back and forth between two technical stances may allow the analyst to avoid the twin dangers of being a "bull in a china shop" on the one hand and "handling the patient with kid gloves" on the other. If the analyst feels free to challenge, question, or confront the patient's point of view, the analyst should also feel free to empathize with what it is like for the patient to work with a challenging, questioning, and confrontative analyst. Wachtel (1993) suggested that clinicians must learn how to reconcile the conflicting poles of affirmation and change without burying the contradictions between the two and without overidentifying with one pole or another. He warned that "without the therapist acting in certain respects as an agent for an alternative point of view, without her challenges—usually gentle, but necessarily persistent—to the patient's familiar, if not always comfortable assumptions, change will at best be slow and precarious and may well be deterred altogether" (p. 136).

The dialectical approach I am advocating might seem at first glance to be an approach that is inconsistently empathic rather than consistently empathic, as though it were acceptable to be alternately empathic and unempathic as long as there is sufficient empathy for one's regular lapses of empathy. I believe that this only seems to be the case if one is content with the standard colloquial definition of empathy: seeing the world from the patient's point of view. This common-sense definition of empathy is a circumscribed one. To say that patients possess a point of view is to imply that they possess a singular and unitary point of view. In discussions of empathy it is not always said that one must empathize with the patient's "points" (i.e., plural) of view. I doubt I will find much opposition to the argument that patients possess multiple points of view—some conscious, some unconscious, and some conflicting. Mitchell (1993) suggested that the most enduring and important discovery of psychoanalysis was that "[a]ll of us have multiple, conflictual perspectives, many of which are unconscious or preconscious; one's perspective on past and present is always context-dependent and changes according to motivational and affective state; and one's perspective varies a great deal depending on the other to whom it is being spoken and the purpose for which it is being expressed" (p. 53) According to Mitchell, consciousness is fragmentary, discontinuous, and much too complex and inaccessible to be captured in a singular, true report.

The implication of patients' possession of multiple viewpoints is not always incorporated in discussions of empathy. The implication is that whenever one is empathizing with one point of view, this approach may be experienced as an implicit lack of empathy for the opposing point of view. For example, to empathize consistently with the patient's experience as a subject could be felt as a lack of empathy for the patient's experience as an object. Thus, to empathize with one point of view at the expense of a different point of view could be felt as taking sides. The classical concept of technical neutrality addresses exactly this issue, that one should have empathy and consideration for all sides of a conflict.

Kohutian self psychology could be said to be taking the side of viewing the person as a subject as opposed to viewing the person as an object. Curiously, though, Kohut drew attention to the fact that the sense of self in part comes from the outside, from the infant's internalization of its reflection in the mother's eyes. The mother as mirror of the infant's

personhood is always filtering that personhood through the
lens of her own preconceived notions. As a developmental
process we learn to see ourselves as others see us—what
sociologists such as Mead (1934) called the "looking glass
self." We are a "me" (i.e., an object) prior to becoming an "I"
(i.e., a subject): "I learn to see my 'self' as others have seen
'me'" (p. 201). The subjective sense of self derives from an
identification with the other's perceptions of the self. Thus
how others see us, how others objectify us, and how others
characterize us become an essential component of self-
experience.

Character analysis in the most general sense (i.e., not
Reich's particular approach) reflects the analyst's *characterization* of the patient, how the analyst perceives the patient from
an external frame of reference. Inevitably the analyst will
characterize the patient, and that characterization will reflect
the analyst's preconceived ways of characterizing people in
general. I would suggest that every analyst possesses as one
important component of their preconceptions an implicit
character typology through which the patient is prereflectively characterized. It is a pretense to believe that the analyst
can somehow relate to the patient in a manner that suspends
such evaluative judgments and that spares the patient the
experience of being characterized by the analyst as being a
such-and-such kind of person. Despite the aspiration to
appreciate the patient as a unique individual on his or her
own terms and from the patient's own subjective point of
view, the analyst as an external observer cannot understand
the patient except through the prism of the analyst's own
objectifying characterizations of the patient.

Everything the analyst says to the patient, every interpretation, either explicitly or implicitly communicates what the
analyst's characterization of the patient is. For this reason, all
analysis is character analysis, a process in which the patient is
confronted with the analyst's explicit and implicit characterizations of the patient's personality. Given this state of
affairs, one should not think of character analysis as some
anachronistic approach to treatment developed in the 1920s
by Wilhelm Reich, an approach that has no relevance to

contemporary psychoanalysis with its relational emphases. From a relational perspective it becomes apparent that the therapeutic dyad is immersed in a process of mutual characterization that is often denied. Character analysis occurs in a relational context and is a relational process. Thus we may speak of *relational character analysis*. To fully grasp the omnipresent character-analytic dimension of treatment, contemporary analysts need to become reacquainted with and learn from old ideas about character analysis (i.e., Reich's work as well as that of other ego psychologists like Fenichel) and rework those old ideas in the light of contemporary developments.

The old focus on character also dovetails nicely with the modern focus on narrative. Story lines are populated by a cast of characters. With all the contemporary discussion of psychoanalysis as a narrative endeavor in which patient and analyst collaboratively co-author the patient's life story, few theorists have considered the fact that developing a narrative requires creating a variety of portraitures of the cast of characters in the patient's life story, the main character being the patient's own self. Thus there is no such thing as narrative construction without character analysis. With all the discussion of constructivism in the contemporary literature, rarely noted is that what is constructed in the analytic situation is primarily characterizations of the characters of the two participants involved.

In attempting to grasp what constitutes empathic character analysis, we must address another problem with the standard definition of empathy (i.e., seeing the world from the patient's point of view). The standard definition assumes that it is possible to clearly differentiate the patient's perspective from the analyst's perspective. After all, the analyst can only grasp the patient's point of view through the filtering lens of the analyst's own preconceptions. The analyst's empathic formulations cannot help but reveal as much about the analyst's own preconceptions as it reveals something about the patient's subjective universe. As Mitchell (1993) put it, a portrait reveals as much about the personal sensibility and vision of the artist as it reveals the character of its subject.

The subjective universe with which the analyst empathizes is also in part evoked by the analyst's interpretive framework and interactive style. The patient's viewpoint with which the analyst empathizes is not something entirely separate from the analyst but rather something that has been shaped in part by the analyst. Similarly, the analyst's point of view is never entirely reducible to the analyst's preconceptions alone, for the patient evokes the analyst's subjective experiences just as the analyst evokes the patient's subjective experiences. The analytic dyad is mutually evocative so that subjective states are interactively constructed. It becomes difficult to differentiate the separate contributions of each party to the structure of the evolving relationship. Beebe and Lachmann (1992) approached the study of the mother–infant relationship from a dyadic systems view in which the dyad is conceived as mutually evocative of subjective states. Subjective experience is understood as cocreated through a process of mutual influence.

If character analysis is broadly defined as the analyst's verbally explicit communication of his or her characterizations of the patient, then character analysis is simply a form of communication that is neither intrinsically empathic nor unempathic. Character analysis entails making explicit what is always being communicated implicitly through the analyst's interpretations and interactive style, the analyst's characterization of the patient. What makes for empathic character analysis is the analyst's willingness to acknowledge possessing characterizations of the patient, to take responsibility for what is evoked in the patient by such characterizations, to acknowledge that those characterizations reflect the analyst's preconceptions, and to be curious about what it is like for the patient to be characterized according to the analyst's preconceived notions. Unempathic character analysis transpires when the analyst denies possessing characterizations of the patient, when the analyst refuses to take responsibility for what the analyst's characterizations have evoked in the patient, when the analyst denies the preconceived notions embodied in the analyst's characterizations of the patient, and when the analyst has no appreciation of what it is like for the patient to be characterized according to the analyst's preconceived notions. According to these criteria, character analysis as it was practiced by Wilhelm Reich could be said to be unempathic. Yet there is nothing intrinsic to character analysis per se that makes it incompatible with an empathic stance if empathy is understood as encompassing attunement to multiple, unconscious, and conflicting points of view within a mutually evocative dyad.

Given this expanded definition of empathy, it is not clear that Kohut's self psychology is consistently empathic despite aspirations to the contrary. Not clear in Kohut's approach is the extent to which the patient is understood as potentially possessing multiple and conflicting viewpoints as opposed to primarily an essential unitary viewpoint. Not clear is the extent to which the analyst is understood as invariably constructing the patient's point of view through the lens of his or her own preconceived notions. Not clear is the extent to which the analyst's preconceived interpretive framework is understood as an interactive style that evokes the patient's self-experiences. If these criticisms have some degree of validity and if they have not been fully addressed by contemporary developments in self psychology that are moving in a more interactive direction, then it could be said that the self psychological approach may be lacking in empathy for some of the patient's multiple, unconscious, and conflicting perspectives and for the patient's experience of the analyst's preconceived characterizations. And when Kohut characterized his patients' selves as strong or weak, cohesive or fragmented, grandiose or devalued, elated or deflated, and so on, he was objectifying their self-experience and therefore implicitly doing character analysis.

The benefit of the character-analytic approach is that it requires the analyst to articulate a verbally explicit formulation of just what the analyst's preconceived characterization of the patient is. The patient is then free to confront, challenge, question, ponder, refute, refine, and/or assimilate the analyst's characterizations, be they flattering or unflattering. The danger of the character-analytic approach is the extent to which the patient does not feel free to confront,

question, or challenge the analyst's characterizations but
rather feels forced to accept them at face value. The character-
analytic approach reflects the Socratic method in psychoanalysis. A questioning and curious attitude as well as a healthy
skepticism on the part of both the patient and the analyst can
generate a thought-provoking atmosphere conducive to appreciating familiar things from novel perspectives. Seeing the
world from the patient's point of view and respecting its
validity versus exposing the limits of that point of view
through confrontation with novel and multiple perspectives
need not be considered two irreconcilable analytic stances
between which an analyst should be forced to choose.
Instead, a dialectic can be achieved in which the analyst
experiences the flexibility and freedom to oscillate between
these polar opposite positions and thereby achieve a dynamic
balance. Overemphasis on one approach or another could be
seen as a sort of cognitive rigidity reflecting an inability to
maintain a dynamic balance between polar opposites. Instead, one pole is valorized as the other pole is devalued.

If the analyst is granted an equivalent metapsychology to
the patient, then it must be stated that the analyst does not
empathize with the patient through the lens of any unitary or
completely coherent set of preconceived notions. Rather, the
analyst possesses multiple preconceived notions—some conscious, some unconscious, and some conflicting. Analysts,
therefore, possess several empathic constructions of the
patient's subjective universe and several characterizations of
the patient as an objective other. Interpretations then reflect
compromise formations between conflicting understandings
of the patient. Analysts are unconscious pluralists despite
some analysts' conscious efforts to strive to be relative pur-
ists. Through what sorts of implicit organizing principles do
analysts prereflectively organize their unconscious pluralism
in which contradictory points of view coexist? Do conflicting
views become polarized, leading to an either/or approach, or
do conflicting views become condensed, leading to a mixed-
model approach? Or are there other options such as a
dialectical approach in which opposites are either juxtaposed

and held in dynamic balance or deconstructed as false dichotomies?

This book is about character analysis, but it is not *only* about character analysis. To some extent I utilize the term *empathic character analysis* as a concrete symbolization that reifies and dramatizes the dynamic tension between empathy and analysis in psychoanalytic theory and practice. To a psychoanalytic audience, the word *empathy* associatively evokes the work of Heinz Kohut, and the term *character analysis* associatively evokes the work of Wilhelm Reich. The names *Kohut* and *Reich* have come to have an emotionally charged symbolic valence among psychoanalysts, deservedly or not—Kohut representing the extreme "warm-hearted" end and Reich the extreme "hard-headed" end of the clinical spectrum. To combine Reich and Kohut into one mixed metaphor, then, is not such an odd hybrid (i.e., an oxymoron) if one is trying to balance the hard and the soft, the warm and the cold, the confrontational and the supportive, the intellectual and the emotional in psychoanalytic theory and practice.

Though at a concrete level this book is about empathic character analysis, at a more abstract level the book illustrates a dialectical method of addressing the dynamic tension between the new and relational in psychoanalytic theory and practice and the old and individualistic. To speak of *relational character analysis* is to attempt to meld one person and two person psychologies. I try to look alternately at clinical issues through conflicting theoretical frames of reference, attempting to juxtapose seemingly opposite and contradictory points of view. I then try to articulate a way of working that is not either/or but that tolerates the dynamic tension of oscillating between alternative and conflicting ways of looking at and working with the same issue. Sometimes I try to sustain if not heighten the paradox; sometimes I try to resolve the paradox by demonstrating that irreconcilable differences are based on false dichotomies. I try to maintain a dialectical tension between tolerating paradox and resolving paradox and between tolerating ambiguity and clarifying ambiguity. I use the mixed metaphor of empathic character analysis as a vehicle for the application of my dialectical methodology.

My mission in this book is to demonstrate how a traditional approach to character analysis is still relevant and necessary to contemporary psychoanalytic practice but to note also that it can be improved by applying some of the innovative ideas of contemporary psychoanalysis. Too often it seems that in discussing the shortcomings of classical psychoanalysis, of which there are many, critics tend to throw out the baby with the bathwater. I believe that traditional character analysis needs contemporary psychoanalysis and vice versa, that each is impoverished without a consideration of the other so that some rapprochement is sorely needed. To me the classical approach to character analysis highlights a rigorous analytical approach to the conduct of treatment that focuses on the intrapsychic, interpretation, and insight. Classical approaches tend to focus on principles of technique that offer a rationale for the orderly sequencing or timing of one's interpretations in order to avoid *wild analysis*.

Contemporary approaches tend to highlight the countertransferential and interactional aspects of the treatment situation that make empathy and new relational experiences more central in the analytic dialogue. Contemporary approaches emphasize the experiential in which the analyst is embedded in the give and take of the therapeutic encounter. Classical approaches tend to require linear and hierarchical clinical reasoning (i.e., working from surface to depth or interpreting ego before id), whereas contemporary approaches tend to highlight analogical and dialectical reasoning (i.e., articulating evolving patterns of reciprocal influence in the transference–countertransference relationship). In addressing the issue of hierarchical versus dialectical clinical reasoning dialectically, it is possible to propose principles of analytic technique and orderly sequences of interpretation while counterbalancing that recommendation with the advocacy of an empathic immersion in the spontaneously arising dyadic relational experience.

I believe it is primarily the move from a one-person psychology to a two-person psychology that has led to contemporary clinicians' declining interest in the classical approach to character analysis, for character analysis may seem almost emblematic of an exclusively intrapsychic one-person approach. The one-person approach of traditional character analysis is both a weakness and a virtue. The strength of the traditional character-analytic approach was that it required the analyst to think through explicitly the nature of the patient's unconscious defensive strategies in all its intrapsychic and interpersonal complexity as it manifested itself as resistance in the transference. The weakness of this approach was in its lack of consideration of the analyst's contribution to the patient's unconscious defensiveness and its insufficient empathy for the patient's narcissistic vulnerability in having this defensiveness interpreted.

Sometimes the analyst's characterizations of the patient as an individual in his or her own right may become less complex as a result of shifting the focus of attention to the analyst's contribution to the patient's behavior in the analytic situation and censoring unflattering characterizations that might offend the patient's narcissism. I believe it is possible to maintain a focus on characterological complexity in an interactive context, one in which the analyst is free to develop both flattering and unflattering characterizations of the patient cognizant of the fact that such characterizations may wound as well as soothe the patient's narcissism (i.e., character affirmation as well as character assassination). If empathy encompasses empathy for the evocative impact of the analyst's unconscious on the patient's self-experiencing in the analytic situation and if one aspect of the analyst's unconscious consists of a variety of prereflective objectifications and characterizations of the patient, then it behooves the analyst to develop as verbally explicit and consciously thought-through characterizations of the patient as possible. The patient can then respond to these characterizations in a more explicit manner.

I believe a secondary reason for the decline of interest in character analysis has been the ascendancy of developmental models of the treatment situation, conceptualizing the analytic situation as analogous to a parent–child dyad, what Mitchell (1988) referred to as the "developmental tilt" (p. 151). In contrast, character analysis tends to focus on interpretation of the patient's character as it manifests itself in the here and now of the clinical encounter. As the patient tends to resist such an analysis, considerable analytic work transpires in the here and now prior to attempting to reconstruct the origins of the patient's character structure in the there and then. It is not possible to reconstruct the origins of something whose present structure is yet to be fully articulated.

Character analysis is unlikely to be construed by some developmentally oriented clinicians as a means of facilitating the unfolding of aborted or arrested development and is likely to be seen as a major impediment to such work. Character analysis can be seen as a "royal road" to the reexperiencing of childhood narcissistic trauma in the transference. Depending on one's outlook, that is either a danger or a virtue. I would suggest that the clinical efficacy of character analysis, especially if it is practiced empathically, is that it can move quickly to the essence of the patient's narcissistic vulnerability. As such, character analysis provides a powerful means of enabling the patient to reexperience and rework childhood narcissistic trauma in the transference in a manner that need not be retraumatizing. Analysis can proceed dialectically between resuming arrested development in a supportive atmosphere and working through narcissistic trauma in the transference. The two therapeutic processes are not mutually exclusive.

I have found that in being explicit about one's characterizations of the patient's character, one is particularly vulnerable to the criticism of being seen as typecasting the patient as though it were possible to characterize a patient without using any preconceived notions that exist independently of the patient. Yet it is inherent in the act of interpretation that the analyst is always characterizing the patient as being some type or other of person. Analysts invariably possess implicit character typologies through which their patients' self-reports are assimilated. It behooves the analyst to make as explicit as possible the nature of the underlying character typology through which he or she organizes an understanding of the patient as a person. An emphasis on the analyst's preconceptions tends to highlight the ways in which the data of analysis are created rather than discovered, and analysts have tended to feel more comfortable in characterizing themselves as discoverers like scientists rather than creators like artists. And each analyst, like each artist, possesses a distinctive style of character portraiture. For a more detailed look at the character typology I employ, the reader is referred to *Character Structure and the Organization of the Self* (Josephs 1992). In that work I conceptualize character structure in terms of a theory of multiple selves in conflict and compromise that I then apply in describing the major psychoanalytic character styles.

My approach to theory reflects a postmodern sensibility. I view each theoretical orientation not as true or false, right or wrong, but as a perspective based on implicit and not unquestionable assumptions, a way of seeing that highlights some issues while minimizing others. Though theories may reflect competing and conflicting points of view, I try to take turns looking at the process of psychoanalysis from alternative viewpoints so that each viewpoint has a voice in the ongoing dialogue. The end result will invariably be somewhat idiosyncratic as it will not be readily categorizable in terms of any of the preexisting schools of thought. Instead, it will reflect a spirited conversation between a wide variety of theoretical voices, old as well as new, with diverse sensibilities. I hope my approach will particularly resonate with the experience of younger clinicians who are confronted daily by the confusing pluralism of contemporary psychoanalysis. Thus my approach to character analysis is relational as it requires an ongoing dialogue between competing viewpoints.

To focus on character analysis will also prove to be a pragmatic focus, for the emphasis is on here-and-now personality functioning and personality change. In an era of managed care priorities, the only justification for long-term dynamic treatment is the treatment of the Axis II personality disorders. Despite the plethora of books on the treatment of borderline and narcissistic pathology, there is little in the recent literature regarding a contemporary psychoanalytic approach to treating personality or character disorders in general, an approach that would be broadly applicable to obsessive, hysterical, and depressive character pathologies as well as borderline and narcissistic conditions. Thus an exploration of the subtleties and intricacies of character analysis in the light of contemporary developments is a must for any clinician hoping to achieve personality change with patients.

In this book I hope to demonstrate the utility of a dialectical approach to grappling with some issues of comparative psychoanalytic theory and technique. When different approaches are presented as irreconcilable and inherently oppositional, the practitioner often feels forced to choose between competing ideologies that demand one's allegiance. The alternative, a mixed-model approach, is often less than satisfying because the mix may seem random and haphazard. In mixing apples and oranges one has a fruit salad, a hybrid or mongrel entity that may have increased clinical flexibility and practical utility but not the elegance or clarity of a pure breed. To be integrative seems pretentious because it implies having achieved some grand synthesis in which all the thorny epistemological loose ends have been tied up once and for all. To be dialectical, though, is to transcend the polarizations of the either/or approach, to have greater internal coherence than the mixed-model approach, but not to be so grandiose as to imply that all is seamlessly accounted for as in an integrative approach.

Of course the dialectical approach I am advocating is a preconceived way of ordering things that will have its inherent limitations, its own tunnel vision. It imposes an oppositional structure on the data in order to discover—or should we say *create*—inherent polarities. In this sense it might seem a little bit like defensive splitting in which issues are polarized in black and white terms in order to avoid seeing the shades of gray. A dialectical approach tends to assume that differences of opinion stand in polar opposition, although there is no reason to assume that difference neces-

sarily implies opposition. It assumes oppositions that may
later be demonstrated to be artificial or false dichotomies.
And assumptions are often made in terms of what are
superordinate oppositions and what are subordinate oppositions. Not everybody sees the same dialectics in the same
material.

For better or worse, I have chosen to pit analysis against
empathy as the superordinate polar opposite around which
my thinking will be organized. And I recognize that the
distinction between empathy and analysis is not always so
clear-cut. Empathy is never pure emotional intuition devoid
of cognitive appraisal, and analysis of another's inner life is
never purely a cognitive act of logical reasoning devoid of
personal emotional involvement. There is no such thing as
psychological analysis without empathy and no such thing as
empathic perception or understanding without psychological
analysis. Yet I believe that the dynamic tension between
empathy and analysis has led to much polarization of psychoanalytic theory and practice.

Though my recommendation in this book could be boiled
down to one simple idea, the need to maintain a dialectical
balance between empathy and analysis in the course of
treatment, it is a suggestion easy to make but difficult to
implement. This book is about the difficulty of achieving this
balance and even the ambiguity of knowing whether such a
balance has been achieved. It is a dynamic balance that is not
attained without struggle, and when it is attained, it will
inevitably be lost. It is a balance that must constantly be lost
and continually reachieved. To some extent, when it is found,
it is found through persistent experimentation, through trial
and error. And given that one person's dynamically balanced
approach may be another person's inherently skewed approach, it might be more apt to say that what we achieve is a
temporary illusion of dynamic balance in our clinical work.
Yet this seems to be the nature of progress in psychoanalysis,
to demonstrate the illusory nature of what had heretofore
been presumed to have been an incontrovertible reality.

To give a brief preview of what a dialectical approach might
look like, I will note the sorts of technical recommendations I

will be making as well as illustrating with clinical examples. In the beginning phase of treatment, it has long been acknowledged that the analyst must develop an alliance with the patient. However, it has also been noted that such an alliance may reflect the patient's unconscious passive compliance, thus constituting a resistance to deeper exploration. To work dialectically is to foster an alliance by empathically understanding the patient yet also to analyze the defensive function of needing to maintain the therapeutic relationship in a state of perfect empathic attunement. For the treatment to progress to the middle stage, it has been recognized that the patient must repeat, reexperience, and work through old traumas in the transference, yet it has also been recognized that the patient may need to have new developmental experiences with the analyst as a new object unlike the patient's parents. To work dialectically is to analyze self-dystonic character traits, thereby precipitating the reexperiencing of narcissistic trauma in the transference, yet also to empathize with the patient's experience of the analyst's empathic failure, thereby allowing the patient a new and healing experience. Throughout the book I will highlight a wide variety of technical controversies in psychoanalysis that could be appreciated as reflecting the dynamic tension between empathy and analysis. I will also propose a variety of dialectical solutions to these conflicting technical recommendations.

I

Psychoanalytic Technique

1

Working from Surface to Depth

In adopting a historical perspective in examining the development of psychoanalytic technique, I hope to be able to illustrate the relativity of what it means to be analytic and what it means to be empathic. Each theory of technique possesses its own conception of what constitutes empathy and what constitutes analysis. Psychoanalysts of all persuasions and all historical eras have believed they were empathic analysts, only to be seen in the light of new developments as having not been quite as empathic or analytic as they had assumed. Thus in telling the story of the evolution of psychoanalytic technique, I will also be describing the changing nature of what constitutes empathic analysis of the subjective life of the individual.

In doing a literature review that summarizes other theorists' work, their theories as well as their case studies, the person writing the summary is also inevitably interpreting those points of view in a manner reflecting his or her idiosyncratic personal perspective. Summarizing is an act of interpretation that is selective in what it includes and omits. And to the extent the summary involves paraphrasing the author rather than quoting the author verbatim, the author is no longer speaking in his or her own words but through the words of the person doing the summation. If the summary is also intended to lay the basis for a critical reading of the theorist's work, it raises the possibility of unconsciously and tendentiously misreading and misrepresenting the original material in order to erect a straw man that can then be unfairly knocked down. There is no way around the dilemma of the potential unfairness of the critic's reading of the original material. In psychoanalysis some theorists have uniformly felt severely misunderstood if not caricatured by their critics. For this reason, I have chosen to quote liberally from original works in order to let theorists speak in their own words and their own voice before I go on to present my reading of the material.

In discussing the case examples of other theorists, one is considering an abbreviated summary of a case report that is already a highly condensed and selective account of an actual treatment. Thus my criticisms of a case report may have little to do with what "actually" happened, as perhaps the issues I raise were well analyzed in the actual treatment but not presented in the case report either for lack of space or because the issue was not the focus of that particular clinical discussion. My point in critiquing case examples is not so much to offer supervisory advice as a "Monday morning quarterback" as it is to illustrate how case reports are entirely consistent with the clinician's theoretical point of view. I hope to demonstrate that the case report shares the same strengths and limitations, emphases and deemphases as does the theory it serves to illustrate. Case reports are not so much "facts" or "evidence" as they are dramatizations of abstract ideas about personality organization and the technique of treatment that the reader might find difficult to comprehend unless presented in concrete narrative form. Case reports thus reflect the dramatization of theoretical preconceptions so that if one employs a different set of preconceptions in examining a case report, one can generate an alternative and equally plausible dramatization of the same material. One can easily review the case reports of classical analysts and plausibly reinterpret the same material in light of the insights of contemporary psychoanalysis and vice versa.

If we examine Freud's papers on technique, we can see that he grappled with the tension between empathy and analysis in a variety of ways. On the one hand, Freud suggested that one should not interpret until rapport had been established through an unobjectionable positive transference. Yet as soon as one begins to analyze unconscious content, one begins to confront resistance and negative transference so that the rapport necessary for the patient being open to interpretation is diminished. On the other hand, if one fails to analyze unconscious content, the treatment remains stuck at the superficial level of the unobjectionable positive transference, which becomes a resistance to deeper exploration.

Freud hoped that if one interpreted from surface to depth and addressed resistance before content, then one would gradually be able to gain access to deeper material. Making the unconscious conscious was analogous to peeling the layers of an onion. Wild analysis and premature interpretation only exacerbated resistance. Yet well-timed and precise interpretation was insufficient, for Freud also recommended using the leverage of the patient's attachment to the analyst as a means of encouraging deeper exploration despite the patient's resistance. Though the emotional leverage of the patient's deference to the analyst's authority was thought of as a temporary expedient, Freud did not seem to be aware of or attempt to interpret the patient's experience of this sort of interpersonal pressure. He seemed to see it as a sort of temporary transference manipulation for a good cause, to make the unconscious conscious. For the sake of the progress of the analysis, Freud seemed to have lost empathy for the patient's experience of the analyst's interpretive authority.

We will examine in more detail Freud's struggle with this issue, how to make the unconscious conscious (i.e., how to analyze) without evoking so much resistance (i.e., loss of empathy) that the analysis founders. Freud's (1911, 1912a, 1912b, 1913, 1914b, 1915) seminal papers on technique, which provide the foundation of classical technique, were written primarily within the framework of his topographic and psychodynamic models, having been published prior to the introduction of the structural model in 1923. The development of the structural model did not lead Freud to reconceptualize or reconsider the fundamentals of analytic technique. Freud defined the goal of psychoanalysis in topographic terms—to make the unconscious conscious. In his papers on technique, Freud elucidated a variety of technical principles that can be summed up by two well-known aphorisms: that one should always work from surface to depth and that one should always interpret resistance before content. These aphorisms can be understood as recommendations concerning how to balance empathy with analysis. Before analyzing what is deep, one must have empathy for what is surface. And before analyzing unconscious content, one must have empathy for the patient's fears of revealing unconscious content, as such fears are expressed in the patient's resistance to self-revelation.

Resistance to free association was conceptualized as the main impediment to making the unconscious conscious. Initially, Freud viewed resistance as a surface phenomenon that prevented access to greater depth:

> The analyst should always be aware of the surface of the patient's mind at any given moment, that he should know what complexes and resistances are active in him at the time and what conscious reactions to them will govern his behaviour. [Freud 1911, p. 92]

> He contents himself with studying whatever is present for the time being on the surface of the patient's mind, and he employs the art of interpretation mainly for the purpose of recognizing the resistances which appear there, and making them conscious to the patient. [Freud 1914b, p. 147]

Resistance analysis was conceived as the primary interpretive technique through which the analyst worked to make the unconscious conscious. Resistance to the uncovering of unconscious content was a ubiquitous phenomenon. Freud found that patients would inhibit the flow of free associations and reject the analyst's interpretation of forbidden wishes and painful memories until the analyst had interpreted the patient's resistance to the awareness of such warded-off unconscious contents. Premature interpretation (i.e., interpreting too deeply) tended to exacerbate resistance and evoke negative transferences. In a paper on "wild analysis," Freud (1910) suggested, "The pathological factor is not his ignorance in itself, but the root of this ignorance in his inner resistances. . . . Informing the patient of his unconscious regularly results in an intensification of the conflict in him and an exacerbation of his troubles" (p. 225). To avoid the deleterious effects of premature interpretations, Freud made the following recommendations:

> First, the patient must, through preparation, himself have reached the neighbourhood of what he has repressed, and secondly, he must have formed a sufficient attachment (transference) to the physician for his emotional relationship to him to make a fresh flight impossible. [Freud 1910, p. 226]

> Even in the later stages of analysis one must be careful not to give a patient the solution of a symptom or the translation of a wish until he is already so close to it that he has only one short step more to make in order to get hold of the explanation for himself. [Freud 1913, p. 140]

Freud discovered that the major form of resistance was to be found in an examination of the transference, so that a consideration of the dynamics of transference became a central locus of analytic scrutiny.

> Over and over again, when we come near to a pathogenic complex, the portion of that complex which is capable of transference is first pushed forward into consciousness and defended with the greatest obstinacy. . . . These circumstances tend towards a situation in which finally every conflict has to be fought out in the sphere of transference. [Freud 1912b, p. 104]

To avoid premature interpretation of the transference or, perhaps to put it more precisely, transference-resistance, Freud (1913) gave this recommendation: "So long as the patient's communications and ideas run on without any obstruction, the theme of transference should be left untouched. One must wait until the transference, which is the most delicate of all procedures, has become a resistance" (p. 139).

Before transference can be interpreted as a resistance, however, a crucial preparatory phase must transpire if interpretation is to be effective.

> When are we to begin making our communications to the patient? . . . The answer can only be: Not until an effective transference has been established in the patient, a proper rapport with him. It remains the first aim of the treatment to attach him to it and to the person of the doctor. To ensure this, nothing need be done but to give him time. If one exhibits a serious interest in him, carefully clears away the resistances that crop at the beginning and avoids making certain mistakes, he will of himself form such an attachment. [Freud 1913, p. 139]

What makes for an effective interpretation is not only the correct content of the interpretation but the nature of the transference at the time the interpretation is made. "The patient, however, only makes use of the instruction in so far as he is induced to do so by the transference; and it is for this reason that our first communication should be withheld until a strong transference has been established" (Freud 1913, p. 144).

Freud's recommendations in regard to transference interpretation can seem contradictory, for Freud seems to pose a paradox: that transference is simultaneously the means of exerting a suggestive influence on the patient by virtue of the patient's attachment to the analyst yet also the major resistance to analysis. Through transference the patient develops an empathic connection to the analyst, yet through transference the patient resists the analysis of deeper material. Do we leave the transference alone to protect the patient's attachment to the analyst and the cooperation derived from that attachment, or do we interpret that transference as a resistance to the emergence of deeper material?

Transference serves as the primary resistance to analysis, since in the transference the patient tends to repeat in action the core unconscious conflicts rather than remember these conflicts and work them through in consciousness.

> We may say that the patient does not remember anything of what he has forgotten and repressed, but acts it out. He reproduces it not as a memory but as an action; he repeats it, without, of course, knowing that he is repeating it. . . . The greater the resistance, the more extensive will acting out (repetition) replace remembering. [Freud 1914b, pp. 150–151]

The "friendly or affectionate feelings which are admissible to consciousness and transference of prolongations of those feelings into the unconscious" (Freud 1912, p. 105) provide the analyst with the power of suggestion so that the analyst's interpretations are taken seriously and therefore can be used in the service of resistance analysis. "Transference to the doctor is suitable for resistance to the treatment only in so far as it is a negative transference or a positive transference of repressed erotic impulses" (p. 105). In summary, the analyst attempts to pit the unobjectionable positive transference, which is conscious, against the negative and erotic transferences, which tend to be unconscious and serve as resistance to free association.

To make the latent transference more accessible to consciousness, Freud (1914b) suggested that the analyst allow a "transference neurosis" to develop.

> We admit it into the transference as a playground in which it is allowed to expand in almost complete freedom and in which it is expected to display to us everything in the way of pathogenic instincts that is hidden in the patient's mind. . . . We regularly succeed in giving all the symptoms of the illness a new transference meaning and in replacing his ordinary neurosis by a transference neurosis. [p. 154]

Despite the intensification of the latent transference through a transference neurosis, the patient is still not particularly receptive to acknowledging this transference neurosis.

> The analyst had merely forgotten that giving the resistance a name could not result in its immediate cessation. One must

allow the patient time to become conversant with this resistance with which he has now become acquainted, to work
through it, to overcome it, by continuing, in defiance of it, the
analytic work according to the fundamental rule of analysis.
[Freud 1914b, p. 155]

At this point Freud's technical recommendations appear to
boil down to an appeal to be patient, tenacious, and persevering in hope that the patient's attachment to the analyst
will outweigh in the end the negative transference neurosis
intensified by the patient's frustrated erotic longings. Freud
depicted the working-through of the resistance as crystallized
in the transference neurosis as the crucial therapeutic process, yet it is a process that paradoxically may possess the
apparently deceiving appearance of a therapeutic impasse or
stalemate: "This working-through of the resistances may in
practice turn out to be an arduous task for the subject of the
analysis and a trial of patience for the analyst" (Freud 1914b,
p. 155). Making the unconscious conscious through the
emergence of the negative and erotic transferences evokes so
much resistance (i.e., loss of empathic connection) that the
analysis seems close to an insurmountable impasse that only
time and patience will alleviate, as the patient is no longer
receptive to interpretation.

With the advent of the structural model in 1923, Freud was
able to refine the technique of resistance analysis with his
discovery of resistance to the awareness of resistance. Although resistance is closer to the mind's surface than wishful
impulses and anxiety-laden memories, the expression of
which resistance serves to inhibit, resistance itself is nevertheless a dynamically unconscious phenomenon for which
there is no ready access to awareness. In the topographic
model, resistance tended to be construed as evidence of the
operation of preconscious censorship and, as a consequence,
relatively accessible to consciousness. In the structural model,
resistance could be understood as a function of the unconscious defensive activities of the ego and therefore relatively
inaccessible to conscious awareness. There is censorship of
the fact that one engages in self-censorship.

> There can be no question but that this resistance emanates
> from his ego. . . . We have come upon something in the ego
> itself which is also unconscious, which behaves exactly like the
> repressed—that is, which produces powerful affects without
> itself being conscious and which requires special work before
> it can be made conscious. [Freud 1923, p. 17]

The technical rule of interpreting resistance before content could be amended to read as a recommendation to analyze ego before id, ego defined as the unconscious mechanisms of defense.

The implication for transference analysis is that there invariably will be transference resistance to the awareness of transference resistance, which is why analysis of the transference neurosis is so arduous. In working from surface to depth, surface-level transferences defend against the awareness of latent transferences. Since the unobjectionable positive transference tends to reside at the surface whereas the negative and erotic transferences tend to be repressed, it is the unobjectionable positive transference that serves as a resistance to the awareness of the repressed negative and erotic transferences. These latter transferences in turn serve as a resistance to consciously recalling original infantile conflicts and traumas. The analyst is placed in somewhat of a double-bind situation, for it is the patient's attachment to the analyst that motivates the patient to participate in the analytic enterprise, yet it is also this attachment that serves as a resistance to the awareness of latent negative and erotic transferences. To interpret the unobjectionable attachment to the analyst as a defensive attitude endangers the rapport that makes treatment possible, yet to not interpret it as in part a form of resistance is to remain blocked at the first obstacle to the awareness of latent transferences to the analyst. Freud's compromise solution appeared to have been to use the emotional leverage afforded by the attachment to the analyst as a means of enabling the patient to overcome his or her resistance to becoming aware of more unacceptable feelings about the analyst.

Freud's theory of therapeutic technique suggests two

worst-case scenarios that could potentially lead to a treatment impasse. First, interpretation of the defensive function of the unobjectionable positive transference could lead to an intractable negative transference resistance as a consequence of the loss of rapport. Second, if in order to preserve rapport the defensive function of the unobjectionable positive transference is never interpreted, the treatment may fail to deepen. Presumably, to the degree that the patient possesses a high capacity for maintaining rapport or that the analyst possesses a high capacity for tact in the service of preserving rapport, the transference neurosis will be worked through and resolved. In order to achieve a therapeutic success, some optimal balance would need to be maintained between preserving rapport and uncovering latent transference resistances.

Given the ubiquity of resistance to the awareness of resistance, how does the analyst ascertain whether the analytic process is successfully unfolding, given that both compliance with and opposition to the analysis may serve as transference resistances? Freud (1937b) posed the problem of the patient's suspiciousness of the analyst's attempts at interpretation:

> "Heads I win, tails you lose." That is to say, if the patient agrees with us, then the interpretation is right; but if he contradicts us, that is only a sign of his resistance, which again shows that we are right. In this way we are always in the right against the poor helpless wretch whom we are analyzing, no matter how he may respond to what we put forward. [p. 257]

A manifest "yes" may hide a latent "no," whereas a manifest "no" may hide a latent "yes." Unwilling to accept the manifest content at face value, Freud (1937b) searched for indirect evidence as confirmation of his hypotheses—evidence beyond symptomatic relief that could result from an unanalyzed transference cure alone, a cure achievable through suggestion and hypnosis. The emergence of new memories, fantasies, dreams, or analogies following a "yes" may be taken as confirmation, as it signifies a lifting of repression. An absence of such associations following a "yes" could be taken as disconfirmation, as it may signify no lifting of repression. Increased defensiveness following a "no" could be taken as confirmation, as it would indicate heightened anxiety as repression has been weakened. Indifference following a "no" could be taken as disconfirmation, as it would indicate that repression has remained undisturbed.

Despite Freud's (1937b) guidelines for validating the correctness of an interpretation, it is easy enough to demonstrate innumerable exceptions to these rules. In terms of the elicitation of new associations, Freud (1923) acknowledged that latent dream thoughts of patients in analysis can be influenced or suggested by the analyst, producing dreams in compliance with the analyst's expectations. Freud's assumption that indifference may reflect a wrong interpretation (proving that wrong interpretations are essentially harmless) neglects the possibility that someone could be so psychologically impenetrable that he or she remains unperturbed by even the most incisive interpretations. Though Freud assumed that increased defensiveness derives from a correct interpretation that the patient repudiates, such defensiveness is also a normal response to feeling misunderstood. Thus, all of Freud's indirect means of confirming or disconfirming a hypothesis are open to multiple and contradictory interpretations. The point here is not to engage in a philosophical debate about the scientific status of psychoanalytic evidence but to note that patients, like philosophers of science, are quite capable of summoning a skeptical attitude toward the analysis of transference resistance. There is no rejoinder to this analysis that will not be experienced by the patient as the analyst's implying "Heads I win, tails you lose," an imposition of the analyst's interpretive authority.

The theory of psychoanalytic technique that Freud elucidated provides the organizing assumptions on which later innovations and refinements in technique have been based or to which ideas have been developed in counterpoint. Freud's model poses fundamental technical dilemmas that it does not entirely resolve and around which later controversies in technique have arisen. The dynamic tension between establishing and deepening therapeutic rapport and uncovering and resolving latent negative transference has remained controversial. The dynamic tension between accepting the patient's subjective point of view and questioning, challenging, and deconstructing this point of view also remains controversial. These two controversies tend to be correlated, as empathizing with the patient's point of view is thought to enhance rapport, whereas questioning the patient's point of view is thought to elicit latent negative transference. Some suspect that overemphasizing empathy and rapport results in a superficial supportive psychotherapy; others believe that overemphasizing interpretation of transference resistance leads to either a negative therapeutic reaction or false-self compliance. Of course, the greatest controversy resides in assessing just what constitutes an over- or under-emphasis in technique.

Freud's (1909) "Notes upon a Case of Obsessional Neurosis" provides a good clinical illustration of the strengths and limitations of his technique. It illustrates how Freud utilized the patient's deferential transference to him as a respected authority figure in the service of overcoming the patient's resistance to making the unconscious conscious. In this paper Freud presented the treatment of the patient who has come to be known as "the rat man." The patient was a youngish single man who was university educated. His presenting problem was that he had obsessive fears that something bad might happen to his father and a lady friend. His fear for his father was unusual as his father had passed away 4 years before treatment began. He also reported impulses to harm himself such as cutting his throat with a razor. The patient felt he had wasted years fighting against these ideas and had already subjected himself to a variety of treatments.

The patient, aware of Freud's interest in childhood sexuality, described his childhood sexual experiences at the beginning of treatment. He recalled being interested in seeing his governess naked, actually seeing her naked, and fondling her. As a child he felt some vague sense of dread in regard to his sexual interests and was preoccupied with thoughts about his father's death. It emerged that a more recent precipitant for his obsessive worries was an incident that had occurred while he was on a tour of duty in the military in which an officer who was fond of cruelty recounted a form of torture. The punishment was that a pot was turned upside down on a criminal's buttocks, some rats were put in the pot so that they would bore their way into the prisoner's buttocks. The patient also admitted that he had thought of applying this punishment to his father.

Though Freud centered his case discussion on the elucidation of the dynamics of an obsessional neurosis, he also revealed many aspects of his technique that are entirely consistent with his theory of technique. Freud described a variety of interventions that can be understood as attempts to build and maintain therapeutic rapport. The patient revealed early in treatment how dependent he has been on a friend for moral support to assure him that he was a man of irreproachable conduct. The patient immediately formed a similar transference to Freud, looking to Freud for reassurance that he is not thought reproachable. Every step of the way as the patient revealed some new aspect of himself, the patient worried what Freud would think of him.

When the patient was reluctant to recite the details of the rat torture, Freud assured him that he had no taste for cruelty and did not want to torment him. Freud educated the patient that overcoming the resistance was a law of treatment with which Freud could not dispense. Freud also explained to him the psychoanalytic theory of the dynamics of resistance. Later, when the patient expressed doubt that his long-standing problems could be modified, Freud assured him that his youth and the intactness of his personality were in his favor. In addition, Freud said a word about the good opinion he had formed of him, which gave the patient visible pleasure.

Alongside these acts of reassurance and education that enhance therapeutic rapport, Freud began to interpret from surface to depth. He interpreted that the patient possessed a "moral self" that was conscious and an "evil self" that was unconscious (1909, p. 177). Freud explained that a self-reproach arises only from a breach of a person's inner moral principles. As it began to emerge that the patient's neurotic guilt derived from his unconscious hostility toward his father, who was seen as a prohibitor of his sexual desires, the patient, protesting this line of interpretation, repeated rather than remembered the dynamic with his father in his transference to Freud. He began heaping the grossest abuse on Freud and his family. The patient would then state in despair, "How can a gentleman like you, sir, . . . let yourself be abused in this way by a low, good-for-nothing fellow like me? You ought to turn me out: that's all I deserve" (p. 209). He would get up and walk around the room avoiding proximity to Freud for fear that Freud might beat him. Freud noted that despite the patient's verbal abusiveness, in deliberate action he always treated Freud with the greatest respect.

It then emerged that the patient's father had a violent temper. This was the turning point of the treatment, the emergence of his unconscious identification with an abusive father. The patient wished to sadistically abuse his father as he had felt sadistically abused by him, and he felt quite guilty about those desires. The horrifying punishment was to suffer the rat torture for wanting to subject his father to the rat torture. After working through the "father complex" in the transference, the patient's "rat delirium" disappeared. Though Freud described the dynamics of the patient's obsessional neurosis in considerably more detail and complexity then presented here, this synopsis sums up the essentials of what Freud revealed about his actual technique.

Freud developed rapport with the patient by allying himself with the patient's consciously maintained "moral self." He did this through reassuring comments and educational advice about the nature of resistance and the dynamics of self-reproach. Freud used this unobjectionable positive transference to Freud as a reassuring father figure as leverage to explore the patient's unconscious anal sadism, of which the patient was mortified. As the patient's anal sadism began to emerge into consciousness, it was manifested as a negative transference to Freud: Freud was either an abusive father or a degraded victim of abusive treatment. The initial rapport allowed the patient to tolerate and work through the negative transference with consequent insight into his conflicted relationship with his father and symptomatic relief. The strength of Freud's approach is his masterful revelation of anxiety-ridden unconscious conflict for which the patient gained symptomatic relief.

The limitation of Freud's approach in this case is that he did not recognize that the patient's imperious need for reassurance involved a repetitive enactment in making Freud into a father-confessor who would either exonerate or castigate him for what struck the patient as morally reprehensible within himself. Because Freud saw himself as a sympathetic but essentially neutral scientific investigator, he did not suspect that he may have been unconsciously enacting the role of someone who would actively expose and then forgive the patient's sins. Freud did not recognize that the unobjectionable positive transference, the patient's need for reassurance, was a form of transference resistance against the patient's fear of being in anything other than a dutiful, deferential relation to Freud. Though the patient was on one crucial occasion insulting and irreverent toward Freud, he was immediately apologetic, ingratiating, and obsequious in reparation, never altering his basically respectful attitude.

The patient's characterological deference toward authority was enacted rather than analyzed in the transference. Though the patient got in touch with his unconscious desire to defy authority and his guilt about those defiant attitudes, he was never able to stand up to authority as an equal. He could never declare and defend his own moral decency without asking for exoneration. The patient's underlying narcissistic vulnerability, his deference to potentially irrational, moralistic, and abusive authority, was perhaps confirmed to the extent the patient treated Freud's more benevolent authority as sacrosanct. Freud, in a sense, exploited the patient's deference toward him as leverage to make the unconscious conscious, to get the patient to own his underlying guilt-ridden resentment of authority.

The liability of not recognizing the defensive function of the unobjectionable positive transference on which therapeutic rapport is based is that it may allow ego-syntonic character resistances to go unnoticed and unanalyzed. Of course, if Freud did not allow himself to function as a reassuring father figure, the analysis may have never gotten off the ground in the first place for lack of sufficient rapport. As Freud's focus was symptom analysis rather than character analysis, the patient's ego-syntonic deferential attitude toward Freud was never specifically analyzed as a transference resistance. As we shall see, this is the sort of analytic focus that Wilhelm Reich (1928) made the cornerstone of his character-analytic approach to treatment.

What I find most useful in Freud's discussions of technique is his topographic perspective. If patients possess multiple perspectives, then an important question in terms of technique is from which perspective among many does analytic work proceed. If we work from surface to depth as Freud recommended, it is from the perspective of the surface of the mind that analytic work proceeds. Freud (1900) suggested that consciousness was like the tip of an iceberg. The analyst must be capable of pinpointing the patient's unique perspective from the "tip of an iceberg" as a starting point for interpretive work. Interpretations that fail to pinpoint the patient's view from the tip of the iceberg lack empathy for that crucial perspective. For Freud, interpretations that bypass the psychic surface are premature. The principle of working from surface to depth can be understood as one way that Freud tried to address the tension between analysis and empathy. In order to analyze what is deep, we must first empathize with what is surface.

Freud also made clear the patient's ubiquitous resistance to interpretations that go any deeper than the tip of the iceberg. The principle of interpreting resistance before content derives from an understanding of the patient's resistance to entertaining any perspectives on the self that go beyond a surface perspective. Yet resistance analysis evokes a characteristic negative transference—the "heads I win, tails you lose" transference that may effectively stalemate the analysis. At this point, Freud's recommendations are to be patient, persevering, and go on analyzing resistance despite the patient's negative transference, and sooner or later the patient will come around.

These recommendations reflect the limitations of Freud's technique as seen in retrospect through the lens of some of the innovations of contemporary psychoanalysis. I believe that Freud felt effectively stymied many times by the patient's intolerance of interpretations from perspectives other than the surface perspective. Freud lacked sufficient empathy for the patient's narcissistic vulnerability in having the surface perspective challenged as a defensive cover of deeper unconscious material. He construed the patient's egocentrism of consciousness as something to be vigorously challenged by rational thought and empirical demonstration just as Copernicus, Galileo, and Darwin challenged the egocentric beliefs of their day through their scientific discoveries. Though Freud was well aware that psychoanalysis was a narcissistic injury, he viewed the patient's narcissism as an infantile illusion in which he had no interest in participating. In fact, to participate in the patient's narcissism was to collude with the patient's denial of painful truths.

Freud attempted to overcome the limitations of his technique by exploiting the leverage afforded by the unobjectionable positive transference (i.e., reassurance to assuage the patient's narcissistic injury subsequent to resistance analysis) and the patient's deference to the analyst's interpretive authority (i.e., in order to enlist the patient's willingness to tolerate in consciousness unacceptable aspects of the self). Freud did not see that utilizing the unobjectionable positive transference in this manner could reflect a transference enactment in itself, as he understood himself as an essentially neutral scientific investigator as long as he maintained a stance of abstinence toward the patient's instinctual yearnings. Viewing resistance as primarily an intrapsychic defense against unconscious content, Freud, working within the perspective of a one-person rather than a two-person psychology, did not see the interactive nature of resistance; that resistance is in part evoked by the analyst's interpretive framework and interactive style.

To make these theoretical issues relevant even for entry-level clinical practice, I will present the case of a college undergraduate whose treatment by a beginning therapist I supervised. We will follow this case through each of the chapters of Part I in order to illustrate the ideas under discussion in each chapter. I view case reports in the clinical literature as illustrating rather than proving a point of view, as case reports are essentially narrative endeavors. Case reports are invariably selective in what they include and exclude, and they are dramatized in a manner reflecting the writer's rhetorical style. For this reason, I do not see psycho-analytic case studies as data or evidence but as a manner of evoking in the reader a vicarious clinical experience that may resonate with and be pertinent to the reader's own experiences as a patient or clinician.

To protect the anonymity of the patients whose treatment I will present in this book, I have significantly altered any identifying characteristics. The treatment of the undergraduate I will present has some composite elements deriving from my experiences supervising the therapy of a number of underachieving young men with narcissistic pathology at a college counseling center. The supervisee is also in part a composite character whose work reflects several common problems that beginning therapists have had in treating such men.

The patient, who will be called Joe, is a 21-year-old undergraduate who has sought treatment because of poor grades, which he attributed to his own laziness and procrastination. During the beginning phase of treatment, Joe gives weekly reports of his academic progress and has little to say when things have gone well. He is 10 to 15 minutes late for each session, attributing the lateness to his busy schedule in which it is difficult to squeeze in his session time. Joe does not seem to mind having an abbreviated session, acts as though the sessions are helpful, and does not anticipate needing extended treatment with his difficulties because he believes they will be resolved shortly.

The beginning therapist, a 28-year-old woman enrolled in a psychoanalytically oriented doctoral program in clinical psychology, hoping to develop a long-term case of psycho-analytic psychotherapy, is already alarmed and frustrated by the way the case is progressing. Viewing the chronic lateness as transference resistance, the therapist begins to inquire whether Joe has any feelings about her that may account for the tardiness. Joe responds that he feels just fine about the therapist and that he is not trying to avoid the sessions; to the contrary, he is trying to get to the sessions as soon as he can and apologizes for any inconvenience. As Joe does not spontaneously offer an underlying motive for coming late to sessions, the therapist, having surmised that Joe tends to be counterdependent, suggests that perhaps Joe does not want to get too dependent on the therapist as Joe would like to prove that he can solve his problems on his own. Joe admits that he strives to be an independent person but that if he has a problem, it is no "big deal" to seek help to fix it. He reassures the therapist that she has been very helpful.

This brief vignette illustrates what happens to the therapist who does not appreciate the technical precept of working from surface to depth. The therapist bypasses the surface in failing to recognize that what she sees as unconsciously motivated avoidance, the patient sees as justifiable and excusable lateness. As the therapist attempts to facilitate an open exploration of unconscious reasons for avoiding the sessions, assuming the primary reason reflects anxiety in relation to the transference, the patient resists that overture in continuing to highlight the essential innocence of his lateness and the unambivalently positive way in which he feels about the therapist (i.e., the unobjectionable positive transference serving as an essential connection to the therapist as well as transference resistance). As an insightful person, the therapist is quite right that Joe is an uncon-sciously counterdependent person who wishes to engineer a flight into health as soon as his defenses are sufficiently bolstered. However, without an understanding of certain basic principles of technique, the therapist is effectively stymied in making any progress in interpreting that unconscious conflict.

To interpret Joe's sense of self from the surface, the

therapist would have to reflect that Joe views his lateness as unavoidable and regrettable. To interpret the transference from the surface, the therapist would have to examine how Joe feels about the fact that she may not see it that way, that she may see it instead as some excuse Joe has concocted to extricate himself from his commitment to being in treatment. In inquiring how Joe feels that the therapist has treated his lateness as possibly avoidant, it emerges that Joe's girlfriend as well as his father have often seen him (unfairly so, from his point of view) as someone who makes excuses to be relieved of accountability for something for which he has assumed responsibility. Joe still does not acknowledge that his lateness is unconsciously motivated, but he does admit that he gets angry at and frustrated with those who unreasonably deny him the credibility to which he feels entitled.

To work from the surface successfully clarified what was turning into a confusing situation that could have become an adversarial stalemate. Joe now feels that his point of view has been understood, which restores therapeutic rapport, and a repetitive and problematic pattern in his interpersonal relations has been recognized. Yet Joe still does not see his lateness as unconsciously motivated resistance and continues to arrive late for sessions. At this point, I would suggest that the Freudian theory of technique leaves something to be desired. If one goes on to interpret the resistance before content—Joe's need to see himself as an essentially innocent, cooperative, and independent person as a defense against his unconscious fears of commitment and intimacy–Joe will feel severely narcissistically wounded. The therapist, just like everybody else, will seem unfairly critical in treating him as some irresponsible person prone to making excuses for his failings, and he will have either to defy or submit to this harsh judgment. In addition, the theory does not address the interpersonal dimension of the situation. Is the therapist plausibly experienced as being intolerant and judgmental of the patient's stated reasons for lateness in treating the patient's chronic lateness as a problem that must be consistently discussed until the patient begins to arrive on time, or is this perception of the therapist simply transference distortion?

Being able to work from surface to depth is essential if there is to be any sense of clarity in the therapeutic situation as to where the patient is at in the moment. Failure to work from surface to depth generates confusion and misunderstanding in which the patient and therapist talk past each other. And it is at the surface level where the crucial resistances to treatment reside. What the theory does not fully address is the question of how to deal with the patient's narcissistic vulnerability in interpreting that resistance and how that resistance may be evoked in part by the therapist's interpretive/interactive stance. If the therapist just accepts the patient's lateness at face value, the patient effects a successful flight into health in several weeks, and treatment is prematurely aborted. If the therapist interprets the defensive function of the patient's lateness, the patient feels wounded and either defies the therapist by quitting or submits to the therapist's authority begrudgingly and becomes a very passive-aggressive patient for whom treatment is like pulling teeth. What is a therapist (or, for that matter, a supervisor) to do in this situation, a common situation fraught with both complexity and ambiguity?

What is implicit in a theory of technique is a theory of what constitutes empathic understanding. Freud made it clear that to have empathy for the psychology of consciousness was only a partial form of empathy, a starting point for a deeper form of empathy that involved appreciation of unconscious wishes and fears. The only problem was that patients did not immediately experience Freudian empathy with unconscious contents as empathic. Quite the opposite, they experienced Freudian empathy as something dangerous to be resisted. Yet Freud assumed that once the resistance had been overcome, in retrospect the patient would appreciate that Freud had indeed been profoundly empathic to the patient's worst fears, deepest wishes, and most traumatic memories. It was unsettling for patients to realize that the analyst may understand quite a bit more about their inner psychic life than they could dare acknowledge to themselves. Freud believed that the insight of psychoanalysis, that the conscious ego is not the master of the human psyche but that the unconscious is, is invariably a severe wound to human narcissism. And this narcissistic injury is one that the patient simply must learn to tolerate and assimilate for the treatment to succeed.

2

Reichian Character Analysis

Freud's theory of analytic technique raised two separate but related questions with which clinicians needed to grapple: (1) How do we analyze transference resistance to the awareness of transference resistance? (2) How do we develop and deepen therapeutic rapport? In other words, how do we analyze and empathize, and how do we balance the two? With the advent of ego psychology (Freud 1923), both of these questions could begin to be answered in a more refined manner than before. Wilhelm Reich in 1928 was the first to develop a systematic approach to the analysis of transference resistance to the awareness of transference resistance that he called "character analysis." Reich believed that Freudian analysis tended toward intellectual compliance on the patient's part along with an avoidance of the latent negative transference, which remained a hidden resistance. As we shall see, Reich made significant innovations in the question of how we can analyze resistance more systematically and effectively but perhaps at the expense of a deeper appreciation of what is involved in developing and sustaining empathic rapport.

Reich suggested that patients are rarely accessible to analysis at the outset because they are not disposed to follow the fundamental rule of analysis in freely discussing all that comes to mind without censorship. Though even in this censored discourse the analyst is likely to discern derivatives of unconscious impulses and defensive efforts to block the awareness of particular impulses, for the analyst to focus on text analysis may be to neglect a crucial form of resistance that may not be revealed in the patient's words alone. Reich (1928) suggested that a crucial but heretofore neglected form of resistance was to be found in the patient's bearing and attitude: "The 'how' is just as important as the 'what' the patient says as 'material' to be interpreted" (p. 135). It is not that Freud had previously neglected the patient's nonverbal communication as a context for assessing the subtle shades of meaning of the patient's verbal productions, for Freud was well aware that nonverbal signals may be incongruent with manifest verbal content and thus provide an additional clue to unconscious content. What Freud did not do, which Reich attempted, was to call the patient's attention systematically to these nonverbal attitudes and make the analysis of these attitudes a primary focus of treatment.

Reich (1928) called these nonverbal attitudes "character resistances" (p. 131). Utilizing the structural model, he noted that every resistance consists of "an id-impulse which is warded off, and an ego-impulse which it wards off, both of these impulses are unconscious" (p. 141). What Reich innovatively added was to go beyond the microscopic approach to conflict-defense analysis to a macroscopic holistic approach— from symptom analysis to character analysis. Neurotic symptoms always derive from a neurotic character structure, and the neurotic character manifests itself in analysis as a "compact defense mechanism," which Reich called "characterological armor" (p. 134). Character armor reflects not so much a particular defense mechanism as an overarching strategy of defense. Attitudes, beliefs, values, ideals, wishes, affects, fantasies, ambitions, or any other conceivable component of the personality can serve as an aspect of character armor. Character armor is not reducible to any single personality trait alone but rather refers to the superordinate organization of personality traits into an overall strategy of defense, a sort of philosophy or style of living that provides protection against any conceivable situation of psychic danger. Character armor provides a virtually impenetrable "protecting wall" (p. 145) against awareness of unconscious content in the form of a tightly organized web of defensive beliefs, attitudes, values, wishes, dreams, and so forth.

Reich (1928) also suggested that character armor served as a "narcissistic protective apparatus" (p. 144). It is narcissistic in a number of respects. It protects the integrity of the ego in preventing a breakdown of the ego in the face of both internal and external pressures. As a narcissistic defense, it serves a compensatory function in restoring injured narcissism and maintaining a homeostatic balance. The narcissistic dimension of character armor also is responsible for the fact that character armor is ego-syntonic.

> The symptom appears to be meaningless, whereas the neurotic character is sufficiently rationally motivated as not to appear either pathological or meaningless. For neurotic character traits a reason is often put forward which would immediately be rejected as absurd if it were applied to symptoms, such as: "He just is that way"—with its implication that he was born so, that this "happens to be" his character, which cannot be altered. [Reich 1928, p. 133]

The individual may have no reflective awareness of even possessing a character style, as it is just a taken-for-granted way of being in the world. Yet when the person is made aware of possessing a distinctive character style, it is conceived as a normal, rational, and adaptive manner of conducting oneself that need not be questioned or examined, for it is not a problem. Moreover, even if it were somewhat of a problem, it cannot at any rate be changed, for that is simply the way one is, always has been, and always will be. This manner of thinking is narcissistic in the sense of being egocentric. There is no apparent ability to see the world from any point of view other than one's own, which is taken for granted. In order to entertain the possibility that one is being defensive, one must be capable of looking at oneself as someone who could be engaged in an act of self-deception and entertain the possibility that the world may not be as it seems to be at face value.

Reich's discussion highlights two aspects of character

structure that must be taken into consideration in the conduct of clinical work. First, defenses are organized holistically so that any aspect of personality functioning as well as the personality as a whole can be utilized defensively. Second, fear of narcissistic injury, compensation for narcissistic injury, and egocentrism serve as resistances to the awareness of the fact that one's character style can be utilized defensively as well as adaptively or rationally. Given these two factors, we may more readily understand why resistance analysis is like trying to penetrate or break through a seemingly impenetrable wall. Reich's approach to analytic technique reflects one method of attempting to address these issues. The basic method consists of calling attention to the patient's ego-syntonic character style and attempting to make it ego-dystonic. "We isolate the character trait and confront the patient with it repeatedly, until he has attained objectivity towards it and experiences it like a distressing compulsive symptom. The neurotic character thus takes on the nature of a foreign body, and becomes an object of the patient's insight" (Reich 1928, p. 139).

The patient resists making the ego-syntonic ego-dystonic, as that constitutes a narcissistic injury in admitting to possessing a psychological problem where none seemed to have existed prior to the analyst's observations. Reich (1928) noted that "the consistent interpretation of behavior provokes the patient's narcissism to revolt" (p. 145). Narcissistic revolt in interpreting the patient's nonverbal attitudes is no problem for Reich, as it provides a ready means of gaining access to latent negative transference resistances:

> The superficial and more nearly conscious layer of every resistance must necessarily be a negative attitude towards the analyst, regardless of whether the id-impulse that is warded off is one of love or hate. The ego projects its defense against the id-impulse onto the analyst, who has become a dangerous enemy. [Reich 1928, p. 142]

Interpretation of defensive attitudes results in a narcissistic injury that is resisted through a transference of the patient's defensive attitude onto the analyst. The analyst is seen as not accepting the patient, whereas unconsciously it is the patient who cannot accept him- or herself. Once the analyst is construed as "a dangerous enemy," the analyst's interpretations can be dismissed as self-serving attempts at character assassination. Since the latent negative transference is what emerges once one scratches the surface, to work on analyzing the negative transference resistance is to work from surface to depth, in Reich's view. This is consistent with the dictum of interpreting ego before id as transference of defense (i.e., ego) is interpreted prior to transference of wish (i.e., id).

Reich was aware that his method has its dangers and is not always effective. In actively inflicting narcissistic injury, there is a danger of "ego breakdown." The patient may terminate prematurely rather than tolerate further narcissistic injury or may remain stuck in a protracted negative therapeutic reaction. Reich, though, was not particularly alarmed by these possibilities. He believed that ego breakdown is necessary to alter a rigid character armor so that a more flexible character style can take its place; that if a patient terminates prematurely, the patient probably is not analyzable anyway; and that a protracted negative transference can potentially be worked through, which is preferable to the sort of chaotic situations that arise when systematic character analysis is neglected and latent negative transference is avoided.

Nevertheless, despite Reich's innovation in the conceptualization of character resistance and structure, his theory of technique is deficient in one important respect in relation to Freud's initial guidelines: it neglects the facilitative role of the unobjectionable positive transference in addressing only its defensive function. Freud made it clear that without sufficient rapport with and attachment to the analyst, the patient would have no motivation to accept and attempt to work through the analyst's interpretations. Reich's approach creates a situation in which rapport is eliminated under the threat of narcissistic decompensation, and the patient will ward off the analyst's interpretations as destabilizing to his or her narcissistic equilibrium. Though Reich's approach demonstrates a refinement in the analysis of unconscious resistances to treatment in comparison to Freud, it is less empathic than Freud's approach in devoting less attention to maintaining rapport, tending to see the unobjectionable positive transference as *only* transference compliance that repudiates hostility, and tending to treat the patient's words as intellectualization in comparison to nonverbal attitudes, which are treated as the "real" material of the analysis.

Reich (1933) presented the case of a divorced 27-year-old woman to illustrate his character-analytic approach of working with the transference (pp. 145–149). This case illustrates his one-sided emphasis on the incisive analysis of resistance to the neglect of establishing an empathic connection. The patient had been divorced twice, and Reich believed that for a woman of her social standing she had had an uncommonly large number of lovers. Despite an active sex life, which Reich characterized as a "nymphomanic trait," she experienced what he called "orgastic vaginal impotence" (p. 145). The patient was described as very attractive, well aware of her feminine appeal, and not at all modest about it. Concurrent with her display of sexual confidence was a certain self-consciousness.

Initially in the analysis, the patient was uninhibited in recounting her sexual experiences and the embarrassing circumstances of her second divorce. Yet after openly recounting her experiences, she grew silent and reported having nothing to say. Reich suggested that perhaps her silence related to thoughts about the analyst. She reported that she was plagued by thoughts that the analyst might hold her in contempt because of her experiences with men. Yet in the next session the patient remained inhibited. When Reich noted that she might be once again warding off something about the analyst, she acknowledged that she was worried that Reich might become sexually interested in her and act on that interest. Reich noted her fears that he might take advantage of the analytic situation in not living up to a professional code of ethics. The patient recounted that in the past, all her physicians had propositioned her sooner or later.

Reich suggested that it was important to interpret her ego fears (i.e., her fears of being seduced) prior to her id wishes (i.e., her own desire to seduce). It emerged that the patient tended to seek relationships with younger men toward whom she behaved seductively. Yet she tended to lose interest in her lovers once they had shown sufficient admiration for her. Once again the patient became silent and inhibited, and Reich interpreted that she was warding off something. She admitted that she had begun masturbating with the fantasy that she was having sexual intercourse with the analyst. Reich interpreted that her pride made it difficult to admit such feelings.

Reich went on to ask whether she ever experienced love or desire spontaneously. She acknowledged that men had always desired her, and she simply acquiesced to their desire. At this point Reich went on to interpret the defensively narcissistic nature of her transference to him. He interpreted that she was irritated to see that Reich was not seduced by her charms and therefore found the situation unbearable. Her underlying desire was to make the analyst fall in love with her. And if Reich did not fall in love with her, she would lose interest in the analysis.

It then emerged that the patient had a scornful attitude toward men in general, especially men who chased after her. She reported that her relationships tended to be superficial and that she was often bored by the dreariness of it all. She admitted that she was not really all that involved in the analysis. Thus in this brief piece of analysis at the beginning of treatment, Reich seemed effectively and quickly to get past a sort of superficial, false-self compliance in which the patient is falling in love with the analyst and offering herself as a sex object as she feels is expected of her. This was a recurrent pattern in her relationships with men. Reich revealed the underlying impoverishment of her relationships with men and the deeper issue of the underlying emptiness of her life in general.

The strength of Reich's approach in this example is that he got quickly to the essence of the patient's narcissistic pathology and the analysis did not get stuck at the level of a sexually compliant false self, which was the patient's typical character problem in her relationships with men. This is no small accomplishment because many analyses could easily enough go on for years without getting to the heart of the patient's character pathology. On the face of it, the patient had not suffered any grievous narcissistic injury in the face of Reichian character analysis and did not seem to have taken offense at any of his interpretations or experienced them as character assassination. Yet perhaps Reich's neglect of the issue of therapeutic rapport and the patient's narcissistic vulnerability in having her character defenses interpreted may have manifested itself in more subtle ways.

The patient acknowledged after her underlying narcissism had been revealed that indeed she was not all that involved in the analysis despite her and Reich's effective character-analytic work. Thus an essential element of rapport was missing in the therapeutic relationship. In addition, it becomes apparent that the reason the patient was not offended or enraged by any of the character analysis was that in part she did not take it too seriously but rather regarded it as just another routine, meaningless encounter with the opposite sex. Implicit in her defensive unrelatedness was the assumption that relationships with men are about seducing and abandoning or being seduced and abandoned. From this perspective, it would seem that Reich had been seduced into pursuing her every time she withheld feelings about him, which she then compliantly handed over to him, and that he had seduced her into the awkward position of revealing her inner impoverishment to a man who did not desire her. Reich, seeing himself as both neutral and abstinent in not responding to her overtly erotic overtures, did not seem to contemplate the possibility that he may have participated more subtly in a repetitive enactment with her.

Her initial verbalized anxiety in the transference was that Reich would have contempt for her because of her sexual experiences with men. What then emerged was material that could have plausibly justified a contemptuous attitude on Reich's part from the patient's perspective: that the patient was a cold, narcissistic woman who seduced and abandoned men once they met her need for admiration. Thus the analysis seemed to confirm an unflattering self-image. Her lack of indignation over this exposure may have related to her tendency to submit to a demeaned role in her relationships with men. Even if she had exploited men, they (i.e., previous physicians, at least, if not others) had also exploited her, without apparent protest on her part. The patient submitted to Reich not sexually but passively, by allowing him as a dominant male to define her sexual behavior in an unflattering light.

Reich was not curious what the patient thought his opinion of her was once he had revealed the fact that she was not only a sexually experienced woman but also one who seemed to use men to flatter her narcissism. Reich seemed to take for granted that he was a nonjudgmental person in sexual matters, as psychoanalysts are supposed to be, so he did not worry that the patient may have seen him otherwise, despite her initial worry about what his opinion of her was. In fact, his rejection of her sexual overtures could have heightened her perception of him as a potentially critical superego figure, perhaps gratifying an unconscious need for punishment for what she may have felt was her contemptible sexual conduct. Though Reich had empathy for her ego anxieties (i.e., her fear he would take sexual advantage of her) and was careful not to interpret prematurely her id anxieties (i.e., her desire to seduce Reich), he tended to minimize her superego anxieties (i.e., her fear that he would condemn her as she may have unconsciously condemned herself). In this sense, Reich was not patiently working from surface to depth and not taking time to build an essential element of therapeutic rapport—confidence in the fact that the analyst is not a moralistic person.

Perhaps greater empathy for the patient's feeling that it was demeaning to confess the full extent of her difficulties with men to a potentially moralistic or exploitative male authority may have diminished the possibility that treatment may have unwittingly confirmed a despised self-image to which she submitted. Her initial fear of being treated contemptuously, though perhaps unconsciously reflecting a masochistic wish to be treated contemptuously, nevertheless reflected a conscious concern about whether she would be treated with respect. The basis of potential rapport would be the analyst's discovering something in her character that could have been a basis of genuine respect, such as a desire for greater honesty and authenticity in her relationships with men. Reich did not seem to see in this patient anything other than someone trying to put one over on him, which he interpreted incisively. It seems that the patient was vulnerable to another sort of compliance besides the overtly sexual kind. She seemed to comply passively with the vision of a dominant male who saw her and perhaps treated her as little more than a "nymphomaniac" who finally met her match in Reich, who would not allow himself to be seduced or castrated by her as had other men more susceptible to her feminine wiles.

Reich's work initiated a controversy in technique over which there is little consensus to this day. How should the patient's narcissism be addressed in treatment? Should the patient's narcissism be confronted or supported? If confronted, should it be confronted gingerly or actively? If supported, should it be supported by bolstering narcissistic illusions or by providing consolation for narcissistic defeats? And—to avoid an either/or type of argumentation—should all or some of these strategies be employed in some optimal combination? Clearly Reich can be seen as advocating a strategy of actively challenging, with minimal support, narcissistic defenses and actively interpreting the ensuing negative transference as a transference resistance. This strategy places Reich at one end of what could be seen as an interpretive continuum, which is a virtue as well as a weakness. Reich addressed unflattering aspects of his patients' characters more forthrightly than most, often to his patients' benefit, but at the expense of being unable to see much of what is adaptive or affirmative in his patients' characters, often to his patients' detriment.

What I find most useful in Reich's approach is his focus on character and on the defensive utilization of character. Character is a holistic concept that addresses the person as an integrated unit. It addresses the person's existence in the world as an object to others. The analyst objectifies the patient whenever the analyst characterizes the patient, and in understanding the patient, inevitably the analyst will characterize the patient as being a such-and-such kind of person. Character analysis attempts to make explicit that objectifying dimension of the analytic process in which the patient exists as an object in the eyes of the analyst. Reich, though, did seem to act as though his characterizations of the patient were authoritative and definitive rather than simply one way of characterizing a patient among many that reflected his own preconceptions. It did not occur to Reich, who thought of himself as a neutral scientific observer, that his characterizations of the patient might also have reflected in part a repetitive transference enactment based on an induced countertransference in which he characterized the patient in the same manner that others in the past had fairly or unfairly characterized the patient.

What is also useful in Reich's approach is highlighting the defensive function of character. Rather than reduce defensive activity to defense mechanisms, one can examine the defensive function of holistic phenomena such as attitudes, beliefs, ideals, aspirations, goals, ideologies, worldviews, and perspectives. Reich's approach to defense analysis is his calling attention to the fact that character resistance is largely ego-syntonic and that to analyze it, the analyst must enable the patient to view his or her own character as ego-dystonic. The ego-syntonic point of view is the surface viewpoint, whereas the ego-dystonic point of view is the deep viewpoint. To work from surface to depth is to work from what is ego-syntonic to what is ego-dystonic.

The patient begins analysis construing his or her self and character from a taken-for-granted egocentric perspective. As analysis proceeds, the patient begins to decenter and develop a capacity to envision his or her self and character from multiple perspectives. The problem with Reich's approach is in his insensitivity to the patient's narcissistic vulnerability in making the ego-syntonic ego-dystonic and his lack of awareness of and empathy for the interactive impact of working with an actively challenging, questioning, and confrontative analyst who is quite explicit and authoritative concerning his characterizations of the patient and apparently unaware of how his characterizations reflect his own preconceptions. As patients can be compliant with even overly aggressive approaches to character analysis, the narcissistic injury generated by such an approach may be more hidden than apparent, as when the character analysis confirms a despised self-image that the patient takes for granted.

To make these issues clinically immediate, I will return to my supervision of the case of Joe. The therapist, having decided that she did not want to simply accept Joe's stated reason for being late at face value for fear that he would drift out of treatment, instead decided to confront his resistance. She interpreted that Joe was finding excuses to avoid the sessions just as he had used excuses to rationalize procrastinating with his school work and that if he really wished to get to the root of his problems, he needed to attend sessions in a more timely manner. To the surprise of the therapist, who was expecting a defiant response, Joe responded rather agreeably, promised to try to arrive for sessions on time, and thanked the therapist for not letting him get away with anything. The therapist experienced a sigh of relief and began to feel some excitement with her new-found sense of therapeutic efficacy. I felt similarly.

Joe began attending sessions punctually and filled the sessions with his usual progress report. The therapist started to feel somewhat bored listening to these progress reports and did not feel inclined to mirror him in the way in which he seemed to be soliciting mirroring. Trying to make the sessions seem more psychoanalytic, the therapist began to ask Joe questions about his childhood relationship with his parents and siblings and tried to make connections between the family dynamics of childhood and his current difficulties. Joe answered her questions perfunctorily, responded to her interpretations politely, and returned to recounting his progress report as soon as she seemed to let him off the hook. From session to session, he never made spontaneous reference to any of the childhood events or any of the therapist's interpretations discussed in the previous session, seeming to imply that he had given no further thought to the matter. The therapist viewed this avoidance as resistance and confronted him with his minimization of the impact of his childhood relationships on his present functioning. Joe responded that all the therapist's interpretations were interesting, plausible, and useful, but he just never happened to think of this "stuff" on his own and was happy that she could think up this "stuff" for him—after all, she was the expert, not him.

From the history that the therapist had been able to garner through questioning Joe, it emerged that Joe's mother treated him rather indulgently. He felt that in relation to his mother he could do no wrong and that she would always be there to cater to him. In contrast, his father was a rather gruff, surly person who often found fault with Joe. He had two older sisters, and in his Italian-American family, as the only boy, he felt that he was treated as a prince by the women in the family. Joe always did well enough in school to get by but never tried to excel, as he never felt he had to. Now in college, Joe felt it was important to prove to himself that he could do well, as his professional future seemed to depend on it. In addition, he wished to reverse the low opinion he thought his father had of him as someone who was spoiled and would not do well for that reason. In discussing his childhood, Joe could easily enough see that his difficulty with academics derived from a combination of feeling that he did not have to perform (i.e., his mother's indulgence) and that he was not able to perform (i.e., his father's derision).

This sort of situation is just the sort of clinical situation for which Reich developed his character-analytic approach. The patient was superficially compliant and agreeable, but all insight seemed intellectualized, and the analytic process did not seem to be deepening. The therapist was overly focused on content to the neglect of process, overly focused on the "what" rather than the "how." With a little probing, it was not all that difficult to discern the family dynamics that shaped his character style and to enable the patient to see that connection. Yet establishing such a connection had no visible impact on the analytic process. The resistance to treatment could be seen as a character resistance. The patient, feeling entitled to the indulgence of maternal women whom he would then take for granted, felt it was easy to slip into the role of a passive but privileged son in relation to the therapist. When the therapist confronted Joe about his lateness, Joe was assured that his therapist was indeed a strong, domineering, and controlling woman, like his mother, who would take charge and take care of him and that she would not be a critical and unsupportive person who would shame him, like his father, for being too spoiled to take responsibility for himself.

For Joe it was entirely ego-syntonic to see himself as a basically decent and likable "nice guy" who could just take for granted the support of a maternal woman. It was quite ego-dystonic to view himself as passive, pampered, spoiled, infantilized, and therefore somewhat emasculated. And he needed constant reassurance that he was not seen as such a person. It was also quite ego-dystonic to acknowledge his rage and humiliation at being seen in such a light. He would go to great lengths to avoid exposing his humiliation at being seen in that manner, expressing his rage indirectly by acting passive-aggressively. His unconscious counterdependence and need for distance reflected his fear of being smothered and suffocated by an overly indulgent and controlling mother. Yet he needed such a mothering presence in his life to reassure him that he was still a male whom a female could love, in contradistinction to the sort of surly, aggressive type like his father with whom he felt he could not compete directly.

For Reich the essence of character analysis was to point out the ego-syntonic character resistance and make it ego-dystonic while interpreting the latent negative transference that character analysis evokes. As the therapist was becoming frustrated with the intellectualized insight emerging from discussions of the patient's past, at my behest she began to confront his character resistances. She noted how in the treatment Joe seemed to keep her at arm's length yet always wanted her to reassure him that he was making progress. Joe acknowledged that he needed reassurance because he was an insecure person and should probably have more confidence in himself, but he did not see how he was keeping her at a distance—after all, he was coming to his sessions on time. After this session, Joe seemed somewhat depressed and deflated, as he seemed to have experienced the therapist's interpretation as a personal rejection. He had apparently felt that he had become a "good" therapy patient who arrived on time, gave upbeat progress reports, and with the assistance of the therapist made interesting insights into his childhood. Given the therapist's as well as my assessment of his character resistances, he felt rejected by the therapist as an unlovable and needy person who could not do anything right.

In discussing the situation in supervision, the negative transference that had been elicited by the character analysis and had damaged the therapeutic rapport had to be addressed. The therapist interpreted that Joe had apparently felt rejected and unappreciated by her when she pointed out his need for distance and reassurance and that she seemed insufficiently appreciative of his progress in their work together. Joe reassured the therapist that he was not angry at her and realized that she was just doing her job and he needed to face his underlying insecurities, something he had been trying to avoid. The treatment seemed to move forward as Joe was able to acknowledge that there were indeed long-standing problems of low self-esteem and emotional insecurity that he needed to address. Yet despite this acknowledgment, the basic process remained essentially the same as Joe resumed his progress reports, only probing more deeply in response to the therapist's initiative.

Unconsciously, Joe re-created and maintained his relationship with his mother in two respects. On the one hand, he became dependent on the therapist for reassurance and support as he was dependent on his mother. He repudiated this dependency to the degree he felt infantilized and emasculated by it in creating distance in the therapeutic relationship. This distance was in part maintained by his adoption of a reassuring attitude toward the therapist in which he treated her as his mother treated him, as though their relationship were one that was completely conflict-free. What was ego-dystonic in Joe's character was not only his dependence on his mother, of which he was ashamed, but also his behaving like his mother in trying to seduce others into the illusion of a conflict-free, blissful relationship that was covertly controlling in not letting others be themselves.

This vignette displays the strengths as well as the weakness of the Reichian approach. In terms of strength, it certainly brought immediacy and affect into the clinical encounter, which it vitalized and personalized. It also went to the essence of the patient's narcissistic vulnerability in a manner that was in part therapeutic. Though somewhat deflated by the therapist's interpretation, the patient was able to acknowledge the deeper sense of narcissistic injury that constituted the underlying reason he sought treatment in the first place. With this insight, he no longer saw himself as someone in short-term, problem-solving counseling but a patient in long-term, insight-oriented psychotherapy. The weakness of the approach was the manner in which it ruptured and damaged to a degree the therapeutic relationship in inflicting a significant narcissistic injury on the patient. Without some of the insights of contemporary self psychology, it might have been difficult to know how to repair that rupture. Yet in repairing the rupture, the treatment seemed on the face of it to have returned to the sort of mirroring relationship that kept the therapist at arm's length and did not seem to deepen from the patient's spontaneous initiative.

The therapeutic dilemma is that to fail to address the characterological issues is to avoid the essence of the patient's pathology. Yet to address the essence of the patient's pathology head-on risks damaging the therapeutic relationship and the patient's self-esteem in a major way. And the patient's pathology is not just in the patient's intrapsychic process alone. To what degree does the therapist's stance evoke the patient's need for distance and reassurance when the therapist has become a potentially dangerous person who has assumed the power and authority to either affirm or assassinate the patient's character? Reich's approach does not address the interpersonal impact of assuming the role of character analyst.

Reich's emphasis on analyzing character style and structure subtly shifts what it means to be empathic with a patient. To be empathic is not simply to appreciate the patient's deepest wishes, worst fears, and most traumatic memories. These are aspects of the whole person but are not equivalent to the whole person. To understand the person as a whole, as a gestalt, one must appreciate the person as a character, as an integrated unit in which the whole is greater than the sum of its parts. Yet much of a person's character is ego-dystonic, is repudiated as incompatible with a more narcissistically edifying ego-syntonic view of the self. To analyze ego-dystonic aspects of character is very unsettling to the patient who experiences analysis as character assassination rather than character affirmation. Yet presumably once those ego-dystonic aspects have been assimilated, the patient in retrospect will appreciate the analyst for having had the courage to confront him or her with those aspects of the patient's character for which the patient had little empathy or tolerance.

3

Defense Analysis and the Therapeutic Alliance

Fenichel (1953) said of Reichian technique, "In so far as these principles are merely elaborations of Freud's views they are 'nothing new'; in so far as they are 'consistent elaborations' of it, they 'are' something new" (p. 337). Fenichel's agreement with Reich's approach was a qualified agreement, for he possessed some concern as to the zealousness with which Reich's principles may be applied:

> I believe that the "shattering of the armor plating" could be done in a very aggressive way, but that the aggression and the consequent disintegration of the armor can be dosed, and indeed, that it is the task of the physician to make this procedure as little unpleasurable as possible for the patient. The first thing we must be clear about is that the consistent tackling of the patient's character traits wounds his narcissism much more than any other analytic technique. [p. 339]

The implication is that the analyst should not avoid making interpretations that would be experienced as narcissistic injuries, but if the analyst recognizes that character analysis is inevitably a blow to the patient's narcissism, then such interpretations can be titrated in a manner that respects the patient's capacity for assimilating narcissistic injury.

Fenichel (1954) suggested a technical rule for the conduct of character analysis: "In order to be treated, character resistances have to be changed into transference resistances" (p. 189). This transformation is easy enough, as the narcissistic injury provoked by character analysis expresses itself as a negative transference to the effect that the analyst has given offense through some sort of slanderous character assassination and is hated as a consequence. Fenichel (1941) cautioned that such negative transferences may prove unanalyzable if they have been evoked by the analyst's overly zealous interpretive efforts:

> When a patient's aggression is mobilized by an aggressive act of the analyst, this aggression is not properly speaking a "negative transference"; or rather, to the extent that it still is one, it loses its ability to be demonstrated as such. . . . Reich's preference for "crises," "eruptions," and theatrical emotions makes one suspicious of a "traumatophilia" that has its roots in a love of magic. [p. 105]

Though the negative transference should not be evaded through assiduously avoiding certain lines of interpretation, neither should it be provoked by adopting a confrontational line of interpretation intended to elicit a strong negative transference.

Sterba (1953) suggested that Reich's approach proved to be unduly provocative because he could only understand the unobjectionable positive transference in terms of its defensive function:

> It is one of Reich's basic errors that he denies the genuine character of positive transference, particularly in the beginning of the analysis. Reich's technique of dealing with the transference seemingly is an outgrowth of his own suspicious character and the belligerent attitude that stems from it. This makes him imply "secret" resistances even where genuine transference love is established. Under the impact of his technique, which is conditioned by the mistrust in the patient's positive transference reactions and by the disbelief in the genuineness of initial and even later transference love, the patient must necessarily feel unaccepted and constantly questioned as to the truthfulness of his positive feelings toward the analyst, so that he finally has to develop negative reactions out of his feeling of being frustrated and rejected. If these negative

reactions finally manifest themselves in dreams or otherwise, Reich is triumphant because it proves to him that the initial transference was not genuinely positive. [p. 9]

Ego analysts developed two strategies of attempting to avoid stalemate in the analysis of resistance: (1) refining the conceptualization of the function of the unobjectionable positive transference in developing the notion of the therapeutic or working alliance and (2) refining the notion of the psychic surface to allow for a more precise and less adversarial form of defense analysis. Kris (1951) suggested:

> Resistance is no longer simply an "obstacle" to analysis, but part of the "psychic surface" which has to be explored. The term resistance then loses the unpleasant connotation of a patient who "resists" a physician who is angry at the patient's opposition. This was the manifestation of a change in what may be described as the "climate" of analysis. [p. 19]

Many of the technical developments of ego psychology can be seen as a counterbalance to what was seen as Reich's adversarial approach to resistance analysis. Ego psychologists attempted to ensure that analysis would be conducted in a benign (i.e., empathic) atmosphere in developing a strong alliance with the patient and in carefully exploring the psychic surface to guarantee that resistance analysis would not be experienced as abrasive character assassination. Ego psychologists attempted to restore an optimal balance between empathy and analysis that seemed to have been lost in Reich's overly confrontational approach to the patient's character resistances. These innovations could be seen as part of an ongoing effort to minimize the use of interpersonal pressure to overcome the patient's resistance to making the unconscious conscious. In 1910, Freud recalled that during the early days of psychoanalytic treatment, the analyst would incessantly urge the patient to say all that came to mind, so that treatment possessed a more "friendly air." It is ironic that clinicians who believed that their innovations led to the creation of a more benign analytic atmosphere might later be critiqued in the light of more contemporary developments as having made the atmosphere not quite friendly enough. Of course, other innovators, like Reich, warned against the atmosphere of analysis becoming too friendly, which would result in a collusion between patient and analyst to avoid exploring the latent negative transference and its attendant anxieties.

Sterba (1934) refined Freud's description of the process through which the unobjectionable positive transference becomes a force that allies itself with the analyst against the forces of resistance. According to Sterba, the analyst forms an alliance with that aspect of the patient's ego that tests reality and develops an objective perception of it. By forming an alliance with the patient's reality testing, the analyst effects a split in the ego, creating an observing ego that examines an experiencing ego as an object of "intellectual contemplation" (p. 121).

> The subject's consciousness shifts from the center of affective experience to that of intellectual contemplation. . . . [T]here must be a certain amount of positive transference, on the basis of which a transitory strengthening of the ego takes place through identification with the analyst. This identification is induced by the analyst. From the outset the patient is called upon to cooperate with the analyst against something in himself. [p. 121]

The analyst induces such an identification not by making any particular educative, suggestive, or moral exhortations or pressures to be rational but rather by making transference interpretations.

> The technique by which the analyst effects this therapeutic dissociation of the ego consists of the explanations which he gives to the patient of the first signs of transference and transference resistance. . . . Through the explanations of the transference-situation that he receives the patient realizes for the first time the peculiar character of the therapeutic method used in analysis. . . . Over against the patient's instinct-conditioned or defensive behaviour, emotions and thoughts it

sets up in him a principle of intellectual cognition. [pp. 120–121]

Loewenstein (1954) noted that "only this alliance with the patient's intact functions permits us to overcome the power of his resistance" (p. 189). Loewenstein believed that a precondition for psychoanalytic work is a certain integrity of the patient's ego, whose alliance with the analyst is essential for the success of treatment. "The intactness of the patient's perceptions, of his memory, his thinking, his reality testing, of his capacity for self-observation and understanding of others, and of his faculty for verbal expression, is indispensable in psychoanalysis" (p. 188).

Freud (1937a) posed a paradox in regard to the alliance concept that neither Sterba nor Loewenstein appeared to have recognized. He too believed that the analyst must enter into an alliance with the patient's ego to subdue certain uncontrolled portions of the id in order to include them in a synthesis of the ego. Yet Freud also recognized that such an endeavor presupposes a normal ego: what if there is no such thing as a normal ego? He suggested that the concept of a normal ego is an ideal fiction. In real life even the healthiest ego only approximates normality and in even the best of situations will resemble a psychotic's ego in some respects.

The reason for this state of affairs is that defensive conflict invariably entails a split in the ego in the service of denying some painful aspect of reality that has frustrated an infantile wish. Thus, ego functions such as reality testing, judgment, logical thinking, and so on, are always compromised as a result of defensive activity, generating what Freud (1937a) called a "modification in the ego." As a consequence of a defensive splitting of the ego, which weakens the patient's reasonable ego, the patient breaks the analytic pact and becomes impervious to logical argument. So it seems that facilitating the ego function of self-observation and forming an alliance with that function is a rather tenuous basis for ensuring successful analysis, for the patient's self-observation is bound to prove an unreliable ally in the face of heightened conflict and defensiveness. Friedman (1969), in his critique of the alliance concept, suggested that although a relatively autonomously functioning observing ego with which the analyst is in alliance may be a result of a successful analysis, it does not appear to provide much of a motive force to oppose the tenacity of resistance to the awareness of resistance.

Zetzel (1956) introduced the concept of the "therapeutic alliance" to focus on some of the unconscious determinants of the unobjectionable positive transference. The therapeutic alliance appears to derive from some fundamental capacity to form a trusting attachment based on the prototype of the nurturing infant–caretaker relationship. The question arises as to whether an alliance based on the patient's infantile dependence provides any more reliable a basis for an alliance than the patient's rational ego. The assumption is that in order to preserve the infantile attachment to the analyst, there will be a strong unconscious motive for the cooperation of the patient's rational ego.

Greenson (1967), who coined the term *working alliance*, suggested that the patient's motivation to overcome illness and sense of helplessness in conjunction with a rational willingness to cooperate and a capacity to follow instructions entail the patient's contribution to the alliance with the analyst. Greenson was well aware that the working alliance could be subverted in the service of resistance. The working alliance can be used as a vehicle of gaining the analyst's love and approval and avoiding separation rather than of acquiring insight. Remaining rational and logical can become a resistance to experiencing primary process mentation and its attendant affects. And, of course, the working alliance can be employed as a resistance to the awareness of latent negative transference.

Greenson (1967, p. 193) provided an example of the defensive use of the working alliance. The patient maintained a persistent reasonableness toward Greenson and the analytic situation. She accepted the frustrations and restrictions good-naturedly, with no trace of conscious annoyance or anger. Nevertheless, her dreams were full of rage. Yet when the analyst pointed out her anger in her dreams, the patient responded that it was "only" a dream for which she was not responsible. If she forgot to attend a session, it was only a "natural" mistake. She took Greenson's interpretations of her underlying hostility as an eccentric's musings that she tolerated gracefully. When her superficial associations eventually petered out and silence reigned, her hostile feelings became unmistakably clear. At that point the patient realized how she had clung to the working alliance as a defensive facade.

Both love of the analyst as well as love of rationality do not seem sufficient to the task of overcoming resistance to the awareness of resistance, for love is fickle (i.e., readily displaced when frustrated), as Freud surmised. Even Hartmann's (1939) postulation of a conflict-free sphere of autonomous ego functioning cannot solve the dilemma, for certainly the ego function of self-observation has very little functional autonomy and would seem to be one of the more easily compromised ego functions. The alliance with the analyst, despite its intrinsic unreliability, appears to provide a necessary but not sufficient condition for the resolution of resistance to the awareness of resistance. Without any sort of alliance, the patient would have little motive to cooperate with the analysis or even to remain in treatment, other than the compulsion to repeat sadomasochistic enactments. Thus the absence of an alliance is a major therapeutic dilemma that must be addressed before treatment can move forward.

What is missing in the idea of developing an alliance with the patient's ego is any reference to the role of the superego in forming a therapeutic alliance. Though the analyst may serve as an auxiliary ego, Strachey (1934) suggested that the analyst also functions as an auxiliary superego. In his view, it is from a transference of the patient's superego onto the analyst that the therapeutic action of analysis derives. Since the superego disapproves of instinctual expression, it is at the behest of superego anxiety that the ego institutes defensive measures. Ameliorate superego anxiety, and the need for ego defense is reduced, which allows for the more open expression of id derivatives. Since one of the major defenses against superego anxiety is projection and since in the therapeutic situation the analyst becomes the natural object of that projection, the superego can be analyzed via its transference to the analyst. Strachey (1934) suggested that as the analyst makes transference interpretations, the analyst is put in the light of a benevolent superego and the projection of the patient's own overly harsh superego is disconfirmed. The patient then identifies with the analyst's apparently nonjudgmental and accepting attitude and develops a more benign superego him- or herself.

A fear of the analyst as a persecutory superego figure may generate resistance to the formation and maintenance of an ego alliance. The patient is not going to trust or utilize the analyst as an auxiliary ego unless the analyst is first experienced as a relatively benign auxiliary superego. Thus superego aspects of the transference may need to be interpreted before ego aspects of the transference to the effect of saying to the patient, "You fear that I will disapprove of you so that you do not feel it is safe to trust me or utilize my interpretations." And, to move on to the id element of the sequence, one might say, "Given that you see me as disapproving and cannot trust my objectivity, it is understandable that you would not feel that it is safe to openly express either your hostility or your love."

The problem with relying on the patient's experience of the analyst as a relatively benign superego figure is that the superego is readily compromised under the pressure of intrapsychic conflict. The superego is "corruptible" and is as a consequence an unreliable ally in the analysis. A manifestly benign superego may serve as a disguise for a latently permissive superego, which lets the patient "get away with murder" (and incest), so to speak. If the analyst simply serves as a reassuring superego figure who assuages the patient's manifest self-blame, the analysis remains at a superficial level that never addresses the patient's unconscious conflictedness. The reassuring analyst as a benign superego may be in unconscious collusion with the patient in suppressing the emergence of the unconscious conflict between overly permissive and critical superego introjects. The patient seduces the analyst into the role of exonerating the patient of all self-criticism in order to maintain the patient's self-esteem. This is the role that Freud seemed to have unwittingly assumed with the Rat Man.

Even though one component of the unobjectionable positive transference is a sense of the analyst as a benign superego figure, it remains a conditional positive transference based on the patient's compliance with the rules and limitations of analysis and the analyst's avoidance of seeming to the patient critical, moralistic, or punitive. Once those rules are broken or the limits tested or once the analyst says something that seems to mirror the patient's self-criticism, the analyst is likely to be seen as a harsh superego figure. Cooperation with the analysis will diminish to the degree that the analyst is perceived as disapproving, critical, unfair, unreasonable, overly demanding, prejudiced, persecutory, and so on. Though analyzing the punitive superego transference would need to be the first order of business, that task simply achieves the necessary but not sufficient conditions for analysis in reestablishing a benign superego transference. The benign superego transference is in part based on a fantasy of being magically cured by a loving protector if only one is a good person (i.e., a good patient). The patient becomes disillusioned with the analyst once it becomes apparent that despite the patient's cooperation with the analysis, "bad things *still* happen to good people."

Alliances with the patient's infantile dependence and helplessness, basic trust, rational ego, or benign superego all constitute necessary but not sufficient conditions for the conduct of analysis, since each element of the alliance can be readily subverted in the service of resistance under conditions of intensified unconscious conflict that invariably ensue as resistance is threatened through its analysis. The question arising from this predicament is how the analysis can proceed despite ruptures in the therapeutic alliance that are inevitable, since the alliance sooner or later becomes a vehicle of resistance that must be analyzed. Infantile dependence and helplessness may serve to defend against fears of separation and self-assertiveness; basic trust may serve as a defense against basic mistrust; rationality may serve as a defense against irrationality; a benign conscience may disguise an overly permissive one that fears punishment.

From a topographic point of view, the therapeutic alliance can be seen as a surface resistance to unconscious content despite the fact that its presence appears to constitute a necessary condition for the progress of the analysis. It would appear that some refinement of the notion of how one works from surface to depth is needed if it is going to be possible to interpret the therapeutic alliance as a form of transference resistance without rupturing a relationship that constitutes a prerequisite for analysis. Both Friedman (1969) and Brenner (1979) recognized the paradox inherent in the alliance concept and for this reason questioned its utility. Perhaps it is better simply to think of all aspects of the therapeutic relationship— whether positive or negative, manifest or latent—as forms of transference that may be utilized by the patient as transference resistance and therefore must be analyzed. Thus, innovation in technique must derive from refining the technique of transference resistance analysis rather than by trying to offset resistance to the awareness of resistance by attempting to strengthen the therapeutic or working alliance.

Despite the need to refine the technique of transference resistance analysis, it is not as easy to discard the alliance concept as Friedman and Brenner seemed to have implied. Friedman (1969) found unappealing the idea of basing a therapeutic alliance on either a "split-off, uncathected, reality-focused ego fragment" or "an indulgent, magical alliance with a fantasy analyst" (p. 145). Friedman responded more favorably to Loewald's (1960) suggestion that the analyst identify with the patient's growth potential. Such a suggestion is in effect forming a narcissistic alliance with the patient's ego ideal. It would seem to be a necessary but not sufficient condition for successful analysis for the analyst to be experienced as supporting a realistically affirmative ego ideal, thereby instilling a reasonable sense of hopefulness about the future as a motivating force for change. Nevertheless, the ego ideal, no matter how realistic, will prove an unreliable ally in the face of disillusionment, as even realistic goals and ambitions are sometimes disappointed. Realistic hope for the future will remain a motivating force for change to the degree that the sense of hopefulness achieves some degree of here-and-now gratification. The frustration of both realistic and unrealistic hopes is bound to be a disincentive for participation unless the analyst can revive some hope that the analysis can be beneficial. Cognizant of the dangers of supporting hopeful illusions, Friedman advocated tolerating the patient on his or her own terms, resistances as well, without settling for the patient's own terms. A paradox remains in that while a hopeless patient may have little motivation to change, especially if he or she is hopeless in regard to the outcome of the analysis, even a hopeful patient who is manifestly motivated to change may utilize the sense of hopefulness to resist exploring depressive or anxiety-laden fantasies or realities.

Brenner (1979) discarded the alliance concept by suggesting that the alliance is simply a form of transference, and as transference it constitutes a compromise formation. Like any other compromise, the alliance reflects a compromise between conflicting forces such as love and hate, wish and fear, defense and drive, and so on. Though all psychic phenomena may be constituted by compromise formations, some compromises result in more proanalytic attitudes than others, even though it is well known that even a proanalytic attitude can function as a subtle form of resistance. Brenner (1979) suggested, "In my opinion, it is not being more or less 'human' that is most important. What is most important, I believe, is to understand correctly the nature and origin of one's patients' transference reactions however one behaves" (p. 148). Yet he added a qualifying statement: "Even when an analyst believes he does understand a resistance . . . interpretation does not always lead to constructive change. Analysis is not a panacea, nor is it universally applicable" (p. 150). Brenner's qualifier begs the rejoinder that if correct understanding and interpretation is a vitally necessary but not sufficient condition for constructive change, it might be possible that the facilitation of a more "humane" atmosphere may be a crucial factor in determining the patient's amenability to analysis.

Brenner (1979) offered the additional caveat:

> If, for example, a patient suffers a catastrophe or a success in life, it is not the best for him and his analysis for his analyst to express sympathy or congratulations before "going on to analyze." . . . There are times when his being "human" under such circumstances can be harmful, and one cannot always know in advance when those times will be. [p. 153]

Similarly, one cannot know in advance when refraining from the common courtesies will be harmful. It is an empirical question, although as Greenson (1967) illustrated, such refrain may result in an error of humanity rather than an error of technique for which the patient may not readily forgive the analyst. Regardless of the question of so-called transference gratifications as a facilitator of the analysis, Brenner did not consider the possibility that the alliance concept might be useful in providing a focus for interpretive work by focusing analytic scrutiny on the patient's resistance to the formation and maintenance of a therapeutic alliance. Perhaps correct understanding and interpretation of this facet of the transference may crucially affect the patient's amenability to analysis. Brenner is certainly correct that being human is not a substitute for correct interpretation. Likewise, correct interpretation cannot substitute for being human or correct for errors of humanity.

Greenson (1967, pp. 219–220) gave this example of an error of humanity from the supervision of a young analyst. The patient was a young mother who spent most of the hour discussing her terrible anxieties about her infant son's sudden illness. The son had a high fever with convulsions, and the mother had been frantic until she reached her pediatrician. After she finished her story, the analyst remained silent; when the patient became silent, he told her after a few minutes that she was resisting. The patient said nothing. The analyst hypothesized to himself that the patient's silence may have related to the patient's repressed death wishes toward her son over which she felt guilty.

The patient attended the next hour and said nothing, tears streaming down her face. From time to time the analyst asked her what she was thinking. The hour ended in silence. That was their last hour of the week. The next week the patient announced she was quitting. When the analyst inquired why, the patient responded that the analyst was sicker than she was. She paid her bill and left. The analyst never discovered what had happened to the baby. Greenson felt that some open concern for the baby's welfare and show of compassion for the mother's plight was essential to maintaining a working alliance.

Despite the innovative technique of considering the state of the therapeutic alliance over approaches that do not, the ego-psychological approach to working with the therapeutic alliance does not offer sufficient empathy for the patient's narcissistic vulnerability or sufficient consideration of the fully interactive nature of the analytic situation. Another example by Greenson (1967, pp. 195–197) illustrates some of the potential limitations of the ego-psychological approach to developing a therapeutic alliance. The patient was an intelligent middle-aged man who had been in analysis for over 6 years in another city. Although the patient had demonstrated some improvement, he remained unmarried and lonely. With Greenson the patient was passive in working with his own resistances and waited for the analyst to point them out to him as his previous analyst had.

The patient was never silent in treatment because he had learned in his previous analysis that this behavior suggested resistance. He responded to whatever Greenson said with an immediate stream of free associations as though he never really pondered what Greenson had said. Once when Greenson asked the patient what his middle name was, he responded "Roskolnikov," the first name that occurred to him. After Greenson "recovered his composure," he questioned the patient's "bizarre" response. Greenson hypothesized that the patient had never formed a genuine working alliance with his previous analyst but had meekly submitted to what he imagined the analyst expected of him, resulting in a caricature of psychoanalysis.

In order to give the treatment a fair opportunity to proceed, Greenson carefully explained to the patient over the first months of treatment what psychoanalysis requires of a patient. Nevertheless, the patient discovered that it was difficult to say what came to mind without knowing what the analyst was looking for. He could not tolerate the silences without fearing some awful danger. In addition, he could not let himself disagree with Greenson for fear the disagreement would kill Greenson. Greenson believed that the patient's ingratiation covered up an inner emptiness, an insatiable infantile hunger, and a terrible rage. After 6 months, Greenson decided that the patient was a "schizoid, as if character" who could not tolerate the deprivations of classical analysis. He referred the patient to another therapist for supportive psychotherapy.

Greenson did not realize that what may have been transpiring was some sort of repetitive enactment: the successful attempt at false-self compliance with the first analyst as well as the failed attempt at false-self compliance with Greenson, followed by termination for being unable to work in the manner Greenson expected a classical patient to work. It is not clear that the patient could not tolerate the deprivation of analysis as there was no report of undue regression, symptomatic exacerbation, or psychological decompensation as a result of the privations of analysis. The patient's major difficulty being in analysis seemed to be a rather entrenched character resistance in which the patient did not know what to say if not advised as to what was expected of him.

The repetitive enactment seems to be that the patient felt a desperate need to comply with what was expected of him or face an intolerable rejection. In the first analysis, compliance spared him abandonment; in the second analysis, it did not. Having thought of himself as making an essentially objective diagnostic judgment about the patient's suitability for analysis, Greenson did not consider the possibility that his diagnostic judgment and decision to terminate could have been effected by an induced countertransference, which led to a repetitive reenactment. Perhaps Greenson played the role of a parent who punishes for failing to accommodate to parental expectations, the sort of parent for whom one would need to develop a compliant false self in the first place.

The narcissistic vulnerability for which Greenson demonstrated insufficient empathy was the patient's painful self-consciousness. The patient was acutely oriented to what was expected of him, worried about the analyst's opinion of him, and dreaded disagreeing with the analyst. Given how lonely and empty his life was, preserving the connection to the analyst through accommodation was perhaps all the more vital to his sense of well-being given that he remained for 6 years with his first analyst, went back for a second treatment experience, and accepted a referral for a third. Greenson seemed to fall into the role of arbiter of the rules of propriety for an analytic patient. He informed the patient that he did not do it right in his first analysis and educated him as to the right way to do it in his second analysis. When the patient was unable to get it right with Greenson, he was sent away for supportive therapy with someone else.

Perhaps empathizing with the patient's fears of not being a "good enough" analytic patient, interpreting how that re-created some childhood scenario of failing to please a parent who put great emphasis on following the rules of propriety, and trying more actively to enable the patient to feel a "good enough" patient may have relieved the patient of his paralyzing self-consciousness and allowed him to associate more freely and genuinely. There seems to have been little empathy for the possibility that the patient might feel quite a failure as an analytic patient, given his experience with Greenson.

As one alternative means of engagement, one might have appreciated the hidden irony of the patient's caricature of analysis. When the patient associated "Roskolnikov" to the analyst's inquiry about his middle name, rather than have viewed it only as a "bizarre" incident from which the analyst needed to recover his composure, one could have appreciated a clever method in the patient's madness. Maybe the patient meant to defy unconsciously Greenson's conventional expectations while being overtly compliant and innocent. There are many ways to engage a patient affirmatively besides educating a patient as to the proper way in which a classical psychoanalytic patient should work collaboratively.

I believe the false dichotomy that ego psychologists such as Sterba or Greenson established between the "real" or "reasonable" relationship with the analyst and the transference relationship leads to a certain loss of sensitivity to narcissistic vulnerabilities. With the patient whose child was ill, Greenson granted that her need for compassion was legitimate and may be gratified. With the patient who floundered when he could not ascertain or meet the analyst's expectations, Greenson seemed to see this as a neurotic need that he was less inclined to gratify except through some initial educative advice. And as it was a need that he believed should be largely frustrated in analysis, he did not feel it was necessary to empathize with the patient's anxiety in not knowing or not being able to do what was expected of him. If the patient could not tolerate the analytic situation as Greenson defined it, he was terminated rather than Greenson perhaps accepting responsibility to experiment with different ways of engaging the patient in order to make the analytic situation more tolerable for the patient.

If it is not possible to clearly differentiate a real relationship from a transferential relationship, the patient's relationship to the analyst can be appreciated as an interpenetrating mix of the real and the imagined that can only artificially be dichotomized. For this reason, Brenner seemed wary of any attempt to gratify a so-called real need for a humane analyst and of any way of dealing with transference that is not primarily interpretive. He seemed to fear that being more human or more freely interactional will make the patient less rather than more analyzable. I would suggest the opposite.

As being more human and freely interactional tends to evoke a transferential atmosphere of safety that lowers the patient's anxiety level and therefore defensiveness, the patient initially is more open to analysis. If over time the patient clings to the comfortable relationship with the analyst as a means of keeping the analysis at a superficial level, the unobjectionable positive transference can be addressed as a transference resistance to deeper work. On the other hand, to begin the analysis in an austere atmosphere of abstinence, poker-faced responsiveness, and careful adherence to the rules of analysis is likely to induce regression to a hostile/ dependent transference paradigm that raises the patient's anxiety level and defensiveness, making the patient less receptive to analysis. As Freud initially noted, successful analysis depends on the fact that the patient's transferential attachment to the analyst outweighs in the end the patient's transferential hate. And the weight of that balance depends to a large degree on not only the analyst's interpretive skill but interpersonal ability to engage the patient skillfully as well.

In summary, the alliance concept is innovative because it highlights the elements of an empathic relationship that are prerequisite for the patient to be open to analysis. The patient must experience the analyst as a benign superego as well as an affirmative ego ideal, identify with the analyst as a rational observer and collaborator, and feel a basic sense of trust in relation to the analyst. Yet each of these elements of the alliance is likely to prove an unreliable ally in the face of resistance analysis, with its attendant intensification of unconscious conflict. In addition, each element of the alliance can serve as a subtle resistance in itself to deeper work, which keeps the analysis at a superficially compliant level. To the extent the analyst sees the alliance as a "real" rather than "transferential" relationship, the analyst is vulnerable to falling into the unwitting role of arbiter of what are legitimate or illegitimate needs to be gratified or frustrated in the analysis. To the extent that certain of the patient's needs are treated as unrealistic and illegitimate, the patient may experience the analyst as lacking empathy for those needs.

One aspect of the ego-psychological approach to making resistance analysis less adversarial is in the refinement of the concept of the psychic surface. It was thought that if analysis proceeded by working from surface to depth then the patient would never feel criticized or attacked by an interpretation because the analyst would always be saying something the patient was just about to say for him- or herself. This would confirm for the patient that patient and analyst were in sync on the same empathic wavelength. It would be almost as if the analyst were reading the patient's mind in anticipating the patient's next thought just as the patient was about to articulate it.

Glover (1955) reported that the concepts of "surface" and "depth" did not have clear-cut definitions. "Deep" could refer to a developmental stage or to the accessibility of a psychic content to consciousness. Is a deep interpretation one that interprets an early developmental experience, such as a primitive fantasy or childhood trauma, or one that interprets an experience that is highly defended against, such as a distressing unconscious perception of the analyst in the here and now? Regardless of the definition of "deep," Glover (1955) seemed to suggest that the antidote to making premature interpretations that go too deeply, too quickly is to adjust the extent of interpretation according to the "appropriate dosage" (p. 282). Of course, the concept of dosage is probably fuzzier than the concept of depth. It seems an overextension of the medical model to assume some analogy between interpretation and medication, although some forms of resistance analysis might be aptly captured by the notion of "taking one's medicine."

Loewenstein (1954) noted that the term *surface* possesses several meanings: *surface* can refer to (1) the patient's current reality situation and present interest; (2) accessibility to conscious awareness, thus including preconscious content and processes; (3) the point of emotional urgency that highlights the state and nature of conflicts between drive and defense at the immediate moment; or (4) those aspects of the patient's mental activity, such as an observing ego, that are at the disposal of the patient's autonomous ego functions. Levy and Inderbitzin (1990) gave four definitions of the psychic surface: (1) the point of emotional urgency in the here-and-now transference; (2) the surface manifestations of unconscious conflict that can be observed and scrutinized by the patient; (3) continuities and especially discontinuities in the process of free association; and (4) the perceptual and experiential world of the patient, especially the patient's experience of discrepancies between the psychic realities of patient and analyst.

In reviewing these conceptions of the psychic surface, some conflicting definitions are evident, and such conflict is of crucial concern if the concept of the surface is going to determine one's focus of interpretation. When *surface* refers to what is going on in the immediate moment, the "moment" may refer to what the patient is discussing in the moment or to what the patient is doing and experiencing at the immediate moment in the relationship with the analyst. Although there is always an immediate here-and-now relationship to the analyst in every single moment of the analysis, the patient is not always consciously thinking about or focusing on that relationship. Gill (1982) noted the ubiquity of the patient's resistance to the awareness of the here-and-now transference. Many aspects of the here-and-now transference, though an immediate experience in the moment, are nevertheless relatively inaccessible to conscious awareness and are therefore far from the psychic surface.

The point of heightened emotional urgency and conflict at the immediate moment may not be the point on which the patient is currently focusing but rather the point from which the patient actively avoids focusing. Surface manifestations of unconscious conflict such as discontinuities in free association or parapraxes available to the patient's observing ego for analytic scrutiny, though accessible to consciousness, may nevertheless constitute content of which the patient would prefer to avoid thinking. Such content therefore may be considered not quite as close to the surface as those psychic contents of which the patient would prefer to think. For example, a patient may prefer to gloss over a slip of the tongue by quickly correcting the mistake and proceeding to make the consciously intended point. The patient may resist the analyst's efforts to draw attention to the slip despite the ready accessibility of the slip to conscious awareness. Thus, the patient's intended point is closer to the surface than awareness of the slip, which might be considered to reside at a point just slightly below the surface.

Perhaps the best way to think of the surface–depth dimension is in terms of levels of defensiveness. "Deep" describes content of which the patient is most defensive, whereas "surface" is content of which the patient is least defensive. To interpret from surface to depth can then be simply defined as interpreting that of which the patient is least defensive prior to interpreting that of which the patient is most defensive. Perhaps the absolute surface of the mind would be constituted by those psychic contents of which the patient is not defensive at all. In terms of interpreting from surface to depth, Fenichel (1941) suggested:

> When an interpretation has no effect, one often asks oneself: "How could I have interpreted more deeply?" But often the question should more correctly be put: "How could I have interpreted more superficially?" . . . For we must operate at that point where the affect is actually situated at the moment; it must be added that the patient does not know this point and we must first seek out the places where the affect is situated. [pp. 44–45]

Here would seem to be a possible inconsistency. If the patient does not know where the affect is located at the moment and is presumably defending against that awareness, then the affective point of urgency is not at the surface.

Fenichel (1941) provided the following criteria for assessing when an interpretation is too deep: "When is an interpretation too deep? When the patient cannot recognize its correctness by experiencing the impulse in question" (p. 45). It seems that one interprets not at the absolute surface (i.e., that of which the patient is not defensive at all) but rather from a relative surface (i.e., that of which the patient is least defensive and would probably therefore acknowledge if brought to his or her attention). Fenichel (1953) recommended that one interprets "when there is a minimum of distance between allusion and what is alluded to" (p. 322) and "when the distance between what is said and what is meant is at a minimum" (p. 324). To interpret at the absolute surface would then be to take the patient at face value in a wholly literal way, to reflect only what the patient consciously intended to communicate. To interpret just below the surface would be to interpret what is most obviously implicit in the patient's communications, though what is most obviously implicit may not be quite what was consciously intended. What is most obviously implicit is preconscious in that it constitutes a meaning that was not immediately conscious but is readily accessible to consciousness.

Fenichel (1953) stated that one never interprets repressed drives directly but rather their preconscious derivatives (p. 341). In regard to unconscious aspects of ego defense, he suggested that in interpreting resistance "one cannot reveal more to the patient than what he is able to discover in himself by self-observation" (p. 341). Thus the analyst attempts to form a connecting link between the absolute surface (i.e., that of which the patient is not defensive at all) and the relative surface (i.e., that of which the patient is least defensive). In topographic terms, the analyst is linking immediately conscious material with preconscious material (i.e., material that is most obviously implicit in the conscious material and of which the patient is least defensive). Material of which the patient is least defensive is material of which the patient would find it difficult to establish a modicum of plausible denial and would therefore be most likely to acknowledge if called to his or her attention.

Despite the modesty of the link that the analyst is attempting to establish in interpreting what is most obviously implicit in the patient's consciously intended meaning, the patient may resist establishing even such a link. The means of disrupting the establishment of such links derives from the fact that there is a fluid rather than static relation between what is conscious and what is preconscious. Material of which one had not been defensive at all may turn into material of which one is at least somewhat defensive once it is subject to analytic scrutiny, and material of which one had been minimally defensive may turn into material of which one is quite defensive once it begins to be interpreted. Perhaps something of which one had been quite defensive may become something of which one becomes quite open in order to avoid becoming aware of some other material of which one is even more defensive. For example, despite having had a positive working alliance in which hostility was denied, one might rather admit one's hatred of the analyst than one's homoerotic love of the analyst if there were some danger of that love being exposed and one felt forced to choose between the lesser of two evils. The point here is that levels of defensiveness are fluid rather than fixed. Orderly stratification of defenses would reflect a rather simplistic defensive strategy. Freud likened the resistance to an opponent in a chess game, an opponent capable of sophisticated strategic thought. Thus, although defenses are layered from surface to depth, those layers are constantly shifting as a clever strategy of defense rather than remaining fixed as an immobile armor plating, as Reich suggested.

The implication of the fact that levels of defensiveness are fluid is that what is surface and what is depth may be reversed as a strategy of defense. Freud, in originating the psychodynamic model, noted that any conscious psychic phenomenon constitutes a compromise formation in that it consists of a compromise between instinctual expression and instinctual inhibition, between defense and wish. In suggesting that resistance be interpreted before content, Freud implied that the defense side of a compromise formation should always be interpreted prior to the wish side of a compromise formation. Fenichel (1941) noted that in the service of defense, there can be a reversal between the defense side and the wish side of a compromise formation. Not only do defenses serve to defend against awareness of defenses, but "instinct serves for suppression of instinct" (p. 57) just like there "are reaction-formations against reaction-formations" (p. 61). Fenichel qualified the two-layer approach of drive and defense and suggested a three-layer approach:

> The problem may be rather more complicated in that there are not only two, but three (or more) "psychic layers": instinct-defense-superficial instinctual attitude. When we interpret we must be quite clear whether an experienced instinctual im-

pulse is original, has passed through a defense, or serves directly defensive purposes. [p. 57]

There exists not only the "three-fold stratification" of (1) instinct (2) defense (3) resurgence of instinct, but also of (1) instinct (2) defense (3) defense against defense. [p. 61]

When drives can function as defenses and defenses can function as a means of drive discharge, determining what is drive and what is defense becomes confusing. This confusion is not so much a conceptual one of the theorist as it is a defensive attempt at obfuscation by the patient that arises as the patient unconsciously surmises the analyst's strategy of interpretation and attempts to resist it unconsciously. Fenichel (1941) provided the example of a man who became passively feminine as a defense against castration anxiety but then assumed an exaggerated masculinity as a defense against passive femininity. Was passive femininity a drive-determined expression of bisexuality or a defensive attitude, and was exaggerated masculinity a drive-determined expression of phallic narcissism or a defense? Obviously the answer cannot be either/or.

Fenichel (1941, p. 57) illustrated the fluid nature of what is drive and what is defense in the instance of a patient who had a dream of incest at the beginning of an analysis. It was clear to the analyst that in the manifest content of the dream there was a return of the repressed incestuous wish into conscious awareness. Yet Fenichel noted that if the patient had been told that he really wished to consummate the incestuous act of which he dreamed, the patient would not have known what to make of such an interpretation. The incestuous act in the dream was experienced as ego-alien in relation to the patient's waking ego so that the patient did not fully identify with the incestuous wish. In fact, the dream may have served a defensive function in relation to the analyst in which the patient preconsciously believed: "If I admit this, the analyst will leave me in peace" (p. 57). The patient's defensive attitude was to oblige the analyst in giving him what he suspected the analyst wanted and in so doing covertly ridiculing the analyst. The incest dream should have then been interpreted first in terms of its defensive function, as a manner of superficially complying with the analyst while covertly defying him before any attempt could be made to meaningfully interpret the patient's incestuous wishes. The open expression of incestuous wishes served as seduction away from noticing certain more subtle attitudes of transference resistance.

Despite the innovation in recognizing that the direct and open expression of incestuous wishes may have served multiple functions such as defense in addition to drive discharge, there are other interpretive possibilities that Fenichel did not consider that may have reflected even more surface-level readings of the material. The patient's attempt to please the analyst by bringing in an incest dream at the beginning of treatment may not have only reflected an outward display of compliance that disguised underlying defiance. It may also have been the patient's manner of engaging the analyst through identification so that to interpret the defensive function of the dream would have been to inflict a narcissistic injury. The patient presented the analyst with a gift as a basis for the establishment of an unobjectionable positive transference, a good analytic patient who generated Freudian dreams. The defense interpretation of the dream was equivalent to a rejection of the patient's gift. An alternative to interpreting either the drive or the defense meaning of the dream would have been simply to acknowledge that the patient had brought in an "interesting" dream to be analyzed and see where the patient took it from there.

Viewing the dream in more interactional terms, one might have inquired about the patient's stereotype of a Freudian analyst and to what degree the analyst seems to fit that stereotype. Fenichel (1941) noted the frequency that his patients were "astonished" at his "freedom and naturalness" as though "they had believed that an analyst is a special creation and is not permitted to be human" (p. 74). He assumed that his patients' perception of his humanity reflected a realistic perception of his actual behavior so that at least initially he did not interpret their "astonishment" as in part a form of defensive idealization or ingratiation. He accepted their gratification at his freedom and naturalness as an essential aspect of building therapeutic rapport. Yet when his patient may have seen him as a stereotypic Freudian analyst in another respect, such as an analyst who might be obsessed with interpreting the patient's infantile sexuality, Fenichel assumed he was dealing with the manifestation of a transference resistance because he did not believe it was a realistic perception of his actual behavior that he would reduce the patient's behavior to its roots in infantile sexuality alone. Thus he could not simply accept the incest dream as a gift in the service of building rapport, as he seemed to accept without initial skepticism his patients' "astonishment" at his humanity. Once again the ego psychologist tends unwittingly to assume the role of arbiter of what is a real and what is an imaginary aspect of the therapeutic relationship.

If the real and the imaginary cannot be differentiated, it does not necessarily mean that the proper analytic attitude should always be one of skepticism on the lookout for hidden transference resistances with which one is attempting to avoid collusion. On the contrary, the proper attitude should be one of a naive observer who takes things at face value until proven otherwise (i.e., the patient is treated as essentially innocent until proven guilty) yet who paradoxically appreciates that in the end the analyst's collusion with repetitive transference enactments is inevitable, regardless of whether the analytic attitude is one of skepticism or naiveté. The naive observer is in a position to have empathy for what is surface, whereas the skeptical observer is in a position to analyze resistances to what is deep.

Anna Freud (1936) had noted that the basic problem for defense analysis is that "All the defensive measures of the ego against the id are carried out silently and invisibly. The most we can ever do is to reconstruct them in retrospect: we can never really witness them in operation" (p. 8). Thus defense interpretations often possess an inferential quality that seems to run counter to the patient's conscious self-experience of being essentially nondefensive in her free associations. As soon as the analyst begins to interpret beyond what is consciously self-evident, the patient begins to feel that the reality of her subjective experience is being undermined by the analyst's speculations in regard to what is defensively concealed beneath the surface of the patient's conscious thoughts and feelings.

Gray (1994) has developed an ingenious method for enabling patients to witness their own defensive activity. Gray suggested that the analyst should not interpret an ego defense until an id derivative reaches conscious awareness and the patient goes on to repress the id derivative that had reached full conscious awareness. The analyst may call the patient's attention to this process, which is fully observable within the patient's stream of consciousness. For example, a patient openly voices his anger at his mother-in-law for being overly intrusive, immediately followed by a self-reproach to the effect that he should learn to be more accommodating. Gray might then point out how the open expression of anger is followed by self-reproach, a self-reproach that seems to eliminate the patient's guilt-ridden expression of anger from conscious awareness. A conscious id derivative, hostility toward mother-in-law, is followed by a consciously expressed ego defense, turning anger against the self. If the analyst calls the patient's attention to the drive/defense sequence, it can be directly witnessed by the patient's observing ego as it has occurred consciously rather than unconsciously.

This approach constitutes an innovative way of working from surface to depth for it calls the patient's attention to the relationship between two conflicting conscious contents (i.e., who is to blame: mother-in-law or self?) that have emerged in the patient's free associations without the necessity of introducing the inference of a deeper hidden content of which the patient is as yet unaware. Nevertheless, the relationship between the two contents assumed by Gray's approach, that self-reproach serves to defend against anger, a standard psychodynamic formulation, is an inference not beyond questioning and is not self-evident in the data. Just as plausible is the speculation that conscious anger at others is a defense against unconscious self-reproach. The sequence of openly expressed anger followed by self-reproach could reflect a failure of defensively motivated anger to effectively suppress the conscious emergence of unconsciously warded-off self-blame. The relationship of the two contents may be ambiguous: as self-blame defends against blaming mother-in-law, blaming mother-in-law may simultaneously defend against self-blame.

Gray tends to assume that an id derivative can be clearly differentiated from an ego defense. If it is appreciated that there is some ambiguity as to what is drive and what is defense, the analyst would be best advised to attempt to maintain a stance of neutrality in regard to the issue. One might utilize Gray's innovative focus by calling the patient's attention to the sequence of free associations and of conflicting conscious contents within those associations. Yet one might keep in mind that what manifestly seems to the analyst to be clearly drive and defense could also reflect exactly the opposite.

In concluding the theoretical section of this chapter, I would like to highlight some of the strengths and limitations of the ego-psychological approach. Though some contemporary analysts do not like the concept of the therapeutic or working alliance for fear of fostering an unanalyzed passive/compliant relationship, I believe it is a valuable idea because it points to the need to establish that the analyst can see the world from the patient's point of view prior to beginning to analyze the defensive functions of that point of view. To begin analyzing the defensive functions of a point of view that has yet to be fully appreciated seems premature. The alliance concept highlights the need for the analyst and patient to establish some preliminary consensus about just what the patient's ego-syntonic/surface point of view actually is prior to subjecting that point of view to analysis. It is also clear that analyzing the defensive function of the patient's ego-syntonic/surface point of view will strain the alliance and that the alliance is a necessary but not sufficient condition for analytic work to continue to unfold.

What I also find of use from ego psychology is its refinement of the topographic model. A liability of the topographic model is if one begins to conceive the mind as organized according to rigidly stratified layers. Ego psychologists noted that the mind may be layered from surface to depth but that those layers are fluid and shifting. Thus, working from surface to depth is not like peeling the layers of an onion in an orderly and set sequence. There is not one unitary, never-changing surface/ego-syntonic perspective but rather multiple, ever-changing surface/ego-syntonic perspectives that may conflict with and defend against each other. In other words, there are multiple views from the tip of the iceberg depending on which direction one is facing. The problem, though, with the concept of working from surface to depth is that once we appreciate that there are multiple, constantly shifting views from the tip of the iceberg, how can we ever be confident that we have actually captured the current psychic surface in our interpretation? What is surface (i.e., conscious or preconscious content) becomes as complex, ambiguous, and controversial to assess as what is deep (i.e., unconscious content). How do we know whether we have articulated what the patient was just about to arrive at by him- or herself, and are therefore in perfect empathic attunement, or whether we are putting words in the patient's mouth to which he or she submits as part of a "compliant" alliance?

The ego-psychological approach demonstrates considerably more sensitivity to the patient's narcissistic vulnerability in being subject to resistance analysis than Freud's or Reich's approaches, but I do not think it is as sensitive as the approach Kohut went on to develop. Though I believe the timing and tact of ego psychologists in relation to the patient's resistance became quite sophisticated in many respects, ego psychologists still tended to view the patient's narcissistic attitudes in the treatment situation as primarily a resistance to deeper exploration. And it was the tendency of ego psychologists to focus primarily on the defensive nature of the patient's narcissism that led Kohut to develop his self-psychological approach in which the self-affirmative function of the patient's narcissism could be appreciated as well.

The ego-psychological approach adds considerable refinement and sophistication to the intrapsychic understanding of the more surface levels of the mind, but it remains relatively oblivious to interpersonal or interactional complexity in the analytic situation. It is more interactional than Freud or Reich in addressing more explicitly the impact on the analysis of the presence or absence of the alliance, an interpersonal dimension of the treatment situation. Nevertheless, transference and resistance are still conceived in primarily intrapsychic terms. In the work of Greenson (1967), this manner of thinking leads to a false dichotomy that is established between the "real" relationship and the transference, as though the two could be clearly differentiated.

In returning to the case of Joe, the insights of ego psychology may be of use. As we left the case in the last chapter, Joe had settled into long-term treatment with the acknowledgment of possessing chronic problems of low self-esteem and emotional insecurity that may underlie his academic underachievement. Yet Joe's approach to treatment was primarily to provide the therapist with weekly updates and progress reports for which he sought the therapist's reassurance when he had had a difficult week and for which he sought the therapist's approval when he had had a good week. On his own initiative, Joe was not inclined to discuss his conflicted relationships with others, his inner conflicts, his fantasy life, or his childhood experiences. If we consider the ego-psychological concept of the therapeutic or working alliance, it becomes apparent that the therapist in many respects had not established a stable alliance with the patient.

When we discuss the presence or absence of an alliance, we must ask with which aspects of the patient's personality is the therapist allied or nonallied. In terms of an alliance with the patient's observing ego, such an alliance was surely not present; in fact, the patient resisted the formation of such an alliance. The therapist tried very skillfully to evoke the patient's curiosity about his internal dynamics, the transference, and his childhood, to which the patient responded with transient superficial compliance and then quickly changed the subject back to his everyday situational concerns. At the level of basic trust, an alliance seemed to have quickly formed as part of Joe's maternal transference. Joe became dependent on the therapist for support and reassurance, and when the therapist confronted him about his lateness, he was assured that the therapist was a strong person who could take care of him. Yet this level of alliance was not without ambivalence, as Joe kept the therapist at arm's length out of his unconscious fear of becoming overly dependent on the therapist and infantilized and emasculated by that dependence.

For the most part, Joe experienced the therapist as a benign if not overly permissive superego from whom he did not anticipate criticism, like his mother for whom he could do no wrong. Yet when the therapist addressed his ego-dystonic character resistances, she was experienced as critical like his father. The other aspect of the therapeutic alliance that was not securely established is what has been called the narcissistic alliance. Joe was seeking treatment to prove that he could be an achiever. Although the therapist had implicitly accepted that goal for treatment and set herself the task of addressing his unconscious inhibitions, which were seen as the cause of his underachievement, the therapist had not explicitly communicated to him that she did indeed see him as someone who had the potential to succeed. The therapist's neutrality on that point was unconsciously taken by Joe to mean that perhaps the therapist had some doubts about his capacity to be an achiever since she had never really allied herself with what he felt were his healthful and realistic narcissistic strivings to succeed academically.

In discussing the issue of the therapeutic alliance, Joe's resistance to it, and the therapist's unwitting ruptures of it, the therapist began to try to form a more explicit, consistent narcissistic alliance with Joe. In reflecting his strivings for academic achievement, his sense of academic potential, and the little weekly signs of progress in that direction, Joe began to perk up and demonstrate greater enthusiasm for the treatment. Joe still did not display an observing ego, but he became significantly less anxious in sessions and began to show a much more openly positive transference toward the therapist. Joe began to compliment the therapist in regard to how helpful the sessions were becoming, commenting that they were really making progress together. Of course, the therapist and I were relieved that things seemed to be going well. But the challenge seemed to remain of how to convert a successfully supportive treatment into a more clearly insight-oriented one.

The ego-psychological refinements of how one might work from surface to depth once the prerequisite therapeutic alliance has been established may be helpful at this point. The basic idea is that treatment must proceed from consideration of that of which the patient is least defensive to that of which the patient is most defensive and to appreciate that that of which the patient is least defensive is fluid rather than fixed. Since patients often enter treatment when their defenses are failing, psychic content that is usually deep is often close to the surface because when defenses fail, it returns from repression. As a result of the blow to Joe's self-esteem derived from his academic underachievement, Joe in a sense regressed and fled to the security of his relationship with his overindulgent and overcontrolling mother (i.e., in seeking treatment) as a defense against his performance anxiety at having to compete as a separate and autonomous individual, which evoked the narcissistic trauma of feeling rejected as a man by his father.

What the therapist responded to interpretively was the evocation and enactment in the transference of his hostile/dependent relationship to his mother. Such an interpretation was premature since it went directly to a highly defended-against issue—his failure to fully differentiate himself from his mother—and it bypassed the more surface-level issue related to performance anxiety for which he was desperately seeking reassurance. When the patient was wanting to be reassured that he was "man enough" to be a successful and competent adult, the therapist was unwittingly reminding him of his fears of getting close to and relying on a maternal woman. What was confusing to the therapist was the fact that Joe was presenting multiple psychic surfaces to the therapist. On the one hand, he was communicating his fear about intimacy with the therapist, which he was enacting in his initial lateness, while, on the other hand, he was communicating that it was really no problem for him to be involved with a supportive woman and that his anxieties really lay elsewhere in relation to his fears of direct competition with other men. Yet the first fear was actually a "deeper" issue that was only evident because of a failure of defense and a return of the repressed, whereas the latter fear was actually the more "surface"-level fear that brought him to treatment and that he was ready and eager to discuss.

As the therapist began to address the extratransference issue of his conflicts and anxieties in relation to competition, performance, and achievement while simply monitoring without comment his ambivalent maternal transference to her, Joe began to evidence some observing ego. He spontaneously expanded the discussion to childhood experiences with sports and competition with peers and was able to discuss in a meaningful way the wound to his self-esteem of his father's derisive attitude toward him as well as his vindictive fantasies of proving his father wrong. The discussions of weekly updates and progress reports began to diminish, while the discussions of his conflicts, anxieties, and defenses in regard to achievement and performance began to increase. The therapist started to feel more like an analyst than a supportive psychotherapist, though feeling somewhat unanalytic in not more directly and vigorously interpreting the transference as she believed would transpire in a "really deep" analysis. She could not easily shed the anxiety that derived from equating the idea of working from the surface with being superficial.

The refinements of ego psychology shift the notion of what it means to be empathic with a patient. It is not enough to empathize with the patient's worst fears, deepest wishes, most traumatic memories, or most ego-dystonic character traits. The analyst must also have empathy for surface-level and preconscious aspects of the patient's personality functioning. The analyst must have empathy for the patient's struggle to adapt to reality, realize healthy narcissistic strivings, maintain a sense of superego approval, and experience a consistent sense of safety and security in the world. In addition, the analyst must have empathy not only for the

patient's deepest anxieties but for the patient's most seemingly superficial worries and everyday concerns. The analyst
must have empathy for the difference between the most
deeply defended-against material that the patient vociferously struggles to keep outside the realm of consciousness
despite the occasional or frequent failure of defense and the
most surface-level issues against which the patient is least
defensive and which are a topic of conscious concern. This
differentiation is not as easy to make as may seem to be the
case at first glance, since what is surface is fluid rather than
fixed so that making such a differentiation requires a highly
discriminating form of empathy.

4

The Principle of Multiple
Function and the
Structural Model

Ego-psychological concepts such as the working alliance and analyzing resistance to the awareness of resistance by working from surface to depth could be seen as demonstrating greater empathic sensitivity to the patient's narcissistic vulnerabilities but perhaps at the expense of analytic rigor. The alliance concept suggests a lack of technical neutrality in exploiting the positive transference in order to obtain interpretive leverage. And working from surface to depth can imply that the mind is rigidly stratified according to layers, a conception of the mind that seems simplistic and overly schematic in neglecting the dynamic and fluid nature of consciousness given a mind that is embroiled in continual conflict and compromise. To focus on Freud's (1923) tripartite structural model of the mind as a whole (i.e., id, ego, and superego) rather than simply on the psychology of the ego alone is to emphasize the psychology of a mind in conflict and compromise.

One of the innovations of the structural model is that it allows for a more balanced emphasis so that one aspect of the mind is not the sole focus, to the exclusion of other aspects. A. Freud (1936) defined analytic neutrality as the analyst's maintenance of an equidistant position from the id, ego, and superego. This sort of neutrality avoids the pitfalls of a one-sided focus on id analysis that bypasses defense analysis, a one-sided focus on ego defense analysis that neglects the adaptive aspects of ego functioning, a one-sided focus on the adaptive aspect of ego functioning that neglects id analysis, or a one-sided focus on realistic anxieties that neglects superego anxieties. The structural model allows for a high level of analytic rigor in clearly delineating the components of intrapsychic conflict so that one can interpret conflict in a balanced manner.

A. Freud (1936) emphasized the point that resistance in the light of ego psychology should not be thought of as being comprised of ego defenses alone, although that is certainly one important component of resistance. There is a resistance of the id derived from its insistence on maintaining both its aims and its objects in their infantile forms. And there is a resistance of the superego derived from the superego's resistance to relinquishing the severity of its demands. Nevertheless, despite such evenhandedness, Fenichel (1954) stated, "I do not find that the formulation that the analyst has to carry on his work from a position equidistant from ego, id, and superego is quite clear. The task is to make the id or the superego accessible by means of analysis of the ego" (p. 190). The implication is that even though any psychic phenomenon can be appreciated from multiple perspectives and interpreted in terms of its multiple meanings, it is through the ego as the organ of self-observation that these multiple perspectives and meanings are apprehended. Whereas A. Freud emphasized analytic rigor in maintaining a stance "equidistant" from the different sides of the patient's conflicts, Fenichel emphasized that unconscious conflict is made accessible through an empathic connection to the patient's conscious ego.

Arlow and Brenner (1964) were perhaps the foremost advocates of the structural model, going so far as to suggest that it serves not so much as an addition to topographic theory but as a replacement for it. Whereas many classical analysts view the two theories as complementary, Arlow and Brenner tended to view the topographic model as anachronistic and the structural model as a more sophisticated replacement. The structural model appears to reflect an innovation in that it allows for the most precise and comprehensive description of the components of intrapsychic conflict and the compromise formations that arise in the process of conflict resolution.

Freud (1900) noted that psychic phenomena are "overdetermined," in that numerous and often conflicting motives go into determining the final outcome of any psychic event. Multiple wishes, fears, defenses, memories, fantasies, and realities are represented in any given psychic phenomenon, which as a consequence must necessarily reflect a compromise between these conflicting forces. Thus any psychic phenomenon represents multiple meanings and is therefore open to multiple interpretations. And unconsciously those multiple meanings are often contradictory, irreconcilable, and opposite yet manage to coexist without canceling each other out. Thus psychic phenomena can never be interpreted in either/or ways but must always be interpreted as reflecting apparent irreconcilables simultaneously.

Waelder (1930) updated Freud's notion of overdetermination in terms of the structural model by introducing what he called the "principle of multiple function." Each agency of the mind is responsible for executing certain functions so that any psychic phenomenon reflects the operations of the multiple functions of each agency of the mind. The id functions to obtain drive discharge, whereas the superego functions to oppose or to at least to mitigate drive discharge. The ego functions as a mediator between these conflicting agencies as well as between these agencies and external reality. The ego is posed with a paradoxical task: to obtain maximal drive discharge and superego compliance yet to defend against instinctual discharge and superego condemnation. The ego may perform more or less successfully at this task of mediation. Poor mediation results in intensified conflict and unsatisfactory compromises, whereas successful mediation diminishes conflict and results in satisfactory compromises in which all parties to the conflict are sufficiently although not perfectly satisfied.

Brenner (1982) criticized Waelder's principle of multiple functioning because it seemed to him to suggest that the ego can function outside of the conflict as though it were a neutral observer whose problem-solving skills assist in conflict resolution. Perhaps the ego is a biased participant in conflict that is thoroughly embroiled in it. Waelder's ego as mediator appears to reflect what Hartmann (1939) later refered to as a "conflict-free sphere of ego functioning." Probably the major difference between what might be called the ego-analytic approach versus the structural model approach is the question of whether aspects of the ego can potentially develop and function independently of conflict. It would seem to be the more analytically rigorous position to suggest that there is nothing in personality functioning that is not a compromise formation deriving from conflict. It would seem to be the more empathic position to assume that there is an ego with which the analyst can become allied that stands outside of conflict as an observer to it.

Perhaps a compromise position is to think of the ego as what Sullivan (1953) termed a "participant observer." The ego is a participant in conflict, as Brenner suggested, but it also attempts to be an objective observer that can serve as a mediator of conflict, as Waelder suggested. When the ego is thought of as a participant in conflict, it becomes apparent that it is simply one participant among many with its own particular viewpoint and therefore does not deserve special attention more than any other participant. When the ego is thought of as an observer and potential mediator of conflict, it deserves special attention as an ally of the analyst.

For Brenner, since every aspect of the personality is a compromise formation imbued in conflict, it does not make sense to form an empathic connection to any particular aspect of the patient's personality. To form an empathic connection is to be seduced into taking sides in a conflict. Yet if a certain aspect of the patient's personality stands outside of conflict as an observer, despite also being a participant, then it is to that aspect of the patient's personality that the analyst is speaking when the analyst interprets conflict. It is to that aspect of the patient's personality to which the analyst must make an empathic connection.

The strength of the structural model is in its evenhanded

description of the various participants in intrapsychic conflict. Brenner (1982) provided the following encapsulation of the components of conflict: "They include drive derivatives, anxiety and depressive affect, defense, and various manifestations of superego functioning. These components interact in ways governed by the pleasure-unpleasure principle. The consequences of conflict are compromise formations" (p. 7).

Brenner (1982) provided a functional definition of defense that expands the concept of defense well beyond any limited repertory of defense mechanisms. He suggested that there are no special mechanisms of defense and that whatever ensues in mental life resulting in less anxiety or depressive affect can be considered to be a manifestation of defense. Any aspect of ego, id, or superego functioning can be used defensively. Thus there is no aspect of personality functioning that does not serve in part a defensive function. And, for that matter, there is no aspect of personality functioning that does not serve drive discharge as well as superego functions. This is the analytic rigor of the structural model— that no psychic phenomenon serves one primary and exclusive function alone, that all psychic phenomena serve multiple functions simultaneously.

No one can argue with the usefulness of looking at the data of analysis from multiple perspectives. The greater the number of perspectives, the richer the interpretive possibilities. The essence of analysis could be thought of as contemplating a phenomenon from one angle and then another, until all possible angles have been exhausted. In reviewing case material in the light of the structural model, one can almost always discover some component of conflict that had been previously overlooked and that may point to a new area of interpretive work. Without doubt the structural point of view espoused by Arlow and Brenner possesses an analytic rigor that stands in contradistinction to less rigorous ego-psychological concepts such as the therapeutic alliance and working from surface to depth. This is the virtue as well as the weakness of the structural approach. What it gains in analytic rigor it seems to lose in empathic sensitivity. Though one aspires to have empathy for all sides of an unconscious conflict, in practice one makes an empathic connection with what is accessible to the patient's conscious awareness. As consciousness is but the tip of an iceberg, empathy is always with one small and selective aspect of the patient's personality. Thus one can only form an empathic connection by taking sides, the side of the patient's conscious ego (i.e., the view from the tip of the iceberg).

Any analysis must proceed in some sequence, focusing on some element initially while temporarily failing to focus on some other element. Although it is important to look at a phenomenon from multiple and conflicting perspectives, it would seem to be impossible to look at things from more than one or perhaps two contrasting perspectives in juxtaposition at a time. The fact that phenomena need to be studied one perspective at a time necessitates some sequencing or temporal ordering of one's focus of examination. The structural model by itself offers no theory for ordering the sequencing of one's interpretive activity other than to fall back on some intuitive sense of what is potentially accessible to analysis at the moment. Fenichel (1941) noted that the aim of analytic theory is to achieve scientific clarity from intuitive comprehension.

A topographic model is necessary for a theory that accounts for the sequencing of interpretations. Loewenstein (1951) suggested, "Interpretations may be characterized by the distance from the surface. The material communicated by the patient may move from the surface to the so-called depths, and it is important for the analyst to make his interpretations conform to this progression" (p. 5). Loewenstein noted that sometimes it is important to reverse the interpretive sequence and interpret "deep" material in more "surface" terms.

> A patient who was familiar with analysis complained repeatedly, in the beginning of his treatment, that his wife's behavior castrated him. I suggested that what he actually wanted to express was his doubt about his wife loving him. Although his remarks about the castrating effect of her behavior might have been genetically correct, it was important at the time when this

interpretation was given to point out the relevant psychic reality—to transpose from a regressive level to a more superficial one. I would like to call this type of interpretation "reconstruction upwards," historically as well as structurally. [p. 10]

The structural model by itself possesses no theory of working from surface to depth and offers no alternative theory (outside of intuitive appraisal) for establishing a sequence or hierarchy of interpretation. Loewenstein (1956) suggested that the concept of the ego in conjunction with a topographic model has the advantage of encompassing conscious as well as preconscious and unconscious phenomena and of uniting them within a common functional organization. As a consequence, the danger is reduced of conceiving of conscious thought processes as mere epiphenomena of unconscious and preconscious processes.

In terms of a topographic construal of the ego, Loewenstein (1956) suggested, "Thus we must conclude that a barrier exists not only between the unconscious and the preconscious and between the latter and the conscious, but also between conscious thoughts or emotions and their verbalization" (p. 463). To work at the surface would be to link conscious feelings and ideas that may be preverbal to words so that conscious experience may be verbalized. Loewenstein noted that patients may resist verbalization of nonverbal experiences that are accessible to consciousness because to articulate the experience to the analyst makes it real, whereas to remain inarticulate allows the reality of the experience to be denied. The analyst serves as a "witness," that is, an auxiliary memory who will remind the patient of certain facts that the patient might prefer to forget.

Though the unconscious mind operating according to primary process thinking is capable of registering innumerable sources of stimuli (i.e., perspectives) simultaneously and combining all of these sources into a unity through processes such as condensation, symbol formation, synthesis, and integration, the conscious mind operating according to secondary process thinking appears to be capable of focal attention to only one or possibly two items at a time, which establishes a figure–ground relationship. Conscious mentation tends to proceed in a logical linear sequence. Although the unconscious functions in a timeless manner, the system consciousness operates according to a linear sense of time comprised of a past, present, and future (Freud 1900). "Timing" (i.e., sequencing or ordering) one's interpretations requires more than a principle of overdetermination, multiple functions, or multiple perspectives; it demands in addition some theory of the hierarchical organization of these multiple meanings, multiple functions, and multiple perspectives.

Loewald (1980) criticized the approach of Arlow and Brenner (1964) for ignoring the distinction between unconscious and preconscious mentation. Primary process mentation operates according to analogical reasoning that is nonlinear, whereas secondary process mentation operates according to logical reasoning that is linear. The analyst cannot simply disown responsibility for ordering the patient's material according to some implicit preconscious theory. The idea that one is simply following the patient's lead in registering the salient themes of the session by using one's unconscious as a receptive organ in a state of evenly hovering attention denies the analyst's own preconscious, theory-derived ordering principles. By definition, the analyst's unconscious, just like the patient's, is beyond volitional control as well as beyond direct introspective awareness since it is repudiated so that the analyst's unconscious cannot be intentionally utilized as a receptive organ. Perhaps it would be more accurate to say that the analyst aims his or her preconscious theory toward the patient's communications and then intuitively surmises something akin to his or her preconscious expectations. That preconscious theory through which one chooses a focus of interpretation may either be refined or simplistic, acknowledged or disclaimed.

One of the challenges and paradoxes of clinical technique is balancing linear and hierarchical modes of thought (i.e., secondary process) with analogical and dialectical modes of thought (i.e., primary process) when the two seem to be mutually exclusive. On the one hand, clinical work is supposed to proceed in an orderly linear sequence as one proceeds from surface to depth. There is an interpretive sequence as resistance is interpreted before content, defense before drive-wish, and an alliance is formed before beginning to interpret unconscious content. Yet on the other hand, how can clinical work proceed in an orderly sequential manner when what is surface and what is depth, what is defense and what is drive-wish, what is alliance and what is misalliance are all fluid, ever shifting, and reversible? To appreciate primary process—that opposite and conflicting positions can simultaneously coexist and are symbolically interchangeable—requires thinking dialectically, in which one attempts to oscillate between polar opposites and thereby achieve a dynamic balance. Much of the clinical process, countertransference as well as transference, is unconsciously shaped by the primary process, which defies linear reasoning and ordering.

In clinical work, one can try to maintain a dynamic balance between hierarchical and dialectical modes of thought rather than reject one or the other as though the two were mutually exclusive. If one thinks *only* hierarchically (i.e., too much secondary process), clinical work is liable to becoming overly prescribed, rigid, and rule bound; whereas if one thinks *only* dialectically (i.e., too much primary process), clinical work is liable to becoming unfocused and lost in ambiguity (i.e., a wild analysis of premature interpretations). Paradoxically, one must maintain a dialectical balance in clinical work between dialectical and linear/hierarchical modes of thought. Clinical work does not proceed in a straight line from beginning to end, nor does it simply go around and around in circles, repetitively alternating between the opposite poles of the circle. Perhaps clinical work proceeds analogously to a descending spiral in which it gradually deepens (i.e., proceeds in a sequence) but follows a circuitous route in oscillating back and forth (i.e., proceeds dialectically) over the same material, but always with an added twist that progresses the work of the analysis. Thus as a principle of technique, empathy should always precede analysis in an interpretive sequence—a hierarchical approach—yet as a spontaneously unfolding intersubjective process, empathy and analysis should always be counterbalanced without overemphasis on either – a dialectical approach.

Often clinicians who think in primarily linear and hierarchical ways are most interested in developing systematic principles of technique that order one's interpretive activity. Such clinicians often view conceptions of treatment that highlight interpreting the spontaneous give-and-take of the transference–countertransference relationship as it is unconsciously enacted as in some way unsystematic. Certainly Freudian/ego analysts have tended to see Kleinian analysts as practicing wild analysis, which will be discussed in later chapters. On the other hand, clinicians who think in primarily dialectical ways often view emphasis on principles of technique as implying a way of working that is overly prescriptive, rule bound, rigid, and insensitive to the unconscious give-and-take of the therapeutic relationship, which is organized according to the primary process.

It should not be thought incompatible to recommend a logical, orderly sequence of one's interpretive activity at the same time that one is advised to intuitively go with the push and pull of the clinical encounter. The analyst is an agent who actively structures the clinical encounter according to his or her own preconceptions and intentional agenda, yet the analyst is also reactive to and molded by the patient's preconceptions and intentional agenda. One cannot help but impose an order and organization on the analytic experience, as one is ordered and organized by the analytic experience beyond one's volitional control. Despite Bion's (1967) recommendation to approach each session without memory or desire, I would suggest that the analyst's memory and desire give rise to preconceptions about the timing and sequencing of the analyst's interpretive activity that the analyst employs to organize the clinical material.

The strengths and limitations of Brenner's (1982) utilization of the structural model can be illustrated through a case presentation he used to demonstrate his approach to the analysis of defense (pp. 82-88). Brenner's neglect of the topographic perspective that requires that the analyst establish an empathic connection to what is surface prior to analyzing what is deep is salient in this case. In addition, Brenner did not seem to consider how his ordering principles seemed to shape what he believed to be the objective facts of the case. Thus he seemed oblivious to some of the underlying transference–countertransference configurations of which he may be an unwitting participant.

The patient was a 29-year-old woman who had been in analysis for 6 years. Prior to analysis, she had had sexual relations only with women. Brenner believed that her homosexuality served a defensive function, to deny (1) sexual feelings for her father, (2) jealous and hostile wishes toward her mother and her older married sister, and (3) her rage and humiliation that she did not have a penis. During the course of the analysis, the patient had sexual intercourse with men for the first time. During intercourse with men, she had the conscious fantasy of controlling her partner's penis or that the penis was part of her body rather than his. These heterosexual affairs were interspersed with homosexual ones that Brenner believed served the defensive function of warding off sexual feelings toward the analyst through identification with the male role in a homosexual relationship.

Brenner described an episode in which the patient was once again involved in a homosexual relationship and was consciously struggling to give up her current girlfriend. He noted that she was obviously resentful of her analyst and was trying to provoke him. She complained with righteous indignation that he behaved unfairly toward her and that he never gave her her due. When she debated with herself whether to give up her girlfriend, she often paused, waiting to hear the analyst's opinion. Brenner interpreted during one such pause that she was trying to get him to order her to give up her girlfriend so that she could rebel, just as she had so often tried to get her parents to take a position she could use as an excuse for rebelling against them. Brenner had already interpreted to her many times in the past that her anger at her parents and her analyst were "really" because she had not been given a penis and because neither her father nor her analyst loved her as she was sure they would have if she had been the boy her father had hoped for before she was born. Brenner hypothesized that the anger the patient attributed to him via projection was a means of evading superego guilt.

Brenner illustrated how subsequent to this interpretation the patient showed the following changes, which he saw as analytic progress subsequent to a correct and well-timed interpretation: she discontinued the homosexual affair; she was more feminine in dress and manner; she began to date a man; she asked an older, male colleague to accept her as a pupil; she was less angry at her analyst and wished to be close to him; she associated to a dream that she might become sexually excited while on the analyst's couch; she became aware of being angry at her mother and sister; she recalled wanting to be close to her father when she was 5 years old.

The strength of the structural model as Brenner employed it is that the patient's homosexuality was understood as a compromise formation serving multiple functions, one of which was a defensive function. The patient's behavior was not understood in any either/or manner. It reflected not only the gratification of endogenous drive wishes (i.e., innate bisexuality and wishes for a penis) but simultaneously a defense against a traumatic sense of the loss of the father's love, a means of identifying with the father in order to undo her sense of loss, and a means of getting close to women in order to repair her hostile conflicted relation with her mother and sister. Her homosexuality was appreciated as an overdetermined, multifaceted, and multidimensional phenomenon that may reflect conflicted and contradictory meanings. When homosexuality as well as heterosexuality are construed as compromise formations, the pitfalls are avoided of viewing sexual orientation and sexual identity as something essential and irreducible.

One problem with Brenner's particular use of the structural model in addition to his neglect of topographic concerns is his particular philosophy of science. Brenner (1982) recognized that clinical examples are schematized and simplified affairs, but he claimed that "they are, nevertheless, faithful to the facts of psychic life" (p. 77). He did not seem to appreciate that facts are created as well as discovered as well as open to multiple interpretations and that case reports are invariably selective in what is included and excluded. In other words, "facts" are compromise formations between conflicting ways of constructing reality.

In addition, Brenner (1982) seemed confident that he could differentiate "pathological" compromises from "normal" compromises (p. 82). In this particular case, he stated, "She became more mature. One can fairly say that she became more normal, since before the interpretation her masculine identification was expressed in a homosexual affair, while after the interpretation it was expressed in her relationship to an older man, her teacher who she planned to emulate in a realistically rewarding and socially desirable way" (p. 86). One of the strengths of the structural model is that it allows for a notion of neutrality in which one attempts to remain equidistant from the components of conflict.

Since questions of normality and pathology, especially the healthfulness of homosexuality, are highly conflictual issues, it is curious that Brenner seemed to take a clear stand on this issue rather than attempt to remain a neutral observer of conflict, though he did not overtly impose his personal opinion on his patient. Seeing the issue in an either/or manner, he did not entertain the option of bisexuality as a possible compromise formation since he framed the issue as perhaps the patient did, as a forced choice, and so he appeared to take at face value the patient's sense that she had to make a choice. Perhaps notions of normality and pathology are also compromise formations that reconcile conflicting ideas about what is "realistically rewarding and socially desirable." Ironically, Brenner was adept at viewing all facets of the patient's behavior as compromise formations but did not entertain the possibility that his behavior, his "facts," his views on normality and pathology, his countertransference, and his clinical interventions based on those views may also have been compromise formations.

In returning to the clinical material, one must wonder to what extent the patient surmised Brenner's personal belief that homosexuality in her case was an immature and pathological compromise formation in comparison to heterosexuality, even though he carefully refrained from ever explicitly telling her what to do in terms of her sexual orientation. And to the degree she surmised his personal position on this issue, how did her perception of his lack of neutrality on this issue impact on the analysis? Given how controversial an issue sexual orientation is, it is probably impossible for any analyst to avoid conveying personal bias, pro or con, in at least subtle ways. Brenner's consistent interpretation of the defensive function of the patient's homosexuality and avoidance of heterosexuality could have implicitly conveyed his personal bias if he failed to raise the equally plausible interpretive possibility that heterosexuality could serve as defensive conformity to the demands of a superego that condemns homosexuality.

Though Brenner gave abundant evidence of her shift toward heterosexuality subsequent to his interpretation, one cannot help but wonder to what degree the patient was finally, after 6 years of analysis, complying with her perception of his expectations in order to win his approval and silence her own superego condemnation (i.e., internalized homophobia). After all, if Brenner's formulation is to be believed, the patient was willing to become the boy she felt her father wanted in order to please him; so it would be entirely in character for her to have become the heterosexual girl she believed her current father surrogate wished her to be, given the patient's desperate need for paternal approval and apparent unconscious guilt over her homosexuality.

Perhaps if Brenner had given evidence of carefully addressing the issue in working from surface to depth, it might be more difficult to dismiss his therapeutic results as transference compliance to a father whose acceptance is desperately needed though often repudiated. What might working from surface to depth look like in such a case? We know from the case report what was deep: the patient's love for the father, anger toward the mother and sister, and masculine identification (i.e., the standard universal oedipal conflict with masculine identification as the attempted resolution).

We do not know from the case report a full account of what was surface (i.e., the unique particulars of the patient's phenomenal experience), so we must infer it.

As Brenner suggested that the patient's defenses could be appreciated as reaction formation, what is surface would be the opposite of what is deep. Therefore, the surface might be anger toward the father, love of the mother and sister, and feminine identification. From her debate about whether to give up her girlfriend, it would seem that neither homosexuality, heterosexuality, nor bisexuality was entirely ego-syntonic for her and that her sexual orientation was an issue around which she was quite conflicted. What was surface in the treatment, not unexpectedly given her reaction formation against love of the father, was her openly stated resentment and defiance of Brenner. Yet we are never informed of the conscious reason for which the patient believed that Brenner treated her unfairly. One cannot help but wonder whether she resented what she perceived, consciously or unconsciously, accurately or inaccurately, to be pressure to become a "normal" heterosexual woman, a violation of neutrality by an analyst who presumes to be neutral.

Thus Brenner's presentation of "facts" was curiously selective, skewed toward presenting comprehensive formulations of unconscious dynamics in standard oedipal terms while presenting quite spotty descriptions of surface-level phenomena. We know very little about the history of her conscious conflicts in regard to her sexual orientation. We are not informed of the quality of her object relations, the degree to which her relationships with men and women were experienced as either superficial or intimate. And we know very little about the history of her conscious conflicts with Brenner in relation to her sexual orientation, history that is crucial to evaluating the degree to which her behavior change reflected transference compliance rather than genuine working-through. Though Brenner did discuss the possibility of a superego transference in which the patient experienced him as condemnatory, he seemed to see her only as defying him as a superego figure but did not report discussing or interpreting the other side of the conflict – her unconscious wish to please him in order to alleviate superego guilt over her homosexuality.

To work from surface to depth would be to recognize that her surface level and ego-syntonic defiance toward father-analyst represented a defense against repudiated ego-dystonic compliance toward father-analyst. In the terms of this defiance–compliance conflict, homosexuality becomes a symbol of father defiance, while heterosexuality becomes a symbol of father compliance. When Brenner interpreted her attempt to provoke a confrontation whereby she would have an opportunity to defy him, it is likely that she experienced his interpretation in terms of a defiance–compliance conflict, as a paternal/superego reprimand to the effect that she should stop being so defiantly provocative if she wants to please her father-analyst-superego. The interpretation brings about a superego-motivated reversal of what was surface and what was depth. She overtly complied with the perceived reprimand but was still perhaps covertly defiant in replacing Brenner with another older man who she hoped would be more appreciative of her and whom Brenner might have regarded as a jealous rival.

Was her defiance worked through or simply driven temporarily underground out of unconscious guilt and a need to please? Did the patient develop any insight into the repudiated compliance side of her defiance–compliance conflict, or did she simply act it out? Since Brenner seemed to see attraction to an older man as a more "normal" resolution of oedipal conflicts than homosexual attraction to female peers, he did not seem to worry about the potentially hurtful consequences to the patient in terms of her sense of personal autonomy of conforming to what was presumed to be "realistically rewarding and socially desirable."

All this is not to say for sure that Brenner did not do good work in this case and that the patient did not make real progress. Without consideration of surface phenomena, it is impossible to know. If it was known that Brenner had empathy for what it was like for her to work with an analyst who she believed possessed a bias in regard to the pathological import of homosexuality, if it was known that the patient had thoroughly worked through her repudiated tendencies to comply with the desires of dominant men as well as internalized homophobia, and if it was known that her sexual relationships with women had been compulsive, impersonal, and sadomasochistic while her sexual relationships with men were becoming intimate, mutual, and equal, then Brenner's argument of analytic progress would be significantly more convincing to an audience who feels that his presentation of the "facts" is highly selective.

The problem in technique, which was raised in the section on ego analysis but which is not solved by the structural model alone, is the question of how one interprets from surface to depth—from that of which the patient is least defensive to that of which the patient is most defensive—when defenses are fluid in their method of operation. When surface and depth, figure and ground, resistance and content, and defense and wish are constantly shifting and reversing, how does one know where and how to focus an intervention, especially when such shifts and reversals are a likely defensive response to one's interpretive activity? (For example, was Brenner's patient simply shifting back and forth from one side of the conflict to the other, from homosexuality to heterosexuality and from defiance to compliance, without ever obtaining a metaperspective on the overall conflict?) If homosexuality defends against heterosexuality as heterosexuality defends against homosexuality, and if defiance defends against shameful compliance as compliance defends against guilt-ridden defiance, how does one do defense analysis?

Kernberg (1984) illustrated in bold relief that in borderline conditions there are often radical reversals between what is defense and what is defended against. The borderline patient may hate the analyst as a defense against loving the analyst, love the analyst as a defense against hating the analyst, and abruptly shift between these two incongruous attitudes when the defensive function of either is in danger of being exposed by the analyst's interpretive activity. Kernberg (1984) cited the need for a moment-by-moment diagnostic decision to assess what constitutes defense and what constitutes defended-against.

> The predominance of splitting over repressive mechanisms permits the alternation in consciousness of the dynamically opposed components of intrapsychic conflict so that access to consciousness per se does not serve to indicate which is the defense and which the impulse aspect of the conflict. Defense and impulse can be rapidly interchanged in the alternating reversals of activated object relations that are typical of part–object relations and conflictual impulses that are conscious and mutually dissociated or split off rather than repressed. Here, consciousness and unconsciousness no longer coincide with what is at the surface and what is deep, what is defense and what is content. But while the topographic approach to interpretation (the ordering of the material from surface to depth) no longer holds for such borderline structures, the moment-to-moment decision of which is the defensively activated ego state directed against which other impulsive ego state is very important. . . . That task often requires relatively rapid, imaginative tracking of what appear to be chaotic interactions. [p. 224-225]

Apfelbaum and Gill (1989) suggested that this assessment can be made by determining what the patient currently experiences as ego-syntonic in contrast to what is experienced as ego-dystonic. What is currently ego-syntonic constitutes defense, whereas what is ego-dystonic constitutes defended-against. Apfelbaum and Gill have innovatively employed a structural concept (i.e., ego-syntonic versus ego-dystonic) to address a topographic question (how to interpret from surface to depth) as well as a structural question (how to interpret defense before drive). What is ego-syntonic could be thought of as reflecting the absolute surface of the mind, as it constitutes content of which the patient is not defensive at all, at least not until it is subject to analysis. What is ego-dystonic constitutes something that is either relatively close to the surface or deep, depending on how incongruent it is with what is ego-syntonic. Thus analysis begins by having empathy for what is ego-syntonic in the moment. And it is from an empathic appreciation of what is ego-syntonic that defenses against what is ego-dystonic can begin to be analyzed.

An assessment of the ego-syntonicity/dystonicity dimension allows for an understanding of the level of defensiveness. The greater the discrepancy, incongruence, or distance between an ego-syntonic perception and an ego-dystonic perception, the greater the need for defense. Conversely, the lesser the discrepancy, incongruence, or distance between an ego-syntonic perception and an ego-dystonic perception, the lesser the need for defense. The implication for interpretation is that one interprets small discrepancies between what is ego-syntonic and what is ego-dystonic before interpreting large discrepancies. One can only begin to analyze ego-syntonic character traits if one makes the syntonic dystonic in small degrees. To work from surface to depth is to work from what is most ego-syntonic (i.e., surface) to what is most ego-dystonic (i.e., deep) in small graduated steps.

The only problem with this approach is in assessing what is syntonic and what is dystonic if the two are constantly shifting as a strategy of defense. For this reason Apfelbaum and Gill (1989) criticized the topographic model for implying a "layer" concept that makes defense seem like a simple cover or barrier on the surface of the mind that must be penetrated in order to go deeper. Rather than visualize defense topographically as an overall pattern of defense, they suggested that defense should be visualized microscopically in the moment as a fluid dynamic relationship between two contents that are interchangeably drive and defense: "What appears clinically to be a covering layer, if looked at in smaller units of experience, will be found to be warded off by another, less apparent content" (p. 1080). They suggested that if a patient rejects an interpretation angrily, it is the id-analytic view that the presence of a warded-off wish is confirmed, whereas it is the ego-analytic view that such a response may be expressive of unanalyzed superego effects. The anger suggests that some aspect of the defense has been overlooked, so that the interpretation is accepted or rejected as a superego injunction.

Apfelbaum and Gill (1989, pp. 1077–1079) illustrated their

approach in discussing a summary of a case by Kanzer (1981). Prior to the session discussed, the previous hour had been canceled because it fell on a holiday 3-day weekend. Kanzer inferred that the missed session was experienced as if it were a cancellation by the analyst, with the patient unconsciously reacting by feeling angry and affronted and wanting to retaliate, a transference repetition of a distant and rejecting father. The patient began the hour by expressing enjoyment of the holiday weekend, which Kanzer thought of as the denial of the loss of the session. The patient also expressed anger at the cab driver making him late to the session. He reported that he wanted to cancel a session at a later date to help his son get settled at college, which Kanzer viewed as a retaliatory tit for tat.

Kanzer's single intervention during the hour was a confrontation to the effect that it was difficult for the patient to swallow that he missed the analyst. The purpose of the interpretation was to prevent a flight from recognition of dependency. As the analysis was advanced and nearing termination, Kanzer felt that given the success of earlier defense analysis, the patient would be able to integrate such a confrontation. The patient responded to the interpretation with a memory at age 8 when he was in the shower with his father and felt close to him. The patient then commented scornfully, "I suppose you would say that I wanted to put his penis in my mouth, and that I want to put your penis in my mouth." As the patient ended the session and rose from the couch he lisped in a little boy voice, "Now I have to make a pee-pee," smiled, and left. Kanzer understood the patient's response to his interpretation as evidence of its success—that the patient was able to tolerate the humiliating fantasy of fellatio with his father and the analyst.

Apfelbaum and Gill (1989) noted that Kanzer was interpreting the presumably ego-dystonic wish directly, the patient's repudiated dependency wishes. They suggested that in Kanzer's neglect of the question of what is ego-syntonic, the interpretation could be experienced as a superego injunction to the effect that the patient should "swallow" the analyst's interpretation. They suggested an alternative interpretive approach that acknowledges the patient's ego-syntonic sense of how dependent or independent a mature adult should be. They proposed saying something along the lines of "There are some hints here that you may have felt affronted by my canceling the last hour, but it looks like you would really hate to feel that. It would make you feel petty and childish, especially since it was a national holiday" (p. 1092). If independence is ego-syntonic and dependence is ego-dystonic, then interpretation of defended-against dependency must always include an initial reference to wished-for independence, with which dependency wishes are in conflict. Independence may defend against fears of dependence, but the reverse may be true simultaneously: that dependence may defend against fears of independence. Apfelbaum and Gill suggested that when the patient responded angrily to Kanzer's interpretation, a follow-up interpretation may have been to inquire whether the interpretation was experienced as an accusation, so that hidden superego effects could be analyzed rather than bypassed and enacted.

The distance between what is ego-syntonic and what is ego-dystonic is determined by the superego. The superego sets the standard by which an evaluation is made in regard to what is acceptable and unacceptable. What is ego-syntonic is more or less what is acceptable to the superego, and what is ego-dystonic is more or less what is unacceptable to the superego. Thus the relation between drive and defense is always going to parallel the relation between the ego and the superego. Drive is determined by that of which the superego disapproves, and defense is determined by that of which the superego approves. As the relationship between the superego and the ego is continually shifting and reversing itself, so too will the relationship between what is ego-syntonic and ego-dystonic and between what is drive and defense. Kanzer's patient may have been ashamed of his wishes to be dependent on his analyst-father, but he may also have been guilt-ridden simultaneously about his wishes to be independent of the analysis as it approached termination and feigned dependency in order to prolong the relationship.

Though the microscopic approach of Apfelbaum and Gill is

illuminating, their rejection of the macroscopic approach that assesses the overall patterning of defense is premature. One of the innovations of Reich's approach to character analysis is that it is holistic rather than reductionistic in some important respects. One could begin to appreciate defensive attitudes and belief systems as well as overarching strategies of defense in contradistinction to the momentary deployment of particular mobile defense mechanisms that inhibit the flow of particular free associations. Nevertheless, one need not think of the overall patterning of defense as a sort of impenetrable character armor, as did Reich, but rather as a sophisticated and clever strategy of defense that is fluid and flexible, though perhaps ultimately self-defeating.

Perhaps Kanzer's patient at a "macro" level alternated between displays of independence and dependence in relation to the analyst as a defense against wishes for a more mutual and equal relationship with the analyst that he feared would be rebuffed. The independence–dependence conflict may have defended against a deeper conflict around hierarchy versus mutuality in a relationship. Maybe the memory of taking a shower with his father reflected not only the wish for a dependent relation with the father but also a wish for a "man-to-man" relationship with the father in which both are their "naked true selves," the sort of relationship he might have wished he could have with Kanzer but may have feared he could not because of an unanalyzed superego transference evoked by the analyst's austere interpretive/interactional stance. This might be an example of what Loewenstein would call "reconstruction upwards."

To remain focused on the microscopic runs the risk of "tunnel vision" in which one cannot see the forest for the trees. Perhaps microdefensive processes constitute simply one element of an overall macrostrategy of defense. For example, the borderline patient who loves the analyst to avoid hating the analyst and hates the analyst to avoid loving the analyst could be understood as employing a more overarching strategy of defense in which the patient, despite being manifestly immersed in loving and hating the analyst, is latently quite unrelated to the analyst and defending against relatedness to the analyst out of a fear that any sort of continuous connection to the analyst is dangerous. To focus only on analyzing the patient's love–hate conflict revealed in microanalysis is to avoid analyzing the patient's relatedness-unrelatedness conflict emerging from a macroanalysis. The patient relates to the analyst in an apparently overly intense manner as a defense against relating to the analyst in a more quietly trusting manner, which evokes fears of traumatic disappointment.

Microscopic events such as reversals of resistance and content, drive and defense, ego-syntonic and ego-dystonic, superego and ego positions, self and other in the transference, and so on, are all elements of an overarching strategy of defense employed as a means of "confusing the enemy," so to speak, by obfuscating the issues to the analyst as well as to oneself. It is defense through a heightening of ambiguity in an attempt to sow the seeds of confusion. The patient may seduce the analyst into exploring only the microlevel as a defense against seeing the macrolevel as well as do the reverse—seduce the analyst into looking only at the big picture to avoid exploring the details. The problem with the topographic model is not that it describes the mind in terms of layers but only that some analysts such as Reich mistakenly conceived of those layers as rigidly stratified. When defense is appreciated holistically as an overarching strategy of defense that operates in a fluid manner, it becomes possible to entertain a topographic view of the mind in which surface and depth are continually shifting phenomena, a view true to Freud's original dynamic conception of the topographic model, as implied by such ideas as the return of the repressed.

Though Hartmann (1951) believed that one of the important innovations of ego psychology is to focus with microscopic precision on the process of ego defense, he also believed that ego psychology leads to the macroscopic study of the patient as a "total personality" (p. 34). When defenses are looked at macroscopically, a character structure emerges as a distinctive gestalt, reflecting an overall pattern or strategy of defensive functioning. This character structure, though

perhaps not a rigid armor plating, does reflect some hierarchical ordering of features that are captured by topographic
concepts. At a macro level, it remains "experience near" to
think of the personality as possessing a surface covering that
disguises while covertly expressing a deeper level. People do
think of themselves as possessing an external public-self
presentation that is manifest to others but that hides an inner
private self that expresses itself only indirectly. The topographic experience of the mind would appear to be rooted in
the development of what Anzieu (1989) called the "skin ego."
The experience of the body becomes a template for the
experience of the mind, so that just as the body possesses a
surface covering, the skin, which protects, hides, and indirectly reveals an inner space, by analogy so does the mind.

The structural model tends to treat the "ego" or the "self"
as a psychic content, a compromise formation, to be dissected
into its component parts rather than appreciated as an
integrated entity possessing a psychological function in its
own right. When viewed as only a product of conflict, the self
becomes an epiphenomenon, an illusion or fantasy formation
that conceals yet indirectly reveals intrapsychic conflict.
Grossman (1982) suggested that though the self as a content
of fantasy life can be appreciated as compromise formation, it
can be seen as an adaptive compromise formation serving an
organizational function; as such, it can be said to possess
structural properties in and of itself. The self, though an
illusion, appears to be a necessary illusion, for we seem to
operate with an implicit concept of a person who experiences
conflict, analyzes conflict, and engages in conflict resolution
and compromise. Experientially, the self is always a
participant-observer in relation to intrapsychic conflict. Thus,
in understanding the self, it can be construed as an object (a
participant in conflict), a subject (an observer of conflict), or
an epiphenomenon (an illusion that arises as a by-product of
conflict).

Without a concept of self as a participant-observer in
relation to intrapsychic conflict, conflict would appear to exist
in a depersonified psyche, a selfless psyche. The structural
model by itself would seem to provide a theory of the mind

without a theory of the person whose mind is conflicted. We need to imagine a person with whom we are in empathic connection in order to feel that someone is listening to the analyst's interpretations of conflict and compromise. It is not clear to me to whom or to what Brenner believed he was addressing his interpretations if he remained "equidistant" from all aspects of the patient's personality in order to avoid being seduced into taking sides in a conflict.

What I find most useful in the structural approach is the emphasis on the principle of multiple function and the concept of compromise formations. Both ideas are consistent with and highlight the need to examine phenomena from multiple and conflicting perspectives. The mind can be seen as an organization consisting of many competing, conflicting perspectives that somehow must achieve a compromise perspective so that the person can attempt to function as an integrated unit. To think of the mind as being organized in such a fashion enables the analyst to avoid becoming over-identified with and taking the side of any specific perspective at the expense of a competing perspective.

The limitations of the structural approach by itself are that it neglects topographic concerns such as the need to proceed from surface to depth and tends to minimize holistic ways of thinking that focus on character and self in favor of dissecting such holistic concepts into component parts. The structural model tends to see the parts as being greater than the whole, whereas I would see the whole as being greater than the sum of its parts. I believe empathic sensitivity decreases if the patient cannot be responded to as a whole person who is consciously at a particular place in a particular moment with which the analyst must be attuned. In addition, the structural model by itself has little to say about interactional complexity in the analytic situation since it maintains a primarily intrapsychic focus. The structural model could potentially make a contribution to an interactional perspective if one were to begin examining countertransference and the resolution of interpersonal conflict as compromise formations that serve multiple functions. This view might bring a greater analytic rigor to an interactional approach.

To return to the case of Joe, treatment seemed to be proceeding nicely as a strong therapeutic alliance had been formed, and the content of the sessions reflected a comfortable blend of progress report and introspective exploration of conflicts related to performance and achievement. To some extent, Joe's academic performance improved from where it had been before the beginning of treatment, but Joe still found it very difficult to focus himself for studying, to pay attention in class, and to prevent himself from procrastinating. Joe wondered whether perhaps he had a learning disability, although intelligence testing in the clinic suggested a person of above-average intelligence with no discernible cognitive deficits, a person who was pretty much above average across the board. Joe seemed to be developing insight but not significant behavior change, and to the extent his performance seemed better, the improvement seemed to derive from the emotional support that the treatment provided.

At this point the insights of the structural model might prove applicable. As the therapist had formed a narcissistic alliance with Joe's desire to achieve, in a sense she was no longer neutral but had taken sides in a conflict. The therapist was on the side pushing Joe to succeed rather than the side that for multiple reasons did not wish to or was frightened of succeeding. The therapist was always analyzing Joe's conflict from a biased angle, the perspective of someone who was personally invested in seeing Joe do well academically and who was invested in seeing Joe make regular progress in that regard. It never occurred to the therapist to take the opposite side: why did he feel he had to do well academically, why did he have to be college educated, or what was so bad about graduating as an average student? My point is not to suggest that the therapist should have taken that side, but to see the other side of the conflict is to bring to light the therapist's absence of neutrality.

As the therapist realized she had fallen into the role of assuming responsibility for promoting Joe's career achievement and as it seemed treatment was becoming less analytic and more like pressure to perform, the therapist attempted to adopt more of a stance of technical neutrality in relation to his conflicts and to express curiosity about the other side of Joe's desire to do well academically. It emerged that neither of Joe's parents had gone to college. He was the first in his family to attend college. His mother was a housewife, and his father was a successful contractor who made a solid middle-class living. His mother very much wanted him to become a college-educated professional, whereas his father was more ambivalent, feeling that Joe could make a good living if he went into the contracting business with him, though business had fallen on hard times because of the declining economy. Since his father was an independent businessman who did not have to go to college and had done well for himself, Joe in part felt that he did not need to go to college or do well academically and that perhaps if he had the courage he would just go into business for himself and skip college.

Joe's behavior could be analyzed as reflecting a compromise formation that attempted to resolve an inner conflict. On the one hand, he wished to play it safe and please his mother by obtaining a college education and becoming some sort of salaried professional with a business degree. On the other hand, he wished to take a risk, skip college, and become an entrepreneur like his father. As a compromise between these two competing sides of a conflict, Joe settled on a compromise—not a particularly satisfactory one in some respects— that he would go to college as his mother wished but he would not totally commit himself to the process, retaining some unconscious loyalty to succeeding in life in a way his father admired and to which he would move on when college did not work out so well.

The therapist interpreted this conflict and the compromise Joe had effected, and Joe responded in an interesting way. He agreed that he suffered this conflict and had come up with a compromise but that perhaps the compromise was not such a bad idea. Why not get a college education and learn a little about business and then after college start his own business? If he was going to start his own business, it did not really matter how good his grades were. Of course, this statement begged the question that if he really did not care about how

good his grades were, why was he having so much performance anxiety that he needed to go for treatment?

The structural model refines in a subtle manner one's
thinking about empathy. It makes it clear that any time one is
allying oneself with one aspect of a patient's personality, one
is simultaneously displaying a lack of empathy for another
side of a conflict. In addition to having empathy for the
different sides of a conflict, the analyst also has to have
empathy for the patient's particular strategy of attempted
conflict resolution, the patient's particular compromise formation. And it becomes difficult to judge the relative healthfulness or pathology of a patient's particular compromise
formation, since in some respects the patient's particular
compromise formation always reflects his or her best effort
given current resources and options. The analyst must be
capable of having empathy for both the pros and the cons of
any particular compromise formation. In essence, the structural model demands that we have empathy for the essential
conflictedness, complexity, and ambiguity of the human
situation and for the compromises we effect in order to cope
with conflictedness, complexity, and ambiguity.

5

From Ego-syntonicity to Self-syntonicity

In developing a structural approach to working from surface to depth, one can begin to develop an analytically rigorous conception of forming an empathic connection with a patient. One forms an empathic connection with what the patient currently experiences as ego-syntonic. Yet to understand what is currently ego-syntonic, one must appreciate the functioning of the superego, which plays a central role in determining what is experienced as either ego-syntonic or ego-dystonic. Loewald (1962) said of the superego, "The superego functions from the viewpoint of a future ego, from the standpoint of the ego's future that is to be reached, is being reached, is being failed or abandoned by the ego" (p. 265). The superego (i.e., conscience as well as the ego ideal) reflects ideal standards of self-appraisal and self-evaluation, a vision not only of who one should be in the present but of who one should become in the future. Any self-perception that deviates from this vision of a future ideal ego is appraised as ego-dystonic and therefore repudiated.

Lewis (1971) defined the superego as the agency of the mind responsible for self-evaluation:

The psychic regulatory agency which functions to monitor and maintain a "balanced" self-evaluation. . . . The superego groups together all the occasions when the person is evaluating himself, either positively or negatively, and whether the context for self-evaluation is moral or nonmoral. . . . The superego concept thus implies a drive-determined sequence such that loss of self-esteem drives the person to repair the loss. [pp. 25–26]

The superego functions as an organ of self-esteem maintenance or, one might say, identity maintenance by attempting to maintain a balanced self-evaluation. Any self-perception that proves incompatible with a balanced self-evaluation is experienced as ego-dystonic and repudiated.

The problem with using the superego as a guide to assessing ego dystonicity is that aspects of the superego are thought to be ego-dystonic. It is well known that aspects of the superego operate unconsciously and are highly repudiated. The reason for this is that, as Brenner (1982) suggested, the superego is a compromise formation made up of conflicting components. Thus there is intrasystemic conflict within the superego. The superego is comprised of conflicting standards of self-appraisal and self-evaluation. The superego envisions multiple and conflicting futures toward which one should aspire. What is ego-syntonic from one standard of self-evaluation is ego-dystonic from a competing standard of self-evaluation. This intrasystemic conflict within the superego accounts for the fluid nature of what is ego-syntonic.

Not only is the superego comprised of conflicting components but so is the ego. Freud (1923) spoke of the "multiplicity of the ego." He observed that in dreams, different figures may be regarded as fragmentations and representatives of various aspects of the dreamer's own ego. Even in the waking state, the ego tends to divide itself into subject and object, an "I" and a "me." In this context, the term *ego* does not refer so much to a constellation of cognitive operations such as defense, thinking, reality testing, judgment, impulse control, and so forth, as it does to particular senses of self, self-experiences, or self-states. In describing superego–ego relationships in terms of multiple superegos in relation to and in conflict with multiple egos, we are using the structural model not so much in the manner in which Arlow and Brenner utilized it but in the manner in which object relations theorists use structural concepts, to describe how multiple and conflicted relationships between self and others become interiorized as internal psychic structure. In this context, it would probably be more precise to speak of self-syntonic or self-dystonic than of ego-syntonic or ego-dystonic. We probably possess as many different self-experiences as there are different frames of reference through which we observe and evaluate ourselves. In identifying with the attitudes of others toward oneself, identification being a major source of superego attitudes, the person develops multiple perspectives toward the self.

Here we see a paradox. The superego functions to maintain a balanced self-evaluation and a sense of self-esteem. Yet paradoxically the agency of the mind that is responsible for maintaining a homeostatic balance in terms of self-esteem maintenance (i.e., a sense of self) is itself made up of a wide variety of conflicting identifications. Mitchell (1991) noted the dialectic tension in psychoanalytic theory between views of the self as unitary and views of the self as multiple. Perhaps the self is paradoxically unitary and multiple simultaneously. When the self is viewed as multiple, the analyst goes in search of repudiated selves and analyzes defenses against recognition of these disowned selves. When the self is viewed as unitary, the analyst's attention is drawn to the homeostatic function, how a stable self-evaluation with positive self-esteem is restored, maintained, and cultivated. The analyst empathizes with disturbances to that sense of unity and the need to restore a sense of homeostatic balance.

From a self-psychological perspective, defense possesses a function broader than Brenner's (1982) limited functional definition of defense as a means of maximizing drive discharge while simultaneously attenuating anxiety and depressive affect. The overarching function of defense is to preserve the sense of identity by repudiating self-dystonic self-experiences. Anxiety and depressive affect are signals of the emergence into awareness of self-dystonic self-experiences that may undermine and spoil the consciously maintained sense of a cohesive unitary self. Defenses not only serve to evade and escape something unpleasant (i.e., the existence of conflict-laden multiple selves) but to maintain, preserve, and achieve something (i.e., a cohesive unitary self with positive self-esteem).

When defense/resistance/character analysis is thought of in terms of analyzing the patient's manner of maintaining a cohesive sense of self in prereflective conscious awareness, in addition to analyzing the patient's manner of resisting the awareness of repudiated, self-dystonic self-experiences, a new and transformative dimension is added to the traditional Freudian ego-psychological approach to defense/resistance/character analysis. Balint (1968) captured the flavor of this shift in emphasis when he suggested that "the patient is running away from something, usually a conflict, but it is equally correct that he is running towards something, i.e. a state in which he feels relatively safe and can do something about the problem bothering or tormenting him" (p. 26). Every attempt to repudiate a self-dystonic self-state is concurrently an attempt to maintain or achieve a self-syntonic self-state.

Atwood and Stolorow (1984) viewed repression as a "negative organizing principle" (p. 35) that prevents certain experiences of self from crystallizing in awareness. Repression operates alongside "the positive organizing principles" (p. 35) underlying the self-states that do repeatedly materialize in conscious experience. For Atwood and Stolorow "the *dynamic unconscious* consists in that set of configurations that consciousness is not permitted to assume" (p. 35). Conversely, *dynamic consciousness* consists of those configurations whose crystallization is achieved in conscious awareness.

In terms of interpretation, the analyst must choose which side of the process to emphasize—anxiety avoidance or identity maintenance. In addition, if the analyst wishes to be thorough and analyze both sides of the process with a balanced emphasis, there is still a decision to be made in terms of sequencing, whether to interpret the anxiety avoidance or the identity maintenance side of the process first. If one were to interpret from surface to depth, the sequence of interpretation becomes clear in that identity maintenance needs to be interpreted prior to anxiety avoidance and that anxiety avoidance must be interpreted in the context of threats to identity maintenance. The effort to maintain a cohesive sense of self with positive self-esteem is more accessible to awareness than the effort to repudiate those self-dystonic self-experiences that might spoil and undermine the conscious self-syntonic view of oneself. For example, most men are more aware of their efforts to prove their masculinity then they are of their efforts to avoid expressing their femininity. Similarly, most women are more aware of their efforts to prove their femininity than they are of their efforts to avoid expressing their masculinity. Here we have the beginnings of a self-psychological theory of working from surface to depth.

Kohut (1977, 1984) articulated a view of defense–resistance analysis that highlighted the self-affirmative function of defense and resistance: "Defense motivation in analysis will be understood in terms of activities undertaken in the service of psychological survival, that is, as the patient's attempt to save at least that sector of his nuclear self however small and precariously established it may be" (1984, p. 115). From this perspective, resistance is no longer necessarily conceived as an obstacle to the analysis but may be considered a pro-analytic force: "The conceptualization of a pathology of the self leads in these cases to the recognition that the patient's resistance against being analytically penetrated is a healthy force, preserving the existence of a nuclear self that had been established despite the parent's distorted empathy" (1977, p. 149). Focusing on the anxiety avoidance and warded-off content aspect of defensive functioning may prove to be countertherapeutic:

> When the analysand becomes enraged in consequence of our attack on his resistance, he does so, not because a correct interpretation has loosened defenses and has activated the aggressive energy that was bound up in them, but because a specific genetically important traumatic situation from his early life has been repeated in the analytic situation: the experience of the faulty nonempathic response of the selfobject. [1977, p. 90]

Stolorow and colleagues (1987) suggested that resistance reflects the patient's expectations and fears that the therapeutic relationship will be traumatogenic. "Resistance is always evoked by some quality or activity of the analyst that for the patient heralds an impending recurrence of traumatic developmental failure" (p. 14). Increased resistance reflects an increased dread of repeating traumatic experiences in the transference (Ornstein 1974). According to Stolorow and colleagues (1987), "Once resistances are recognized not as malignant opposition to the analytic process, but as efforts by the patient to protect the organization of his self-experience from encroachment and usurpation, then it becomes critical to explore as fully as possible, how, from the patient's perspective, the analyst has come to embody such a threat to the patient's essential selfhood" (p. 51).

What begins to emerge from Kohut's perspective is a theory of why it is that one interpretation rather than another is experienced by the patient as empathic. If we assume that all interpretations are given with sincere empathic intent and tact by the analyst, it is nevertheless apparent that not all interpretations given in such a manner are experienced by the patient as the analyst intended. From the patient's point of view, an interpretation is experienced as empathic to the extent that it stabilizes and bolsters the sense of self and will be experienced as unempathic to the extent that it destabilizes and undermines the sense of self.

The problem, though, with Kohut's approach is that he does not address the question of how one assesses which sense of self from among many to bolster and avoid undermining. When Kohut (1977) referred to a "nuclear" self or Stolorow and colleagues (1987) referred to a patient's "essential" selfhood, they appeared to have assumed that everyone possesses some sort of core or unitary self no matter how insecurely established. Kohut's self psychology, as Mitchell (1991) suggested, appears to be a psychology of a singular, unitary self that is more or less cohesive.

In contrast, the self psychology being developed here is a psychology of multiple and conflicting selves out of which a compromise sense of self is established as a form of conflict resolution. The compromise sense of self, though a potentially integrated entity, is by its very nature a loosely integrated entity that attempts to reconcile conflicting self-states and achieve some sort of homeostatic equilibrium. Since consciousness may be characterized by a variety of shifting self-states, there may not be any nuclear or essential self with which one might consistently empathize. What is empathic to one self-state may be unempathic to a contrasting self-state. Whatever is currently experienced as self-syntonic reflects a precarious and most likely temporary homeostatic balance that could easily become self-dystonic as the balance of conflict and compromise shifts. Thus all self-experiences are potentially syntonic in some respects and dystonic in others. At moments of transition between shifting modes of maintaining a homeostatic balance, self-experiences may be felt to be both syntonic and dystonic simultaneously.

The question arises that if the psyche is comprised of multiple selves, with which self-experience does the analyst empathize? Of course, in developing a working model of the patient, the analyst should privately attempt to empathize with all variety of self-experience whether conscious or unconscious, admirable or despicable, passive or active, loving or hating, and so on. Nevertheless, in interpreting the patient's self-experiences, the analyst must sequence interpretations somehow. The patient is not going to experience all interpretations as equally empathic despite their empathic intent. Interpretations that affirm the currently activated self-syntonic self-state will most likely be experienced as empathic, whereas interpretations that destabilize the currently activated self-syntonic self-state will most likely be experienced as unempathic. Given the fluidity of self-experience, any consistent line of interpretation could be experienced as empathic at one moment and unempathic at the next. What strikes the patient as empathic in one frame of mind may strike the patient as unempathic in another state of mind.

A single woman in her early forties comes for treatment because she feels depressed and ashamed of not being married when she would like to be. The patient also wonders if she is now too old to marry because she has come to value her independent lifestyle and may be too set in her ways to accommodate living with another person. When the therapist tries to empathize with her discouragement about getting married and her pride in living independently, the patient accuses the therapist of pessimism about her marital prospects and trying to reconcile her to permanent spinsterhood. When the therapist tries to empathize with her determination to develop a successful long-term relationship with a man despite her disappointments, the patient accuses the therapist of trying to set her up for further disappointment and blaming her for failing to be married already. The patient is conflicted between two shifting perspectives on her situation that she cannot seem to reconcile. On the one hand, she feels she is a strong and independent woman who is yet to meet her match and would rather remain single than settle for less. On the other hand, she feels that she is a desperately dependent person who would have married already had it not been for the fact that men have rejected her for being too clingy and now for being too old. When the therapist affirms her independent self, her dependent self panics at the thought of never getting married; when the therapist affirms her determination to marry, her independent self is offended at the idea that she is to blame if she does not.

The conscious compromise sense of self is an ever-changing and evolving entity as it strives to maintain a dynamic balance between opposing perspectives on the self. Thus, empathy involves a continual assessment of the patient's evolving efforts to achieve a stable compromise, a state of self-syntonicity as devoid as possible of self-dystonic elements. Kohut (1971) suggested that the crucial curative process is the working-through of the patient's experience of the analyst's failures of empathy, so that working through empathic failure constitutes as much of a proanalytic force as empathic success. One reason that empathic failure may constitute a proanalytic force is that it may reflect the analyst's witting or unwitting evocation of a self-dystonic element that the patient repudiates. It forces the patient to address and assimilate conflict between what is self-syntonic and what is self-dystonic. Empathic failure is not necessarily only an inadvertent, countertransference based accident; it is a regular and predictable occurrence every time an attempt is made to expand the boundaries of the self through the introduction of a novel (i.e., self-dystonic) point of view that would be experienced as a challenge to the patient's currently activated (i.e., self-syntonic) point of view. At these times the analyst could be said to be intentionally and strategically unempathic in an effort to decenter the patient from a predominantly egocentric perspective (i.e., an effort to make the self-syntonic self-dystonic).

If the patient's efforts to develop a stable conscious compromise sense of self are based on maintaining a stable repudiation of self-dystonic elements, a paradox arises in regard to the traditional psychoanalytic aim of making the unconscious conscious. How can the unconscious be made conscious without destabilizing the sense of identity? And, should the unconscious be made conscious if destabilization of the sense of self is the result? Kohut (1984) suggested, "Although the step toward cure that self psychology considers to be decisive is usually preceded by, accompanied by, or followed by a broadening of the area that is accessible to introspection, this increase in the scope of consciousness does not always occur, and it is not essential" (p. 64).

Cure can be thought to arise from two forms of strengthening the sense of self: the self can be strengthened by making its boundaries more secure so that it would be less threatened by repudiated self-experiences; or the self can be strengthened by loosening and expanding its boundaries to make it more inclusive, so that it may assimilate into its structure formerly repudiated self-experiences. Of course, the self can be strengthened in both respects, and this need not be an either/or proposition. The first form of cure would not necessarily entail making the unconscious conscious, although a stronger self may be less threatened by repudiated self-experiences, which it may learn to tolerate as an ego-alien element. The second form of cure would necessitate making the unconscious conscious as it involves expanding the boundaries of the self to include self-dystonic elements.

Strengthening the boundaries of the self tends to be experienced as supportive, whereas loosening and expanding the boundaries of the self is necessarily anxiety laden.

The first form of cure has tended to be associated with supportive psychotherapy, whereas the second form of cure has been associated with "the pure gold" of psychoanalysis. Strengthening the boundaries of the self results from empathy, whereas expanding the boundaries of the self results from analysis. For this reason, the first form of cure has been seen as an inferior form, only supporting the patient's defenses. Yet in terms of the expanded functional definition of defense, which includes the function of identity maintenance, it would seem that strengthening the boundaries of the self is an essential feature of any curative effort. To see this form of cure as *only* strengthening the patient's defenses by avoiding confrontation with unconscious conflict is simplistic, as it ignores the fact that enabling the patient to become a more securely integrated person is a form of structural change. And a more securely integrated person may be better able to tolerate unconscious conflict than an insecurely integrated person. The question is, Which comes first, the chicken or the egg? That is, does awareness of unconscious conflict lead to better psychological integration, or does better psychological integration lead to greater awareness of unconscious conflict? As usual, the answer does not have to be either/or.

Perhaps the boundaries of the self need to be strengthened before they can be loosened and expanded. Therefore, interventions designed to strengthen the boundaries of the self may need to precede interventions designed to stretch and expand the boundaries of the self. Wolf (1988) suggested that the ultimate aim of treatment was to strengthen the self and noted a variety of processes through which that aim might be achieved. In terms of the timing of an interpretation, strength, flexibility, and resilience of the boundaries of the self can be assessed via the patient's level of defensiveness in response to the interpretation of a self-dystonic element of the patient's personality. The greater the defensiveness is, the more insecure are the boundaries of the self. Conversely, the greater the receptivity to self-dystonic elements is, the more flexible and resilient are the boundaries of the self.

The strengths and limitations of Kohut's approach can be illustrated in his classic case study "The Two Analyses of Mr. Z" (Kohut 1979). We shall see that affirming and stabilizing Mr. Z's phallic narcissistic sense of self proved to be an extremely therapeutic experience for Mr. Z, yet it simultaneously bolstered Mr. Z's defenses against unconscious feminine identifications, thereby enforcing a degree of characterological rigidity that diminished his capacity for intimacy.

Mr. Z initiated analysis with Kohut when he was a graduate student in his mid-twenties. The patient was socially isolated as he was unable to form any relationships with women. His sex life consisted of masochistic masturbatory fantasies involving submitting to domineering women. In addition, he suffered from a variety of mild somatic symptoms. Although he did well in graduate school, he felt that he was not functioning up to his potential. Mr. Z lived with his widowed mother in comfortable financial circumstances. His father, who had been a highly successful business executive, had died 4 years earlier.

Kohut understood the beginning of the analysis as the revival of a regressive mother transference that reinstated the narcissistic bliss of being catered to by a doting and admiring mother over whom Mr. Z possessed exclusive control. Kohut believed that this maternal transference served a defensive function that warded off the patient's fears of competition with his father, castration anxiety, and hostility toward his father. His masochism was understood as a sexualization of his guilt about possessing the preoedipal mother and his rivalry with his father. The fantasy of the domineering phallic woman defended against castration anxiety in viewing the mother as someone who would protect him against his father as long as he submitted to her.

The therapeutic tack that derived from this dynamic formulation was that Kohut would interpret the defensive function of Mr. Z's narcissistic transference to Kohut in order to help him become aware of his unconscious conflicts and anxieties in relation to the dangers of masculine self-asser-

tiveness. The cure would be that in overcoming his unconscious fears of masculine self-assertiveness, he would be
enabled to overcome his social isolation, establish better
relationships with women, and function up to his full potential professionally. Kohut found that interpretation of the
defensive function of Mr. Z's entitlement, arrogance, and
narcissistic demands was met with intense opposition and
rage. This did not change until Kohut suggested to the
patient, "Of course, it hurts when one is not given what one
assumes to be one's due" (p. 5). After this intervention, the
climate of the analysis became calmer and more cooperative,
and Mr. Z began to demonstrate symptomatic and behavioral
improvement. Nevertheless, there remained an emotional
shallowness to the treatment outside of the rage, shame, and
then the sense of vindictive triumph in response to blows to
his self-esteem and its restoration. Mr. Z terminated after 4
years of treatment.

Mr. Z returned to treatment for his second analysis 4.5
years later. His complaint was that his relationships remained
emotionally shallow and that his work seemed a burdensome
chore. He was alarmed by his increasing sense of social
isolation. In the meantime his mother had developed a
circumscribed set of paranoid delusions. After a brief idealizing transference at the initiation of his second treatment,
Mr. Z developed a mirror transference of the merger type in
which he became self-centered and demanding and reacted
with rage to the slightest misunderstanding. Rather than
interpret the defensive function of this narcissistic transference as he had done in the last analysis, Kohut now treated
it as the revival of an important childhood relationship with
the mother that needed to be appreciated in greater depth
and with greater empathy. This change in attitude diminished the patient's rage reactions and alleviated the potentially adversarial climate of analysis.

The understanding that emerged from this shift in analytic
attitude was that the patient had become enmeshed in the
pathological personality of his mother. The mother gratified
the patient's narcissism under the condition that he submit
to her total domination. As a result, Mr. Z was unable to

develop a firm and independent sense of self as an agent. To emerge from enmeshment in the mother's covertly paranoid psychotic personality evoked fears of disintegration, anxieties that his enfeebled self would be annihilated by her icy revenge for daring to differentiate himself from her. Resistance analysis focused on analyzing Mr. Z's fears of acknowledging his mother's craziness as though the illusion of her normality was sacrosanct. In retrospect, Kohut speculated that in the first analysis Mr. Z complied with the regimen of analysis just as he had accepted as reality his mother's distorted outlook while growing up.

As issues with the mother were worked through, what emerged in the transference was Mr. Z's need for a strong, idealizable father figure. Between the ages of 3 and 5, the father was initially hospitalized and then fell in love with and went to live with his nurse. When the relationship did not work out, the father returned home. Mr. Z had experienced his father as weak and absent. In the analysis, Mr. Z began to recognize aspects of his father that appeared strong, independent, and masculine and saw the analyst in that light as well. Through merger with these images of masculine strength, Mr. Z began to experience himself similarly. As the patient consolidated this newfound sense of himself, the analysis came to an end after 4 years. Mr. Z at the time of termination was not involved in any significant relationships but was enthusiastically immersed in his work. Kohut heard through an acquaintance that several years later Mr. Z married a warm-hearted woman unlike his mother, with whom he had a daughter.

In the first analysis, it could be said that Kohut unwittingly undermined the boundaries of the self by challenging and destabilizing the patient's self-syntonic archaic grandiosity. The patient eventually accommodated to such destabilization through false-self compliance. In the second analysis, Kohut mirrored the patient's self-syntonic archaic grandiosity and had empathy for the trauma of being exposed to self-dystonic elements such as the humiliation and emasculation of being subservient to the mother's omnipotent control. As a result, the patient began to display a higher level self-syntonic phallic narcissism that Kohut allowed to unfold unchallenged, as he empathized with traumas to the patient's phallic narcissism such as his unrequited father hunger. This enabled the patient to affirm a significantly more firm, strong, independent, initiating, and masculine sense of himself, a significant and genuine therapeutic accomplishment. There is no doubt that the boundaries of Mr. Z's self were significantly strengthened.

Yet I would suggest that this outcome is a limited therapeutic result. The emotional shallowness and social isolation that were his primary reason for seeking analysis on both occasions were never specifically analyzed and not clearly ameliorated. Even though we know that Mr. Z married and made a healthy object choice, we have no information concerning how related or unrelated Mr. Z was in relation to his wife and daughter. Given his family history, one might wonder whether he re-created his family of origin in which an illusion of normality hides a deeper lack of relatedness. If one of Mr. Z's primary characterological complaints was social isolation and emotional shallowness, then where is his emergent capacity for intimacy, attachment, caring, and nurturance? Kohut noted this issue in passing. But in wishing not to impose a mental health maturity ethic that valued mature object love over mature narcissism, Kohut felt comfortable noting that interpersonal relations would never play the dominant role in Mr. Z's life that they do for many people.

Perhaps Mr. Z went as far as he was able to or needed to in his analysis. But if the therapeutic process is understood as expanding as well as strengthening the boundaries of the self in order to encompass self-dystonic aspects, other analytic events may have been possible that might have addressed the unconscious sources of his characterological social isolation and emotional shallowness. Once his independent phallic narcissistic sense of self had been stabilized, it might have been possible to begin wondering about what had happened to his apparently self-dystonic dependent self that may have had unrequited needs for intimacy, attachment, and nurturance in relation to women. And given that he was apparently raised by a controlling and domineering mother and a distant and rejecting father, one might wonder what has happened to his identifications with those parents. Perhaps his social isolation and emotional shallowness reflect an unconscious self-dystonic identification with an icy paranoid psychotic mother and a distant, emotionally rejecting father, fueled by his global hostility toward the interpersonal world for having been emasculated by his mother and abandoned by his father.

It is not that these issues did not arise in the analysis but that Kohut did not see them, wedded as he was to his mission of validating and affirming the patient's unitary, essential, independent, and separate masculine sense of self. In both analyses, Kohut always conceptualized himself in the transference as either the mother or the father. He never entertained the possibility of a reversal of roles in which Mr. Z treated Kohut as his father or mother had treated him. When Mr. Z responded coldly and ragefully whenever Kohut challenged his need for omnipotent control, was he not punishing Kohut as his mother had punished him for daring to differentiate himself from her? And when Kohut complied with the patient's need for omnipotent control, did he then not reward Kohut through idealization as his mother had rewarded him for submitting to her? When Mr. Z terminated his first incompleted analysis to pursue a falsely independent existence, might not Mr. Z have been abandoning Kohut as his father had abandoned him? And when Mr. Z terminated his second analysis to pursue a genuinely independent and masculine existence, might not he still have been abandoning Kohut as his father had abandoned him, in order to avoid uncovering deeper fears of intimacy, attachment, caring, and nurturance in the analysis?

Perhaps the analysis of these self-dystonic elements, which may have been expressed as unconscious role reversals in the transference, may have enabled Mr. Z to develop a capacity to be not only firm and independent but caring, nurturant, and intimate as well. Though the boundaries of Mr. Z's self were strengthened, they were not expanded to include the incorporation of self-dystonic elements such as negative maternal and paternal identifications. As a consequence, Mr. Z seemed to finish his second analysis with a degree of characterological rigidity that diminished his capacity for intimacy, attachment, caring, and nurturance.

Whereas Kohut's (1971, 1977, 1984) approach to defense-resistance analysis seems to have emphasized strengthening the boundaries of the self (i.e., empathy), Schafer's (1983) "affirmative" approach to defense/resistance/character analysis seems to have emphasized loosening and expanding the boundaries of the self (i.e., analysis). Schafer, like Kohut, noted that defense is not only a form of anxiety-avoidance but a form of self-affirmation as well. From an affirmative orientation, Schafer (1983) recommended "[T]o approach it not as resisting or opposing but as puzzling or unintelligible behavior that requires understanding" (p. 168). This affirmative approach focuses largely on what resisting is for rather than simply what it is against (p. 162). "By emphasizing character's value to the analysand in his or her psychical reality this orientation avoids the kind of adversarial orientation on the analyst's part which centers on the ways in which character functions as resistance" (p. 148).

Despite an affirmative orientation, Schafer (1983) recognized that an adversarial relationship was inevitable if repudiated aspects of self were ever to be made conscious. The hope is that the negative transference that will emerge will be in an analyzable form. The function of an affirmative approach is not so much to avoid negative transference as it is to create a climate in which the negative transference is analyzable.

> If one recognizes that an analysand is unconsciously conflicted, then one must expect the analysand to respond angrily to any intervention that highlights one or another unrecognized constituent of conflictedness. For the analysand, it is as if the analyst is taking sides in the conflict by pointing out one of its denied elements. . . . The analyst's highlighting resistant strategies will be particularly threatening and therefore angering. There is no way around hostile activity on the analysand's part. There is only seduction away from this activity, as when the analyst treats the analysand as a fundamentally preconflictual being. This is the approach that Kohut recommend-

ed. . . . In this way Kohut did seem to increase the chances of seducing the analysand into repressing or rerepressing some of the origins and meanings of the hostile actions and reactions that require extensive analysis. To some extent, Kohut seemed to be taking sides—specifically, the side of the analysand's narcissistic sensitivities. [pp. 78–79]

Schafer's criticism of Kohut for siding with the patient's narcissistic sensitivities, as though this were a lapse in terms of a stance of technical neutrality, implies that there is no good reason for selectively siding with the patient's narcissistic vulnerabilities. There are good reasons for granting greater emphasis to the patient's strivings to establish and maintain a sense of self or identity and therefore for granting greater emphasis to what is disruptive to the patient's sense of self or identity. Lichtenstein (1977) made the strongest case for viewing the principle of identity maintenance as a superordinate psychological function:

Psychoanalytic evidence makes it also probable that the maintenance of identity in man has priority over any other principle determining human behavior, not only the reality principle but also the pleasure principle. [p. 59]

The "identity principle": it is meant to refer to a fundamental biological phenomenon, more basic, more drive-like than the pleasure principle. [p. 114]

Identity establishment and maintenance must be considered basic biological principles—principles defining the concept of living matter itself. As soon as a living organism ceases to maintain its identity we speak of its decay. [p. 114]

Although all psychic phenomena can be understood in terms of their multiple functions, some functions might be considered superordinate as other functions are considered subordinate.

It would be legitimate to give interpretive precedence to a function like the principle of identity maintenance if it were considered a superordinate function over some other functions such as wish fulfillment or defense if these functions were considered subordinate though ubiquitous. To arrange psychic functions hierarchically in terms of their superordinate organizational importance can seem to be relinquishing the stance of technical neutrality in which one remains "equidistant" from the various agencies of the mind. Certainly to interpret exclusively in terms of one superordinate function to the neglect of all other functions would be a skewed approach. Yet to recognize that in working from surface to depth there may be a need to address the various psychic functions in some sequential order is not necessarily to relinquish a stance of technical neutrality. It is simply to recognize that certain sides of a conflict may need to be addressed prior to addressing another side of a conflict. To the extent Kohut gave *primary* consideration to the patient's narcissistic vulnerabilities, I believe his approach is innovative in relation to those who do not. To the extent Kohut gave *exclusive* consideration to the patient's narcissistic vulnerabilities, I believe his approach is unnecessarily limiting in relation to those who address other dimensions of personality functioning that may be unsettling to the patient's narcissistic equilibrium.

Though the analysis of the patient's underlying hostility is important and should not be avoided by undue concern for the patient's narcissistic vulnerability, as Schafer suggested, I believe such an analysis is less crucial for the progress of the treatment than consistent respect for the patient's narcissistic vulnerabilities. Though the two issues do not always conflict with one another, when there is a conflict of interests, respect for vulnerability should usually though not necessarily always take precedence over exposure and analysis of covert or overt hostility. Of course, one person's respect for vulnerability is another person's seduction into re-repression, and one person's neutral analysis of conflicted hostility is another person's insensitivity to vulnerability.

Schafer did not seem to recognize that his affirmative approach could also be reasonably construed as a form of siding with the patient's narcissistic sensitivities. Schafer's affirmative approach is indeed a very powerful and subtle form of siding with the patient's narcissistic sensitivities, as is Kohut's approach, both approaches constituting a form of establishing a narcissistic alliance with the patient. A narcissistic alliance, like any other form of alliance, is a necessary but fragile element of the treatment situation, an element allowing for a prerequisite "atmosphere of safety" (Schafer 1983, p. 14). Yet as soon as an element is introduced into the analytic situation that is self-dystonic to the patient (intentionally or unintentionally by the analyst), the patient feels that the analyst is taking sides against him or her and therefore being unempathic. Thus, Schafer, like Kohut, noted the inevitability that the patient will experience the analyst as unempathic, resulting in negative transference.

At the point in which negative transference emerges openly in the therapeutic relationship, Schafer seemed to advocate returning to the more traditional approach to defense analysis in continuing to point out the patient's disavowal of the self-dystonic element despite the patient's negative transference, in the hopes of expanding the boundaries of the self. In contrast, Kohut arrived at a novel and in a sense paradoxical approach, by suggesting that the analyst empathize with the patient's experience of the analyst's lack of empathy. Kohut suggested that empathy with the patient's experience of the analyst in the negative transference takes precedence over analyzing the patient's negative transference in terms of its multiple functions.

Schafer seemed to see the patient's negative transference as *primarily* the patient's defense against taking responsibility for claiming the self-dystonic element, which is projected onto the analyst instead. Schafer, wanting his patients to own their unconsciously repudiated sense of self-agency and intentionality, was reluctant to empathize with their consciously self-syntonic sense of being anything remotely resembling a passive, reactive, fragile, and innocent victim. When it comes to negative transference, Schafer, given his technical stance, seemed more likely to emphasize its defensive function rather than its affirmative function. Kohut, on the other hand, emphasized the affirmative function of the negative transference in being more willing to empathize with the patient's sense of helpless vulnerability, of being a "preconflictual being," as Schafer put it. What Kohut's approach allows for, for which Schafer's does not seem to allow, is an intermediate sequence in the process of reclaiming repudiated self-dystonic elements in which the analyst takes responsibility for containing the patient's self-dystonic element, which has been attributed to the analyst in the transference. The self-dystonic element is not repressed or re-repressed when the analyst empathizes with the patient's experience of empathic failure, but rather it is tolerated in consciousness as a projection onto the analyst who seems to embody and contain what the patient is not yet prepared to tolerate or accept as an aspect of the patient's self.

A case example in which Schafer (1983, pp. 176–177) demonstrated his approach to the analysis of resisting illustrates what I believe to be the absence of an intermediate sequence in which the analyst assumes responsibility for the self-dystonic element prior to expecting the patient to assume responsibility for it. In this example, Schafer seemed to treat the patient's negative transference primarily in terms of its defensive function without appreciating its possible affirmative function. Despite Schafer's affirmative approach to character analysis, he did not seem to convey empathy for those self-syntonic experiences of self in which the patient disclaimed responsibility for unconscious wishes.

The patient was a female college student. After the analyst inquired into some hesitant associating early in one session, the patient reported that she decided not to tell the analyst about a pleasant time she had had with her boyfriend. Previously she had only complained about her boyfriend. She had imagined that the analyst would either merely "grunt approval" or that he would "analyze the shit out of it." Either way she would be angry at the analyst, and she dare not get angry at him. And, in addition, she would be disappointed because he would not react jealously.

Schafer interpreted the resistant implications of her comments: "[s]ecretly she would take his analytic interest in the pleasant time she'd had as an expression of jealousy, she would then get mad at him in order to disguise her gratification, and she would then suppress her anger in order to protect him and take the resulting misery on herself, as she characteristically did in other relationships" (p. 177). Thus the negative transference to Schafer was interpreted as serving as a defense against her conflict over her wish to make Schafer jealous. Her complaint that he was underwhelmed by her positive experience with her boyfriend hid her conflicted wish that he would be aroused by the experience.

Schafer had previously understood in the analysis that her tendency to report affectless, unproductive, and wandering associations reflected a manner of sadistically tormenting the analyst in unconscious identification with her "tight-assed" father. Her tendency to take most of what the analyst said as a critical attack and refusal to take anything good from the analyst reflected an anal-sadistic emotionally withholding attitude. Thus, in his formulations and interpretive approach, Schafer went right to the essence of her unconscious and self-dystonic anal-retentive character trends.

The intermediate step that seems to be missing in his interpretive sequence is a step I believe most self psychologists would take, although they then might fail to go on to address the deeper level of self-dystonic cross-gender identifications, which Schafer did address. This step consists of empathically exploring her experience of Schafer as someone who only "grunts approval" or who will "analyze the shit out of it"—in other words, her experience of Schafer as a "tight-assed" father figure. Perhaps she dreaded that Schafer, like her father, would not enthusiastically or approvingly mirror her pride in having finally achieved a positive experience with her boyfriend. To avoid that disappointment, she did not wish to tell Schafer about the experience and probably felt guilty about that act of withholding.

Perhaps her desire to make Schafer jealous was an attempt to obtain a vital response from him: if she could not obtain his approval, at least she could make him jealous. Schafer's serious and incisive interpretation of her unconscious character dynamics at a time when she may have wished for simply a sign of enthusiasm on his part may have been experienced as a reenactment of her difficulty getting a spontaneously approving response from her "tight-assed" father. At a time when she was hoping to be affirmed as a feminine woman who might be appealing to a man, she was instead seen as an anal-retentive man who presumably many men would find unappealing.

Probably Schafer did not take this intermediate step because he did not wish to treat the patient as a "pre conflictual being" (i.e., as an innocent victim of her father's selfobject failures) and thereby encourage the "re-repression" of her conflicted hostility toward Schafer. Schafer's emphasis was on the patient assuming responsibility for claiming her unconscious intentionality and thereby becoming more fully an agent in her own right. But, if we are both subjects and objects simultaneously, this emphasis is also a form of taking sides. The patient was an object of her father's treatment and was reactive to that treatment at the same time that she was also an independent center of initiative who may have been conflicted in regard to her desires toward her father. Since the patient could use the analyst's empathy with her experience of herself as an innocent victim of her father's "tight-assed" conduct defensively to ward off recognition of her own conflicted desires toward him, I believe Schafer was less inclined to offer empathy for her experience of injury at the analyst's hands than are self psychologists. Conversely, self psychologists appear less likely to interpret defenses against self-dystonic cross-gender identifications (e.g., the case of Mr. Z) than Schafer, who would assume that conflicted cross-gender identifications are a standard feature of everyone's character structure that require analysis sooner or later.

The patient treated the self-dystonic element (i.e., identification with a "tight-assed" father) as if it were the analyst's perspective alone, a perspective with which the patient disagreed (i.e., the only "tight ass" in the room was the analyst, and he should not be that way). The patient's negative transference remained intact, for the patient could not accept the analyst as long as the analyst seemed to accept a perspective that the patient could not acknowledge or accept in herself (i.e., the patient was going to continue seeing the analyst as a "tight ass" as long as the analyst was going to see the patient as emotionally withholding). As the patient struggled to assimilate the fact that the analyst may have had a different perspective than herself, then the patient in identification with the analyst may have begun to tolerate multiple and formerly self-dystonic perspectives within herself (i.e., over time the patient came to accept that perhaps she did not need to hate the side of herself that was a "tight ass" like her father). Empathizing with the patient's experience of the analyst's empathic failure is what makes for an analyzable negative transference and also what allows ruptures in the therapeutic alliance to be survived and surmounted (i.e., empathy for the patient's experience of the analyst as a "tight ass" and how that re-creates a narcissistic injury in relation to her father). Empathic failure does not necessarily imply that the analyst was being insensitive or tactless but rather that the patient had correctly assessed that the analyst possessed a different viewpoint from the patient's own self-syntonic point of view. Recognition of that fact creates cognitive dissonance, perhaps because the analyst's viewpoint reflected a self-dystonic aspect of the patient. In other words, the analyst did not necessarily have to smile approvingly at the patient's report of a positive experience, but the analyst should have had empathy for the patient's experience of that lack of demonstrative approval. To reiterate what I believe to be Kohut's subtle innovation in technique is his suggestion that one have empathy for the patient's experience of the negative transference (i.e., analyst as unempathic) prior to analyzing its multiple and conflicting unconscious meanings.

Bion's (1967) idea that the analyst must contain repudiated aspects of the patient's self without prematurely interpreting the patient's projection is relevant here. Premature interpretation of the projection reflects a failure of containment and is experienced by the patient as a rejection of an aspect of the patient's self as well as a persecutory attempt at character assassination. Containment, though, need not be thought of as simply a passive-receptive attitude toward the patient's projections that are then silently processed, since the analyst can actively empathize with the patient's experience of the analyst in the negative transference without interpreting the unconsciously defensive or wish-fulfilling functions of the negative transference.

According to Atwood and Stolorow (1984):

> Experienced therapists know that clarifying the nature of a patient's resistance has no discernible therapeutic result unless the analyst is also able to correctly identify the subjective danger or emotional conflict that makes the resistance a felt necessity. It is only when the analyst shows that he knows the patient's fear and anguish and thereby becomes established to some degree as a calming, containing, idealized selfobject, that the patient begins to feel safe enough to relax the resistance and allow his subjective life to emerge more freely.
> [(p. 63]

The analyst comes to be able to correctly identify the patient's fear and anguish by containing it in the counter-transference at the moment of empathic failure. I believe that the analyst's nondefensive attitude toward the negative transference, willingness to empathize with the patient's experience of the negative transference, willingness to treat the negative transference as a plausible interpretation of the analyst's behavior, and interpretation of the affirmative function of the negative transference are what allows for the patient to own the self-dystonic aspect that has been projected onto the analyst.

Even in contemporary intersubjective and relational approaches to treatment, controversy arises around the issue of when to affirm the self-syntonic sense of self and when to question it. When does the analyst silently contain the countertransference, and when does the analyst use the countertransference as the basis of an interpretation that might be experienced by the patient as confronting the patient with repudiated self-dystonic aspects? When does the analyst simply empathize with the patient's need for self-affirmation, which supports the patient's sense of self, and when does the analyst confront the patient with repetitive enactments of self-dystonic issues? Self psychologists tend to emphasize the empathic facilitation of new selfobject experiences in the attempt to avoid the dreaded repetition of traumatic selfobject failure. In contrast, object relations theorists, especially of the Kleinian variety, tend to emphasize the inevitable unconscious repetition of self-dystonic pathological object relations in the transference–countertransference relationship, an unconscious repetition requiring rigorous analysis.

Trop and Stolorow (1992) presented a case that exemplifies the strengths and limitations of the principles of defense analysis from a self-psychological point of view. As in the case of Mr. Z, it illustrates how in strengthening the patient's delineated masculine self, the patient failed to assimilate self-dystonic identifications with his mother, which limited his capacity for intimacy.

Alan was a 34-year-old attorney who had been in analysis for 10 years. He sought treatment because he felt deeply depressed in regard to his uncertainty whether he was homosexual or heterosexual. He had had few sexual experiences with women and had isolated and infrequent homosexual experiences with different partners.

Alan was an only child born when his parents were quite old. He described his mother as both intrusive and distant as well as weak and fragile. He described his father as absorbed in his career and distant from his son. The father was invested in his son's academic achievement and died when the patient was 20 years old. Alan tended to be socially isolated and suffered from low masculine self-esteem. He experienced women as domineering, controlling, and emasculating.

In the transference, Alan experienced the analyst's enthusiasm for Alan's dating women as pressure to become heterosexual, as though that were the analyst's agenda for him. Alan feared that the analyst would think that his negative perceptions of women were wrong and that women were nicer than he portrayed them, repeating his experience of his mother undermining the validity of his own perceptions. Alan also feared that the analyst would see his problems with women as an enormous setback and be disappointed with him, thereby jeopardizing the therapeutic relationship. As the analyst demonstrated empathy for the patient's experience of the analyst as potentially disrespectful of the patient's reliance on his own feelings and for the patient's need for the analyst's unfailing support, the patient became more decisive and assertive. As the patient felt more accepted by the analyst, he and the analyst were able to establish that homosexual experiences served to bolster a fragmenting sense of self after experiences of feeling undermined by his mother or women he dated. Over time, the patient's homosexuality was interpreted as serving as a substitute for the father he never had who should have protected him from his intrusive and critical mother. As the analyst began to serve a self-delineating selfobject function, Alan's homosexual activities diminished, and he began to think of himself as a heterosexual male.

Treatment involved working through perceived failures of the self-delineating selfobject function when Alan felt that the analyst had sided with the woman's viewpoint rather than his own in his recounting of his conflictual relationships with women. Dates did not turn into long-term relationships, as Alan tended to find fault with the women he dated. Selfobject failures often triggered severe depressive reactions, sometimes with suicidal ideation. In the eighth year of treatment, a dramatic shift in the transference transpired. After Alan recounted being rejected by a female colleague and the analyst interpreted how Alan experienced criticism as a sign of defect, Alan became angry at the analyst, threatened termination, and stated that he needed a dating service, not an analyst.

It was understood that Alan had developed confidence in the validity of his own perceptions and was no longer as reliant on the analyst to serve that function. The analyst interpreted that the analyst was now needed to serve a new function, that of enabling Alan to overcome his fears of immersion with women and that Alan used faultfinding defensively as a way to avoid involvement. The analyst would now serve as an idealizable father whose strength, support, and encouragement would help him overcome his fears of heterosexual intimacy. In the tenth year of treatment, Alan developed an intimate long-term relationship with a woman in which he began to reexperience and attempt to work through, with the analyst's help, his fears of being controlled by women. Eventually Alan and this woman decided to marry.

In discussing the case, Trop and Stolorow suggested that the first 7 years of the analysis required that the analyst serve a self-delineating selfobject function in which the analyst never challenged the patient's perception of reality. Yet after the seventh year, once the self-delineating function was strengthened, the patient was able to tolerate interpretations of the defensive function of being faultfinding and in fact experienced such confrontations as acts of empowerment from an idealizable father figure.

Mitchell (1992), in discussing this case, suggested that Trop and Stolorow posed the clinical options in this case as an either/or choice between an assault on the patient's perceptions and the validation of the patient's developmental needs. Mitchell hypothesized that Alan learned in his family that relationships boiled down to controlling others or being controlled by others so that differences in perspectives become dangerous battlegrounds for struggles over who is in control. Perhaps Alan unconsciously identified with his mother and controlled the analyst through manipulative weakness as his mother controlled him. Mitchell suggested that this dynamic could have potentially been introduced earlier in the treatment and not necessarily have been traumatic. If it is appreciated that in addition to a need for confirmation of one's own perceptions, there is also a need for the stimulation of exposure to the different perspectives of different subjectivities, then it is possible that Alan could have learned that difference can exist in a mutually respectful relationship in which neither party need play a controlling role.

Stolorow and Trop (1992) responded to Mitchell's critique by suggesting that it was Mitchell who had engaged in either/or thinking in which the possibility of entertaining the real fragility of the patient's self-experience was minimized in favor of seeing the patient as primarily trying to control the analyst. They suggested that interpreting the patient's attempt to control the analyst as the patient's mother had controlled him could have been devastating to the patient and completely have undermined his belief in his own subjective reality. A strengthening of Alan's capacity for self-delineation had to be achieved before he could make use of defense interpretations.

Who is "really" thinking dialectically, and who is "really" making the false dichotomy? Trop and Stolorow have been cast as "walking on eggs" with the patient, while Mitchell has been cast as the "bull in the china shop." Is there some alternative to either diving right into the essence of the patient's unconscious repetitions at the beginning of treatment or not addressing some aspects of those unconscious repetitions even after 10 years of treatment?

I believe that looking at the case example in terms of working from surface to depth may shed some light on the technical controversy. Since it would seem that in the patient's conflict in regard to his sexual orientation that the homosexual side of the conflict was self-dystonic, the self-syntonic sense of self that Alan was attempting to stabilize was that he was a normal heterosexual male with clear self-definition. His feelings of rejection by women were a severe blow to his masculine self-esteem, which was restored through homosexual activity, even though it was apparently somewhat self-dystonic to restore his self-esteem in such a manner. Even if Alan was unconsciously acting like his weak and controlling mother, to think consciously of himself as a weak yet controlling person like his mother would most likely have been highly self-dystonic and just a further assault on his felt lack of manliness as well as his sense of reality. It is difficult to conceive how early in the treatment or perhaps even in the middle of the treatment, a man who was so uncertain of his masculinity could have been helped by confrontation with or exposure to what may seem to have been a hated feminine aspect that was split off, repudiated, and enacted in the transference. The firmly delineated masculine self, be it heterosexually or homosexually oriented, is often loath to acknowledge seemingly feminine aspects of which it may be deeply ashamed.

On the other hand, even after the seventh year of treatment when Alan's self-delineating function had been strengthened, it did not occur to the analyst to interpret Alan's faultfinding in terms of an unconscious identification with his controlling mother, a mother who controlled through her imperious vulnerability. At this point one might think it would have been helpful to attempt to expand the boundaries of the self by helping Alan get in touch with and develop more acceptance of his hated feminine aspect. After all, it would seem that as a background phenomenon in the transference, Alan had been unconsciously controlling of the analyst or felt controlled by him throughout the treatment. Either Alan had placed the analyst in the role of mirror of his perceptions who was allowed no independent perceptions of his own, or the analyst had become the strong father who challenged him to confront his fears of women.

Though after 10 years of treatment Alan's capacity for intimacy had been greatly enhanced, he continued to work through his fears of critical and controlling women, with apparently little insight into how controlling he could be in a relationship through his extreme sensitivity to being controlled or criticized. It is possible that Alan's sense of vulnerability as a compromise formation may have served multiple functions, such as preserving a needed tie to his mother through identification and defending against overt expressions of his desire to dominate while expressing it covertly through manipulative weakness. Perhaps discussion of Alan's sadomasochistic conception of relationships and how it was re-created in the therapeutic relationship, as Mitchell suggested, would have facilitated the process of working through his remaining fears of intimacy at the point in treatment when the patient did not need to be quite so protective of his delineated masculine self.

Stolorow and colleagues (1987) suggested a "bipolar conception of transference" (p. 101) in which the selfobject and the repetitive, conflictual dimensions of transference exist in a figure–ground relationship to one another. The patient's experience of selfobject failure tends to bring into the foreground the patient's repetitive experience of childhood selfobject failure in the transference. The experience of selfobject attunement tends to keep the repetitive dimension of the transference in the background. If in the foreground the patient is experiencing selfobject attunement while in the background experiencing a repetitive reenactment, the possibility does not seem to be entertained by Stolorow and colleagues that the experience of selfobject attunement can serve multiple functions other than self-restorative ones. Perhaps the experience of selfobject attunement as a compromise formation serves in part as a defense against exploring the background repetitive dimensions of the relationship, and at some point in the analysis the defensive function of needing a perfectly attuned relationship with the analyst could be interpreted.

Self psychologists tend to assume that if they are being empathic and are overtly experienced by the patient as meeting selfobject needs, they are probably not covertly participating in the enactment of a pathological object relation from childhood. Perhaps while overtly experiencing something genuinely new, the patient could still be covertly reexperiencing something old as well as the reverse. Conversely to self psychology, Mitchell, aware that meeting the patient's need for perfect attunement could serve a defensive function and thereby obscure the analysis of an underlying repetition, was less likely to see the patient's need for near-perfect attunement as a legitimate need to which the analyst should have attempted to respond affirmatively rather than challengingly. Apparently suspicious of the idea that the analyst could have genuinely met the unmet childhood developmental need of an adult patient, Mitchell seemed wary of allowing or providing that type of presumed experience for fear of patronizing if not infantilizing the patient. Mitchell tended to see primarily the repetitive aspect of the transference to the neglect of what was new and different in the therapeutic relationship.

Another controversy surrounding this case has arisen

around the issue of the patient's sexual orientation and sexual identity. Blechner (1993), Lesser (1993), and Schwartz (1993) all raised the possibility of transference compliance to the analyst's implicit interpretive biases and noted the absence of discussion of the patient's experience of what the analyst's biases may have been. Stolorow and Trop (1993) replied that the patient's report of a vital, intimate, and enduring relation with a woman, in marked contrast to his brief impersonal sexual experiences with men, seemed inconsistent with false-self compliance. They stated that they would have considered a vital, intimate, and enduring relation with a man a successful outcome. In addition, they noted that understanding the impact of the analyst's preconceived notions on the therapeutic process is a key element of their intersubjective approach but not the focus of their case presentation, which was defense analysis.

This controversy relates to the question of what one considers to be a healthful organization of the self. Are selves that are essentially, unambivalently, and "truly" (as opposed to falsely) male or female, homosexual or heterosexual to be considered "healthy" selves, or might they perhaps be seen as defensively constricted and incapable of experiencing the richness and diversity of greater role flexibility? Might such defensively constricted selves arise from either anxious conformity to or defiant rebellion against certain societal prejudices and conventions that have been internalized? On the other hand, are selves that are flexibly and freely male or female, homosexual or heterosexual to be considered "healthy" selves that have been liberated from the shackles of internalized sexism and homophobia, or might such selves perhaps reflect a rationalization and enactment of identity diffusion?

And should the capacity for intimacy in a lasting relationship be the criterion by which the healthfulness of either an essential unitary self or a flexible multiple self is assessed, or might that criterion perhaps reflect anxious conformity to or rebellion against societal moral condemnation of relations that are neither romantic nor monogamous? These are questions toward which any analyst would be well advised to aspire to a stance of technical neutrality. Yet one should be well aware of the inevitability of personal bias that will surely be expressed in the implicit structure of one's interpretive framework. Perhaps to the extent that one lives in a prejudiced society and that those prejudices are invariably internalized, character, then, is always in part a compromise between compliance to and defiance of those internalized social strictures. Those strictures may be softened with the aid of analysis but never transcended as long as we must live within the framework of a social structure in which prejudice is embedded as a relatively permanent feature.

In summary, what I find useful in Kohut's approach is his appreciation of the self-affirmative function of the patient's defenses and resistance. The affirmative approach, which Kohut as well as Schafer delineated, allows one to interpret the patient's defensive strategies with respect for the patient's narcissistic vulnerabilities. Kohut also provided an interactive understanding of resistance in analysis. To the extent the analyst interacts with the patient in a manner that stabilizes the patient's sense of self, resistance is diminished. To the extent the analyst interacts with the patient in a manner that destabilizes the patient's sense of self, resistance is exacerbated and negative transference is evoked. Whatever the analyst says or does that destabilizes the patient's sense of self is likely to be experienced as a lack of empathy for the patient's sense of self. Thus negative as well as positive transference are understood interactively as something the analyst did that impacted on the patient's sense of self. Kohut's genius as a clinician was to turn the analyst's empathic failures into an opportunity for growth and healing. He recommended that the analyst respond to empathic failures with empathy for what it is like to work with an analyst who has lacked empathy for certain aspects of the patient's self-experience. Empathy for the analyst's empathic failures proves to be a key therapeutic experience in which childhood narcissistic trauma is relived and worked through and a ruptured therapeutic relationship is repaired.

What I find limiting in Kohut's approach is his overemphasizing the self's strivings toward unity rather than giving equal emphasis to the multiplicity of the self in conflict and compromise. I believe that a person can grow through confrontation with his or her own multiplicity and confrontation with the novel, multiple perspectives that others possess. I believe the boundaries of the self can be stretched and expanded to be more inclusive of what is self-dystonic. Kohut's approach tends to spare the patient an awareness of the patient's own egocentrism and in so doing deprives the patient of the self-enriching process of connection, confrontation, and interpenetration with that which is different from the self. It can be infantilizing of the patient to assume that he or she may be too fragile to usefully assimilate perceptions of the analyst's difference. I have found in clinical work that it is sometimes the more disturbed patient who benefits the most from confrontation with that which exists beyond the omnipotent control of the self.

Inherent in both Freudian and object relations approaches to the self is an appreciation that the self is comprised of conflicted identifications with different aspects of both parents as well as others that have been repudiated but may be enacted in the transference. These repudiated identifications are threatening to a more consciously maintained self-syntonic sense of self; for this reason defenses against the acknowledgment of self-dystonic identifications require careful analysis. Though both Freudian and object-relational analysts aspire to work from surface to depth in doing such analysis, it can be demonstrated that to the extent they fail to empathize with the patient's consciously maintained self-syntonic sense of self, they do not work from surface to depth. In this sense, self psychologists are adept at working from the surface, but it is not clear that they always make it to what is deep (such as a self-dystonic identification with the hated side of a parent of the opposite sex).

Returning to where we left off with the case of Joe, the treatment had taken an ironic twist. Initially Joe had presented himself to the therapist as someone who was intensely motivated to do well academically and extremely upset about not being able to do as well as he would like. He seemed to be full of self-doubt, performance anxiety, and neurotic inhibition in regard to this issue. Yet in questioning the dilemma as Joe had posed it, in order to avoid taking the side of someone who is expecting and pressuring Joe to perform academically, the therapist evoked and discovered another side of Joe, a side uninterested in college and academic performance that would rather be an independent, entrepreneurial businessman like his father, a building contractor. The therapist, perplexed by this turn of events, immediately noted the incongruity and contradiction to Joe of these two sides of himself, one intensely invested in academic achievement and another indifferent to academic achievement. Joe responded with a shrug of the shoulders as though there were nothing so remarkable about such a revelation, and he went on talking about his desires to make a lot of money in business for himself someday.

At this point, a psychology of the self may have an important contribution to make. Joe was clearly having difficulties establishing for himself a cohesive, coherent sense of self on which to base a sense of positive self-esteem. The therapist had been serving mirroring selfobject functions in bolstering that sense of himself that aspired to have a sense of positive self-esteem on the basis of high academic achievement. His father did not support or value that sense of himself, and his mother, although supportive, left him feeling that he was overly dependent on her for support and could not obtain his aspirations on his own initiative. To the extent the therapist was experienced as mirroring his potential for academic achievement, Joe's self-esteem was stabilized, his anxiety and depression were alleviated, he became more productive in his schoolwork, and he felt enthusiastic about the therapy and the therapist. When there were ruptures in this mirroring relationship, Joe became deflated, depressed, and avoidant. When these ruptures were repaired, the relationship to the therapist became more genuine and authentic.

Nevertheless, despite the unfolding and working-through of the mirroring selfobject transference, there was a latent subtext in which a repudiated self-dystonic sense of self demanded expression, a self that was disinterested in academics and just wanted to be an independent entrepreneur who makes a lot of money. To own this self-dystonic sense of self would have been quite destabilizing to the stability, coherence, and positive affective coloration of his more self-syntonic sense of self, which was to be a high academic achiever, a man his mother would love and admire. To maintain the stability of his sense of himself as a potentially high academic achiever, Joe had to repudiate his sense of himself as an entrepreneurial businessman disinterested in academics.

When the therapist suggested the possibility that there might be other sides of himself than the one that placed great emphasis on academic achievement, the self that had been mirrored began to seem like a false self based on compliance with the mother's expectations, unlike the repudiated self that began to seem in comparison a vital true self in its unabashed expression of the phallic, narcissistic desire to be independent, self-made, and rich. A new form of mirroring transference began to emerge in which Joe looked to the therapist to confirm that he can become a successful entrepreneur and that perhaps he need not be so worried about his grades after all.

The treatment continued to take an unexpected turn. Joe began to do an about-face in his attitude toward schoolwork. He started discussing his newfound attitude, attributable by him to being in therapy, that perhaps he should not take college so seriously. Why not just have fun and be a "party animal," like most of his friends? College seemed a good time to enjoy his freedom from responsibility while he had the opportunity. Maybe he should break up with his girlfriend, whom he just kept around for emotional security, and begin to sow his wild oats. His grades were not really all that bad; after all, he was passing and sure to graduate. As Joe expressed these sentiments in a relatively cocky manner, he hardly seemed to need a response from the therapist at all, taking her mirroring presence for granted without her having to provide much in the way of a response. It seemed as though Joe was now going to base his sense of self on a different aspect of himself. It was now the side of him that was overly invested in getting good grades that needed to be repudiated, as it seemed a sign of weakness to think that grades were really so important, when all that counts is just going out into the world to make lots of money.

The therapist, somewhat taken aback by Joe's about-face in his attitude toward academic achievement, raised the possibility that perhaps this change of heart may have been a defensive retreat from his performance anxiety. Perhaps since he assumed he would not do well in the long run, why keep beating himself over the head about his underachievement? Maybe he would just as well not care about something that he feared he just could not achieve. Joe responded defensively and indignantly that college was not necessarily the answer for everyone and that he had even been thinking about dropping out to get a job so he could have some spending money. The therapist, having by now learned from experience how to recognize and repair a rupture to the therapeutic relationship, backed down from her defense interpretation and reflected Joe's desire to prove himself by establishing his independence and ability to fend for himself. Joe responded with an attitude of "You're damm right, I'm going to be independent, and I'll show you what I can do on my own!"

What seemed to have been re-created was the wound to his narcissism of feeling that his mother was overindulgent and overprotective because she did not see him as someone who was capable of becoming an independent man like his father. His father, too, did not see Joe as being able to follow in his footsteps, because in the father's eyes Joe seemed too much of a coddled "mama's boy." In the transference, Joe was defiantly asserting his formerly repudiated wish to be a virile man in the image of his father and responded to the therapist's challenging defense interpretation in a somewhat surly manner, as his father would have responded to a challenge to his masculinity. Thus Joe was trying to stabilize the coherence and positive affective coloration of his new-found phallic, narcissistic sense of self that did not so much need reassurance from the therapist as deference, if not homage. Unconsciously, Joe may also have been repeating a version of the relationship with the father with the roles reversed. Just as Joe felt that he had to defer to his father's phallic superiority with which he could not identify or compete, the therapist found herself being treated inconsequentially. Maybe like the girlfriend, the therapist was just being kept around temporarily for emotional security and would be discarded shortly.

Self psychology is once again useful in enabling the therapist to recognize the emergence of an archaic grandiose self that required a mirroring transference in which the therapist was barely a separate person in her own right. To maintain the coherence, stability, and positive affective coloration of his grandiose phallic narcissistic sense of self, the patient required a silently mirroring presence who did not intrude with any deflating commentary. And to intrude in such a manner is experienced as a retraumatization. Where self psychology is less informative is in addressing the issue as to which self-structure was the patient's core essential self, the potentially high academic achiever or the independent entrepreneur. Perhaps neither was the patient's "true" self. Each represented one side of a conflicted sense of self of which the therapist should have been careful not to take sides, despite the fact that the patient solicited the therapist's support for both sides of the conflict in order to help him overcome his ambivalence. And there were also self-dystonic aspects of self that had yet to emerge into consciousness but had been enacted unconsciously, aspects that were like his reassuring but controlling mother as well as his critical, superior father.

Though self psychology has made empathy a central construct of its theoretical edifice as a special mode of perceiving the entire subjective life of the individual through "vicarious introspection" (Kohut 1959), I would suggest that self psychology highlights a very particular type of empathy, a form focusing on a particular aspect of personality functioning. Self psychology requires that the analyst be able to empathize with the patient's struggle to achieve self-unity, to achieve a coherent, integrated, and positively affectively toned sense of self. And self psychology requires that the analyst possess empathy for the fact that the patient's need to maintain self-cohesiveness is a superordinate psychological function that takes precedence over all other psychological functions. This form of empathy seems essential to healing ruptures of the therapeutic relationship; without such empathy, treatment runs the risk of retraumatizing rather than healing the patient.

Self psychology's empathic focus on the unity of the self is a weakness as well as a virtue. I would suggest that an empathic focus on the self's strivings toward integration and wholeness can unwittingly lead to diminished empathy for the degree to which the self feels hopelessly split and conflicted. Patients often try to resolve such conflict by positioning the therapist to support one side or another of a conflict. And when a patient is soliciting mirroring for one aspect of the self as though that aspect constituted the patient's essential self in its entirety, it is often in the service of enabling the patient to successfully repudiate another aspect of self that seems incompatible with the aspect that has been deemed essential. Yet when the balance of a conflict shifts, one may be surprised to see a sudden reversal of values in which what was formerly deemed essential to the self's survival has become secondary and what was formerly deemed secondary has now become essential to the survival of the self. The paradox must be tolerated that as the self strives toward unity as a superordinate organizational aim, it is nevertheless hopelessly conflicted and divided.

6

The Analysis of Transference

How do we differentiate what is facilitative (self-syntonic) from what is repetitive and resistive (self-dystonic) in the patient's transference to the analyst? And what is the analyst's role in evoking either facilitative or repetitive/resistive aspects of the transference? When does analysis of resistance derail what is facilitative in the transference, and when does empathic facilitation subtly play into repetitive transference enactments in which the treatment remains mired? I would suggest that if transference is understood as a compromise formation serving multiple functions, identity affirming as well as defensive/repetitive simultaneously, then it becomes apparent that these questions can never be answered in simple either/or ways. Instead, I would recommend a dialectical approach in which empathy for the affirmative function of transference proceeds yet is counterbalanced by the analysis of the defensive function of transference.

Every self-experience involves an experience of self in relation to an other as well as an experience of self in relation to itself. Whereas the basic insight of object relations theory is that self and other reflect an indissoluble functional unit, the basic insight of self psychology is that this functional unit of self and other constitutes the template for the self's relationship to itself. Individual self-experience is construed as an intersubjectively constituted phenomenon rather than an exclusively intrapsychic affair. As Stolorow and Atwood (1991) noted, the notion of an isolated individual mind is a myth that reifies the experience of distinctive selfhood.

Given that intrapsychic experience is intersubjectively constituted, all transference could be considered in part what Kohut (1984) called "selfobject" transference. Kohut defined a selfobject relationship as referring to that dimension of our experience of another person that relates to this person's functions in shoring up our sense of self. All transference serves an identity maintenance function as one of its multiple functions. The analyst in the therapeutic situation is always explicitly or implicitly experienced by the patient as reflecting some aspects of the patient's self so that the patient will necessarily have thoughts and feelings about how the analyst is reflecting the patient's selfhood. As the patient must construct and infer how the analyst sees him or her on the basis of the patient's observations of the analyst's nonverbal and verbal behavior, the patient's perception of how the analyst sees him or her will reflect the operations of the characteristic organizing principles that the patient utilizes to construct, infer, and imagine how other people feel about him or her. As these organizing principles derive from past experience, they echo if not repeat in the here and now the formative experiences of childhood. According to Stolorow and colleagues (1987), "Transference, at the most general level of abstraction, is an instance of organizing activity—the patient assimilates (Piaget 1954) the analytic relationship into the thematic structures of his personal subjective world" (p. 36).

Just as we speak of multiple selves, we must speak of multiple transferences that correspond to each sense of self. For every self-experience, there is a corresponding transference that either validates or invalidates, confirms or disconfirms, supports or challenges that particular sense of self. To the degree that the analyst's assessment is experienced as invalidating and threatening to the patient's self-syntonic self-assessment, it will be discredited and repudiated. It will be experienced as unempathic and evoke resistance. To the extent that the analyst's assessment is experienced as validating of the patient's self-syntonic self-assessment, it will be accepted, constituting an unobjectionable transference. It will be experienced as empathic and affirming. Thus the patient tends to accept the analyst's assessment to the extent it confirms a preexisting self-syntonic view of self, and the patient discredits and repudiates the analyst's assessment to the extent it challenges and undermines the patient's self-syntonic self-assessment.

From this frame of reference, positive transference is therapeutic to the extent it strengthens the boundaries of the patient's sense of self. It is antitherapeutic to the extent it seals the boundaries of the self and makes it impermeable to repudiated self-dystonic elements. Negative transference is therapeutic to the extent it expands the boundaries of the patient's self by facilitating exposure and contact with self-dystonic elements. It is antitherapeutic to the extent it destabilizes the boundaries of the self, leaving the patient feeling fragmented. Given this intrinsic ambiguity, how do we assess the balance of positive and negative transference required to both strengthen and expand the boundaries of the patient's self? How do we avoid the twin dangers of increased self-rigidity as a result of too much positive transference and of increased self-fragmentation as a result of too much negative transference? How do we balance empathy with analysis in working with the patient's transference to the analyst? How do we balance empathy for the identity maintenance function of transference with analysis of the defensive function of transference given that transference serves multiple functions?

To say that the analyst should simply remain neutral in regard to this issue is to deny the analyst's personal participation in the transference. Although the analyst is supposed to remain neutral and neither approve nor disapprove of the patient's self-syntonic or self-dystonic views of self, the patient, nevertheless, does not experience the analyst as neutral but always as either a validating or invalidating presence to varying degrees (i.e., experiencing character affirmation or character assassination). And, though the analyst may refrain from overt expressions of approval or disapproval, the analyst soon develops a preconscious appraisal of which lines of interpretation the patient will experience as approving or disapproving of different facets of the self. Once the analyst has acquired a working model of what is self-syntonic or dystonic for a particular patient, the analyst is then implicitly and in a sense intentionally approving and disapproving of different aspects of the self through the adoption of an internally consistent line of interpretation.

Here we see the intersubjective nature of transference in action. The analyst's contribution to the patient's experience of transference is that the analyst will be implicitly validating and invalidating different aspects of the patient's self-experience through the adoption of a consistent line of interpretation. The patient's contribution derives from the patient's predisposition to experience different lines of interpretation as either validating or invalidating. The analyst appraises the patient's predispositions, whereas the patient appraises the values implicit in the analyst's line of interpretation. Transference analysis entails the verbal articulation of the patient's experience of this intersubjective process. The patient experiences the analyst as possessing an opinion of him or her that exerts a formative influence on the patient's sense of self, and the patient has some feeling toward the analyst in regard to the anticipated effects of this influence.

Presumably the analysis of transference—like the analysis of defense, resistance, and character—should proceed from surface to depth in order to maintain an empathic connection. The manifest transference residing at the surface of which the patient would be least defensive would be the experience of the analyst as implicitly or explicitly validating the patient's self-syntonic view of self. The latent transference that would need to be defended against would be the experience of the analyst as invalidating the self-syntonic sense of self and/or validating the self-dystonic sense of self, for this would undermine the consciously (or preconsciously) maintained sense of self that is self-syntonic. Transferences that undermine the syntonic and confirm the dystonic must be repudiated, whereas transferences that support the syntonic and undermine the dystonic are unobjectionable and can be acknowledged. Here we have the beginnings of a relational model of working from surface to depth in which we recog-

nize the analyst's contribution to either evoking or suppressing the emergence of various self-states.

Gill (1982) distinguished between two types of transference resistance: resistance to the resolution of transference
and resistance to the awareness of transference. Reframed in
terms of working from surface to depth: the patient will resist
the resolution of transferences that support the self-syntonic
view of self, whereas the patient will resist awareness of
transferences that undermine the self-syntonic view of self.
The patient attempts to hold onto transferences that support
the self-syntonic view of self as a defense against the awareness of transferences that would undermine the self-syntonic
view.

Given the affirmative approach to resistance, to understand what resisting is for rather than against, it is important
to understand that resistance to the resolution of transference
as well as resistance to the awareness of transference serve a
self-affirmative function in preserving the stability, cohesiveness, continuity, constancy, and positive affective coloration
of the self-syntonic sense of self. Thus the self-affirmative
function (i.e., selfobject function) of transference should be
interpreted prior to articulating its defensive function. The
sequence of transference interpretation would run as follows:
"It is important that you feel that I can accept you as you are
before you can acknowledge your fear that if I didn't accept
you as you are, you would not be able to accept yourself as
you are, nor would you be able to accept me for not accepting
you." The defensive aspect of transference reflects a strategy
of avoiding an anticipated selfobject failure, an anticipation
derived from a dread of repeating the trauma of prior
selfobject disappointments (Ornstein 1974). The dread of
repeating prior selfobject failures functions as an anxiety
signal that triggers unconscious defenses against the emergence into awareness of archaic selfobject needs that might
not be met.

The self-affirmative aspects of transference are always
closer to the surface than the defensive aspects of transference, and the defensive aspects of transference are closer to

the surface than the warded-off dread of selfobject failure. The dread of selfobject failure in conjunction with the desire to achieve, maintain, and evolve a stable self-syntonic sense of self constitute the underlying motives for defense. A two-sequence approach to transference analysis can be articulated. First, interpret the affirmative function of the self-syntonic manifest transference, and empathize with the sense of selfobject failure when the analyst is experienced as invalidating the self-syntonic sense of self. Second, interpret the defensive function of the self-syntonic manifest transference in terms of warding off an unconscious dread of repeating in the transference prior traumatic selfobject failures. The self-syntonic manifest transference serves multiple functions, both selfobject and defensive functions, that need to be interpreted sequentially.

Understanding the multiple functions of the manifest/unobjectionable/explicit transference makes it more apparent why it is so difficult to overcome the patient's resistance to awareness of the latent/objectionable/implicit transference. The manifest transference functions as a transference resistance to the uncovering of resistance to the awareness of the latent transference. The analyst who attempts to overcome resistance to the awareness of the latent transference will be seen as a spoiler who does not accept the patient on his or her own terms and who may inflict on the patient what the patient most dreads. Thus the analyst who attempts to overcome resistance to the awareness of the latent transference will be experienced as unempathic. Interpretations that support the affirmative function of the manifest transference will be experienced as empathic, whereas interpretations of the defensive function of the manifest transference tend to be experienced as unempathic. An assessment of the openness of the self to self-dystonic elements is the gauge by which the analyst assesses whether to interpret transference in terms of its affirmative/selfobject or defensive/repetitive functions.

Kohut (1984, pp. 74–75) provided a case example he believed illustrated the self-psychological approach to the use of confrontation. The case showed the dynamic tension between addressing the self-affirmative selfobject dimension of transference versus the defensive repetitive dimension of transference. The case also illustrated the liability of an approach that views the patient's self as only essential rather than as also multiple and therefore views transference as only singular rather than as also multiple.

The patient, who was a psychiatric resident where Kohut gave occasional seminars, was in his third year of analysis. He arrived 25 minutes late for a session, tossed his leather jacket on the chair, and crashed onto the couch. He began talking rapidly and, with what seemed a trace of challenging arrogance, related that he had once again been stopped for speeding on the expressway. He had responded belligerently to the police officer, who would have let him off because he was a physician but because of the patient's provocative manner gave him a ticket. The patient reported this event and similar events in the past in an unrepentant, angry tone of voice. After listening 5 minutes in silence, Kohut stated in utter seriousness that he was going to give him the deepest interpretation he had received so far in his analysis. After several seconds of silence, Kohut stated very firmly and with total seriousness, "You are a complete idiot" (p. 74). After a second or so of silence, the patient burst into warm and friendly laughter.

Kohut then discussed his concern about the patient's reckless driving and other forms of tantrum-like behavior. It turned out that the trigger of the patient's narcissistic rage was that Kohut had not responded to the patient's remark in a seminar but to another resident's remark. His associations led him to memories of his father's unresponsiveness. The father would work with tools in the basement with his older brother while the patient was left in his mother's care. The patient had been the young genius with brains from whom the father felt estranged. The patient felt excluded from the company of men.

Kohut used the case example to demonstrate that self psychology is not incompatible with the use of confrontation when necessary to address self-destructive behavior the import of which the patient denies. In addition, self psychology considers the underlying narcissistic vulnerability from which narcissistic rage and self-destructive acting-out arise as well as what may prove to be the triggering event within the transference. Kohut addressed the defensive function of the patient's self-syntonic arrogance and grandiosity, which denied the seriousness and dangerousness of his reckless and provocative behavior. As a result, the patient began to assimilate the repudiated injury to his masculine self-esteem of having felt rejected by his father.

Despite the attempt to enable the patient to expand the boundaries of his self-syntonic sense of self beyond its typically contemptuous, entitled attitudes to include self-dystonic feelings of need for paternal approval as well as feelings of humiliation and rage subsequent to feelings of disapproval, other aspects of the patient's self-dystonic sense of self might have been enacted rather than analyzed. Kohut framed the discussion of his confrontation to imply that he was being the caring and concerned father who strongly set limits on his son's potentially self-destructive behavior, a son who is defiantly provoking authority in order to obtain the fatherly attention he never had. The patient's positive response to Kohut's intervention suggests that he was not offended by being called a "complete idiot"—quite the contrary, apparently.

Yet one unanalyzed effect of Kohut's intervention may have been to achieve a role reversal in the therapeutic relationship. It was usually the patient as the young arrogant genius who treated others as though they were "complete idiots." Now it was Kohut's turn to assume the intellectually superior role in pronouncing dramatically and from on high that the patient was essentially intellectually inferior, the opposite of the patient's sense of himself as a young genius. Yet the patient was pleased rather than humiliated by this reversal of fortunes. Perhaps the patient had turned passive into active. He had initially felt rebuffed by Kohut in the seminar when he was attempting to gain intellectual affirmation. Now he actively re-created that trauma in having seduced the aggressor, having provoked Kohut into openly calling him a "complete idiot," a sentiment that the patient may have felt was implied but not openly stated in Kohut's failure to respond to his remark in the seminar.

The other side of the patient's self-syntonic defiant grandiosity may well be self-dystonic compliant masochism whereby he achieved a spurious victory in defeat. In seducing the aggressor, he won a kind of moral victory over the aggressor whose presumably authoritarian, moralistic, and punitive attitudes have been exposed. What remained unanalyzed but enacted in the transference were the patient's repudiated desires to ingratiate himself with Kohut in order to get his approval as well as getting revenge on Kohut, not so much by being openly superior to him but by being covertly morally superior in seducing Kohut into going tit for tat with the patient, to say something that at least in manifest content would be conventionally characterized as glib, contemptuous, and superior. Perhaps the patient did not need to envy Kohut, feel inferior to him, or competitive with him if he could expose Kohut as a pretentious and pompous authority figure. This formulation of the underlying dynamic is consistent with the way in which object relations theorists such as Klein, Rosenfeld, and Kernberg have typically conceptualized narcissistic psychodynamics, theorists who might well see in Kohut's case example a good illustration of the analyst's failure to contain a projective identification.

Kohut's intervention may have been experienced by the patient as paternalistic as well as paternal. Certainly many clinicians have confronted more severely narcissistic, self-destructive, and acting-out patients without recourse to telling them that they were "complete idiots." One could have tried interpreting that the patient seems to be so routinely dismissive of the analyst's comments that it could seem as though one would have to hit the patient over the head with an interpretation in order to have a serious discussion with him about his reckless driving. If the patient responded dismissively once again, one could have tried to interpret how the patient treats the analyst's concerns about his self-destructiveness as though they were the nagging worries of an overprotective mother not to be taken too seriously. Perhaps the patient seduced the aggressor by trying to attack Kohut's masculine self-regard in treating him dismissively as the overprotective mother in whose care he was left, thereby provoking Kohut to assert his paternal authority through an act of domination to which the patient covertly submits while feeling a vindictive triumph in defeat.

I believe that these interpretive possibilities did not occur to Kohut, not because it is not in the material, since the interpretation of a role reversal in the transference is certainly at least plausible given the manifest content of having called an overtly arrogant patient a complete idiot. Kohut, being wedded to the idea that both his patient as well as himself possessed essential and unitary selves, was less likely to consider the possibility that what he saw as an essential self was simply one side of a conflict, the other side of which may have been repudiated and perhaps projected onto the analyst. Kohut saw the patient as essentially grandiose and the transference as essentially mirroring. The problem in treatment was primarily a failure of mirroring with narcissistic rage as a disintegration product. Yet the patient could be simultaneously defiantly grandiose as well as compliantly masochistic, though one aspect may have been self-syntonic as the other was self-dystonic. Kohut may have been simultaneously paternal and paternalistic as well as maternal and maternalistic in the transference, though certain aspects may have been self-syntonic and others, self-dystonic. Perhaps both Kohut and the patient were alternately unconsciously masochistic and arrogant in their relationship to each other. To envision such a possibility requires an openness to viewing the self as multiple and conflicted.

How does one discover whether such hypotheses are warranted by the material? Apparently Kohut's patient did not complain that Kohut was being paternalistic in handling the patient's reckless driving, but as far as we know, the patient was not asked whether he may have felt that way. Maybe if on reflection Kohut entertained the possibility of role reversal in the transference, he might have made such an inquiry, and different sorts of analytic material might have emerged. Empathic inquiry cannot help but be guided by one's preconceptions, and in psychoanalysis one usually discovers what one looks for. If one looks for unconscious role reversals and repetitive enactments in the transference, one is sure to find them, just as if one is looking for selfobject transferences, one is sure to find them as well. And if we look for both types of transferences simultaneously, we will be sure to discover both simultaneously. In terms of gaining validation from the patient, the analyst can usually more easily obtain direct confirmation for hypotheses that are self-syntonic to the patient than direct confirmation for hypotheses that are self-dystonic. Psychoanalysts of all persuasions are quite adept at collecting indirect validation for a wide variety of hypotheses. The same material can usually be used by those with sufficiently sophisticated interpretive skills to draw plausibly opposite conclusions.

Freud (1900) noted that repressed content continually seeks expression and gains access to awareness in disguised form, a process he called "the return of the repressed." Self-dystonic elements and the transferences that correspond to those self-dystonic elements also return in disguised form. Gill (1982) noted that the latent transference is often expressed in allusions to the analyst. When the text of the session is the patient's discussion of extra-analytic interpersonal events that are conflictual, the subtext of that discussion might allude to conflictual experiences with the analyst in the here and now that are denied access to awareness and direct expression. Thus the patient's repudiated self-dystonic transference to the analyst is always present but is expressed covertly through indirect allusions to the analyst. This was illustrated in Kohut's case in which the patient's grievance with the policeman alluded to the patient's grievance with Kohut for not responding to him in the seminar. Kohut's failure to respond to him in the seminar was the here-and-now interpersonal trigger of the patient's narcissistic rage in the transference.

Reich (1928) noted that self-dystonic latent transference is also indirectly revealed in nonverbal characterological attitudes toward the analyst that are repudiated. If Kohut did not get the allusion to himself in the guise of the policeman, he certainly got the message in the way the patient tossed his leather jacket, crashed onto the couch, and recounted his narrative in an unrepentant tone of voice. The patient's nonverbal behavior could be said to have been "oozing" with arrogance, contempt, and smug superiority aimed at Kohut. Thus the self-dystonic transference was expressed simultaneously through two avenues: symbolically through allusions and nonverbally through body language. And it is likely that these two avenues of unconscious communication would impact on the analyst's countertransference. In this case, the impact was to be unconsciously provocative and challenging of the analyst's authority, evoking rage in the analyst at the patient's reckless disregard as the policeman had been provoked to write the patient a ticket despite having been initially disposed to let him go without punishment.

In their ideas about projective identification, induced countertransference, and role reversal in the transference, Kleinian analysts have made an important clinical contribution to understanding how self-dystonic aspects of the patient's personality are expressed in the clinical situation. At a manifest level the patient experiences the analyst as implicitly treating the patient as the patient's parents treated or mistreated the patient. Yet at a latent level the patient being identified with the parents treats or mistreats the analyst as the parents treated or mistreated the patient. The latent experience of the transference involves a reversal of roles from the manifest experience of the transference. The analyst comes to represent and enact the self-dystonic aspect of the patient's personality. The patient treats the analyst in the same manner in which the patient treats the self-dystonic aspect of his or her personality. Kohut's patient treated Kohut as his despised inadequate self until Kohut could no longer take it and reversed roles with the patient in calling the patient a complete idiot. A more empathic intervention might have been to ask the patient what it was like to work with an analyst who was experienced as a complete idiot despite the analyst's excellent reputation, an analyst who seemed compelled to defend his threatened dignity by turning the tables on the patient.

A form of premature transference interpretation may arise when the analyst attempts to interpret resistance to the awareness of the latent transferential subtext of the patient's narrative prior to interpreting a more surface reading of the patient's narrative. For example, when the patient is telling a narrative about an extra-analytic interpersonal encounter, we may assume that the subtext is a hidden allusion to the analyst as the analyst may be represented in disguised form as one of the characters in the narrative. Nevertheless, at a manifest level the analyst always plays himself in the analytic situation, assuming the role of audience (i.e., selfobject) to the patient's unfolding narrative. At a manifest level, the patient as narrator is always attempting to gauge audience/selfobject reaction to the part that the patient plays as a character in the narratives. The patient is a storyteller who tells narratives in which he or she is the main protagonist. As far as the patient is consciously concerned, the analyst is not an implicit character in the extra-analytic narrative but is, instead, an omnipresent character as a here-and-now audience to the storytelling, constantly evaluating the patient's performance as a storyteller as well as his or her conduct as the main character in the story.

Shapiro (1989) noted that the therapist is only sporadically the subject of the patient's interest but continuously the object of the patient's communications. Thus, to follow the patient's lead and overtly expressed interest is to focus on the content of the patient's narrative, reading that narrative on its own terms not in terms of hidden allusions to the analyst.

> Transference interpretations based solely on the patient's allusions to other figures. . .cannot be reliable. . . .The reactions to the boss and to the therapist may well be similar not because one is a displacement of the other but because both derive from the same general attitude toward figures who stand in a certain relation to the patient. . . . A misinterpretation as a displacement of reaction what is merely a similarity of reaction may retain a degree of plausibility, but it misidentifies the object of the patient's interest or concern. Such an interpretation may gain the patient's "acceptance," but it will not enlarge his self-awareness. [p. 108]

The patient tends to spontaneously make the analyst an explicit subject of his or her narrative interest when the analyst's role as audience (i.e., as selfobject)—that is, as object of the patient's communicative interest—is disturbed. As long as the analyst is experienced as a "good-enough" receptive, affirmative audience, he or she can be taken for granted as a sort of background phenomenon. When the patient begins to become concerned that the analyst may not be such an accepting audience, then the patient becomes preoccupied with audience reaction.

When Kohut's patient recounted the story with the policeman, it is quite likely that the patient assumed that Kohut would take the policeman's point of view rather than his own. His defiant attitude was a defense against the condemnation he probably expected. After listening to the patient's story, Kohut might have inquired which side, the patient's or the policeman's, did the patient assume Kohut took in listening to this vignette. Kohut might have discovered that the patient did not experience him as a neutral or empathic audience but as an audience with a particular point of view who tended to identify with certain characters more than others in the patient's narrative. In this case, Kohut rejected the patient's omnipotent control and grandiosity and identified with the viewpoint of someone concerned about "realistic" dangers to self and others, like a policeman, as opposed to someone thinking they can get away with anything, like the patient.

A consideration of the analyst as an audience who confirms or disconfirms the patient's self-syntonic sense of self that is put forward in his or her narratives brings us back to the alliance concept. The analyst as an attentive, validating audience to the patient's narrative performance constitutes an unobjectionable positive transference. The alliance with the analyst is dependent on the analyst's provision of a favorable review of the patient's performance. Such an alliance will prove to be unreliable once the patient feels that the analyst as an audience has given a critical review that is unsupporting of the patient's performance. Kohut's approach provides a method of repairing these ruptures to the therapeutic alliance; the analyst may attempt to empathize with the patient's experience of the analyst as an inattentive, disapproving, and unappreciative audience. Thus Kohut's confrontation was an active breach of the mirroring transference that the patient demanded for his archaic grandiosity, yet in repairing that breach the treatment was moved forward.

Sometimes even manifestly negative transferences that are devaluatory, dismissive, accusatory, blaming, indifferent, counterdependent, and so on, may serve a self-affirmative function. Wolf (1988) discussed how adversarial selfobjects function to define and sustain the self through opposing it. If the self is defined in contradistinction to the other, then the analyst might have to embody all that is negative so that the patient can embody all that is good, or vice versa. Thus, a kind of alliance can be formed with the patient on the basis of an unobjectionable negative transference that should not be prematurely disrupted. Eventually though, this transference will have to be broached as a transference resistance to an underlying positive transference of which the patient is frightened for fear that it may undermine a sense of self formed on the basis of defiance and opposition rather than on a basis of trust and cooperation. Rosenfeld (1964) discussed the "lavatory transference" in which narcissistic patients make themselves feel better by using the analysis as an opportunity to ventilate all their grievances that they resist analyzing.

Whereas Kohut's approach could be characterized as one that has great sensitivity to the self-syntonic level but is sometimes oblivious to certain dimensions of the self-dystonic level, especially those reflected in role reversal, Rosenfeld's Kleinian object relations approach to narcissistic patients could be seen as the exact opposite. Rosenfeld (1964) demonstrated great sophistication in explicating complicated unconscious dynamics while being relatively oblivious to surface features. Greenson (1974) believed that Kleinian analysts in general did not work from surface to depth, blurred the distinction between resistance and content, and did not pay sufficient attention to the working alliance.

Rosenfeld (1964) presented a case illustrating his approach

to working with the "lavatory transference" that many narcissistic patients form. This case seems to demonstrate how
the analyst bent on interpreting the patient's resistances to
acknowledging the patient's underlying hostility and devaluation toward the analyst seems to lack empathy for the
patient's experience of the analyst as an unappreciative
audience for whom his or her productions will never be good
enough, no matter how hard the patient tries to be a perfect
performer. It illustrates the liability of addressing the "lavatory transference" entirely in terms of its defensive function
to the neglect of its self-affirmative function (pp. 333–337).

The patient was the son of fairly wealthy parents. He had
superficial relations with people with whom he generally got
on quite well. He was bright and had done well at school. He
came for treatment because he had recently married and
found himself jealous of his wife's relations with other
people. Nevertheless, he blamed his wife for any difficulty
that arose and did not believe he really needed analysis. He
maintained a vaguely superior and patronizing attitude,
which he tried to disguise. He thought of himself as the
perfect patient.

Contrary to the patient's experience of himself as the
"perfect patient," Rosenfeld saw him as the opposite, a
patient who could make very little "proper" use of the
analysis. He seemed to project all his problems onto other
people. Despite his externalization of responsibility, he took
interpretations without resentment, took them up quickly,
discussed them, and felt self-satisfied with his knowledge.
Rosenfeld experienced the patient's narcissistic resistances as
a "stone wall" behind which was hidden the patient's omnipotence, hostility, and envy. These underlying attitudes were
completely denied by the patient and difficult to demonstrate
in the material.

The patient did bring in a number of dreams that Rosenfeld was able to utilize to illustrate the patient's underlying
dynamics. In one dream, the Russians were going to attack
some hotels in England with names like Royal, Majestic, and
Palace. There was a food shortage that led to a number of girls

prostituting themselves in order to get food. He approached one of the girls as a customer, but she laughed at him and he felt disappointed. Rosenfeld interpreted the Russian attack as the patient's hostile omnipotence based on envy of the English parents. The prostitutes reflected a devaluation of the maternal breast by which the patient felt rejected. The patient reversed this injury in dreaming that it was the prostitutes who were hungry, not him. Rosenfeld believed he was represented in the dream by the prostitutes. The patient wanted to get close to Rosenfeld but feared rejection so devalued him in turning him into a prostitute.

Rosenfeld interpreted these dynamics directly, and the treatment unfolded as the patient presented a series of dreams that Rosenfeld interpreted similarly. He noted how the patient wanted to depend on him without ever admitting that dependency. Instead, the patient maintained the illusion of self-sufficiency. The patient was reported as withdrawing from Rosenfeld whenever an interpretation came close to touching him. The patient was described as maintaining this distance through role reversal in imagining himself as the analyst with all of the answers, while Rosenfeld had none. Rosenfeld suggested that even though it was deflating for the patient when the illusion of self-sufficiency was interpreted, it was essential to interpret the patient's defensive self-sufficiency if "real" relations with others were ever to be established.

Gradually over time the patient acknowledged feeling inferior in relation to Rosenfeld. The patient admitted his resistance: "I want to feel good and have a perfect relation with you. Why should I admit anything bad which would spoil the good picture I have of myself, which I feel you must admire too" (p. 336). Rosenfeld noted that narcissistic patients rigidly preserve this idealized self-image, a self-image requiring constant nullification of the work of the analysis. Rosenfeld ended his discussion on a somewhat somber note concerning prognosis. "Often the attempt at integration fails because mechanisms related to the omnipotent narcissistic self suddenly take control of the normal self in an attempt to divert or expel the painful recognition. However, there are patients who gradually succeed in their struggles against narcissistic omnipotence, and this should encourage us as analysts to continue our research into the clinical and theoretical problems of narcissism" (p. 337).

One cannot help but wonder, if Rosenfeld experienced the patient's narcissistic resistance as an "impenetrable stone wall" that frustrated his dedicated efforts at analysis and that undid the effects of any hard-won analytic insights, whether perhaps his experience was in part an artifact of his interpretive approach that bypasses analysis of the self-syntonic in favor of exclusive analysis of the self-dystonic. I have no problem with Rosenfeld's formulation of the narcissistic character's underlying psychodynamics, but Rosenfeld did not demonstrate much appreciation of how one might approach the analysis of a narcissistic character in working from surface to depth. At a self-syntonic level, the patient construed himself as a "perfect patient" whom Rosenfeld admired, resulting in a mutual admiration society in which they were "perfectly related."

Rosenfeld was probably experienced as rejecting the patient's invitation to a mutual admiration society in constantly interpreting its defensive function in masking the patient's underlying devaluation of him. Yet the patient would consciously repudiate such a sense of rejection in order to maintain the idealized relationship in which his idealized self-image was embedded. The patient angrily responded to his unconscious sense of rejection through self-dystonic devaluation, a devaluation Rosenfeld experienced through the patient's nonverbal patronizing tone, superficial relatedness, and allusion to the transference in the dream in which Rosenfeld was portrayed as a prostitute. In sum, the patient was overtly appreciative but covertly devaluatory, perhaps feeling conflicted between a desire for mutual affirmation and a desire to revenge a narcissistic injury.

The patient resisted Rosenfeld's interpretation of his covert devaluation of the analysis in trying to assimilate all of Rosenfeld's interpretations. The patient resolutely attempted to prove that he was indeed a "perfectly" appreciative and cooperative patient, notwithstanding Rosenfeld's interpretations to the contrary. Rosenfeld interpreted the patient's facile assimilation of interpretations as a subtle form of rejecting his interpretations. There seemed to be the enactment of an adversarial relation in which the patient was bent on proving one way or another that he was a "perfect" patient, with Rosenfeld bent on proving the opposite. The result was a stalemate. Could this have repeated his relationship with his wife in which he felt unappreciated despite his efforts to prove that he was the perfect husband in seeking analysis? Could this have repeated a situation with his parents in which he never felt quite good enough to please them? Could the patient have been someone whose self-syntonic sense of self was to be a perfectly dutiful, polite person who overtly respects and honors authority while denying that aspect of himself that was the opposite—a dismissive and arrogant person with contempt for authority?

Rosenfeld addressed only the defensive function of the patient's self-syntonic sense of self as a perfect patient in a perfect relationship. He only seemed to treat as relevant to the analytic process the exploration of the self-dystonic aspect of the patient that was devaluatory, hostile, envious, and counterdependent. Perhaps if one had explored with the patient what it meant to him to be seen as a perfect patient in a perfect relationship, one might not have been met with an impenetrable stone wall but a patient eager to discuss what it was like for him to be perfect. It might be appreciated what a struggle it was for the patient to maintain a perfect relationship with an analyst who was constantly challenging his perfection by pointing out aspects of his personality that were less than perfect, as perhaps it was a struggle to prove to his wife that he was the perfect husband and to his parents that he was a perfect son. Did the patient ever experience his perfection as something other than glorious? Was it ever something oppressive, something that others envied, something that made him unique, something that others failed to appreciate, something unreal, or something perfectly normal and ordinary? These are the sorts of issues that might have been raised if one were working from surface to depth.

While at the level of the manifest transference the patient

is experiencing the analyst as either validating or invalidating the self-syntonic sense of self, at the level of the latent transference the patient is unconsciously experiencing the analyst as either validating or invalidating the patient's self-dystonic sense of self that has been repudiated. The patient engages in an unconscious form of reality testing in order to assess whether the self-dystonic sense of self represents an objective aspect of the self. Confirmation of the self-dystonic sense of self is analogous to confirming one's worst fears and may lead to a return of the repressed in terms of an exacerbation of neurotic symptomatology. Disconfirmation of the self-dystonic sense of self brings with it a sense of relief that allows for a more conscious acknowledgment of the self-dystonic element as it no longer constitutes a destabilizing threat. Weiss and Sampson (1986) discussed the patient's "unconscious test" of the analyst, whereby the patient unconsciously carries out a plan to test the reality of his or her pathogenic beliefs in relation to the analyst. The self-dystonic sense of self constitutes a "grim belief" about the self. Unconscious content becomes conscious as the analyst passes the patient's unconscious test and disconfirms the patient's grim beliefs about him- or herself.

Rosenfeld's patient may have been testing him through being unconsciously provocative. The patient was covertly devaluatory to test Rosenfeld unconsciously, to see how his analyst managed relating to an arrogant, devaluatory, and smugly self-sufficient person. His grim belief may have been that there was no way genuinely to engage such a person beyond turning the tables on him. If relations with others boil down to no more than the relation between a superior and an inferior, why not placate one's superiors in being manifestly polite and deferential while unconsciously acting superior to them? The patient's unconscious grim belief about relationships may have been confirmed to the extent the analyst seemed bent on breaking through the patient's impenetrable stone wall in order to make him a "proper" analytic patient who did something more with his sessions than unconsciously "evacuating" his bad objects into the analyst as a "lavatory."

What I find useful in Kohut's idea of selfobject transference is that it allows for a more interactional model of understanding the patient's transference toward the analyst. The transference can be seen as in part an evoked phenomenon, evoked by the analyst's functioning as a selfobject. The analyst's interpretive framework and interactive stance serve selfobject functions that regulate the patient's sense of self. The analyst is never neutral but always having some qualitative and quantitative impact on the patient's self-experience, validating some self-experiences while invalidating others. The analyst also always stands in some relationship to what is self-syntonic and self-dystonic in the patient's self-experience, either validating the syntonic while invalidating the dystonic or validating the dystonic while invalidating the syntonic.

What I find limiting in Kohut's approach to working with selfobject transferences is his assumption that selfobject transferences should always be left to unfold silently and undisturbed and that the inevitable disturbances of selfobject transferences that arise over the course of treatment are due primarily to the analyst's unwitting failures of empathy. I believe that it is helpful for analysts to at times encourage, facilitate, and challenge the patient to function at higher levels of functioning, such as transcending egocentric modes of thought. Wolf's adversarial selfobject transference addresses this issue in recognizing that it can serve a crucial developmental function for the analyst to be experienced by the patient as an adversarial, oppositional, and confrontative other who is clearly different from the patient. This enables the patient to establish a more clearly differentiated and firmly bounded sense of self, a self more capable of assimilating self-dystonic elements. I believe many pivotal moments arise in the therapeutic encounter when the patient as representative of all that is self-affirmative successfully opposes the analyst as the representative of all that is anathema to the patient's sense of self. It seems that the technique of self psychology may be avoidant of just such moments of triumph for the patient if the self-psychological analyst were studiously to avoid making interpretations that the patient might construe as anathema to the patient's sense of self.

What I find most useful in the object relations approach to transference is the notion of unconscious role reversal in the transference. Self-dystonic elements are brought into the therapeutic relationship unconsciously in repetitive enactments with the roles reversed. What I find limiting in the object relations approach is what can be an insensitivity to the more surface-level, self-syntonic selfobject dimension of the transference for which there may be a lack of empathy. In addition, viewing the therapeutic relationship as primarily repetitive and countertransference as primarily induced seems to minimize what the analyst brings to shaping the nature of the therapeutic interaction. In many respects all transference is iatrogenic—that is, evoked by the analyst's particular technique and particular personality.

In returning to the case of Joe, it may be illustrative to conceptualize his transferences to the therapist in terms of their self-syntonic and self-dystonic aspects. The self-syntonic transference was the mirroring transference in which the therapist served as a reassuring, supportive maternal or perhaps paternal presence who validated Joe's capacity to be either a high academic achiever or a successful entrepreneur. The self-dystonic transference that Joe repudiated was his fear that the therapist would either be an overprotective and infantilizing mother or a derisive and belittling father, either of whom could undermine his confidence in himself. Another aspect of the self-dystonic transference could be Joe's fears that the therapist is like a despised aspect of himself, a person who would give in to an infantilizing mother and a belittling father.

Picking up where we left off with Joe's treatment, Joe decided that he need not worry so much about academics after all, as his plan was to try to go into business for himself after finishing college. In the meantime, his plan was to enjoy himself and take it easy while he had the opportunity. To do this, Joe felt he needed to break up with his steady girlfriend so that he could be free to sow his wild oats. Yet Joe found that it was difficult to end the relationship. He felt guilty about rejecting a girlfriend who had no desire to reject him and worried that perhaps he would be giving up a good thing that he would later regret. Joe's ambivalence about his relationships with women was emerging more directly in his relationship with his girlfriend, although it remained a latent subtext in his relationship with the therapist.

At this point in the treatment, Joe began to ask the therapist what she thought he should do as he was finding it difficult to make a decision. The therapist, initially taken off guard by his question, asked why he was asking her opinion. Joe responded defensively, as though he felt that the therapist had implied he was not supposed to ask her questions. The therapist went on to ask Joe what he imagined her opinions were on the matter, to which he replied that he did not have the slightest idea, which was why he asked her in the first place. Seeing that he was not going to obtain a direct answer from the therapist, Joe went back to obsessing about the pros and cons of staying with or leaving his girlfriend. The therapist, feeling that an important transference issue was being enacted, ventured the interpretation that maybe Joe was also having some thought about whether he should continue the treatment with her. Joe responded that he would continue until the end of the school year when the therapist would be finishing her practicum and he would leave for summer vacation, adding that hopefully his problems would be solved by then.

It would seem that Joe had created a bind for the therapist. On the one hand, he solicited her support, reassurance, and advice and seemed to experience it as a rupture to the therapeutic relationship whenever she was not forthcoming with support, reassurance, and advice. On the other hand, Joe made it clear how important it was to him to prove his independence and demonstrate what he could do on his own to the extent of maintaining a certain emotional distance in the therapeutic relationship. Now that Joe was deciding he no longer needed to worry about his grades, was this to be understood as a defensive avoidance of his performance anxieties or as an expression of him finally deciding for himself what was genuinely important for him? Was breaking up with his girlfriend a defensive flight from fears of intimacy or a positive step in the direction of separation-individuation?

If the therapist mirrored his desire to assert himself by not worrying about grades and by breaking up with his girl-friend, was she implicitly being the indulgent mother who did not expect Joe to assume adult responsibilities? Or if she suggested a defensive function for such desires, was she undermining his fledgling steps in the direction of independent initiative and self-agency?

In clarifying the nature of the bind in supervision, it seemed that perhaps it was time to make a conflict interpretation in the transference. The next time that Joe solicited the therapist's advice about the girlfriend problem, the therapist suggested that, on the one hand, Joe would like the therapist to point him in the right direction in life and keep him on the right course, but, on the other hand, he would like to make these difficult decisions concerning career and love life for himself. Joe responded that he knew he had to make these important decisions for himself and that the therapist did not have all the answers. The therapist went on to interpret that if she gave him the answers, she was being like his mother, who did it all for him, and that if she did not give him the answers, she was being like his father, who faulted him for not being able to do it all on his own. Joe responded that this was his problem in life in general and not just with the therapist in particular. If left to his own devices, he became bogged down in ambivalence, indecision, and self-doubt; but if he got other people to tell him what to do, he did not feel sure he was doing what he really wanted to do. They agreed that this was an important problem that they could try to understand together and perhaps make some progress on before the end of the year when they would terminate their work together.

The therapist's conflict interpretation enabled Joe to begin to develop a metaperspective on his self as well as his relationship with the therapist. The problem was not simply one of low self-esteem and lack of confidence in his ability but a conflict in regard to not really knowing what he wanted because his wants reflected seemingly conflicting desires—to be studious yet be entrepreneurial, to be guided yet make his

own decisions, to be in a relationship yet be free, to accommodate his mother yet accommodate his father when they
had conflicting expectations of him, and so on. That the
conflict interpretation addressed conflicts in the transference
was especially important in relation to Joe's unconscious fears
and unconscious tests in relation to the therapist. The unconscious test in the transference was whether Joe could rely on
the therapist without his autonomy being undermined by the
therapist becoming infantilizing like his mother or critical like
his father. These were two eventualities the repetition of
which he dreaded as blows to his narcissism and against
which he needed to maintain a certain distance in the
therapeutic relationship in order to protect himself from those
potential situations of danger.

The therapist also had to bear an element of role reversal in
the transference as the patient alternately and unconsciously
treated her as his mother and father had treated him. Initially
the patient treated the therapist as though everything she did
was fine with him. The therapist felt very uncomfortable in
being treated this way, as everything did not seem fine in the
therapeutic relationship given the patient's initial lateness
and filling the sessions with weekly updates and progress
reports. Just as the patient felt patronized and infantilized by
his overprotective mother for whom he could do no wrong,
the therapist would have felt more comfortable with a more
critical and demanding patient than Joe, who was often
blandly if not falsely reassuring. Yet Joe was the opposite of
reassuring when he put the therapist on the spot in asking
her direct questions and soliciting her advice about what to
do with his girlfriend. This may have paralleled the way Joe
felt put on the spot in relation to his father, to whom Joe had
difficulty proving his competence. Joe's self-dystonic identifications with an overprotective mother and an overly critical
father were elements of his personality that would have been
difficult to acknowledge at this stage of the treatment. Joe was
struggling with the issue of establishing that he is his own
person who will make his own independent decisions in life,
a process that for Joe seemed to center around his efforts to

disidentify with his parents' expectations of him, his parents' perceptions of him, and his identification with them as role models.

Consideration of the transference to the therapist means that the therapist cannot empathize with what is going on in the patient's inner experience without having empathy for what is going on in the patient's experience of the relationship with the therapist. The patient's character structure in the clinical situation is expressed as a particular form of relationship to the therapist, and in understanding this relationship, one is also understanding the patient's character structure. Thus, empathic character analysis is also relational character analysis. To have empathy for the patient's relationship to the therapist means recognizing that the patient does not have simply one unidimensional relationship with the therapist but a multidimensional relationship reflecting both syntonic and dystonic aspects.

7

The Analysis of Countertransference

The phenomenon of countertransference raises a controversial dialectical issue in the psychoanalytic situation: how is the patient's contribution differentiated from the analyst's contribution to the analytic relationship? If the analytic couple are a mutually evocative and regulating dyad, how are the respective contributions of the individual characters of the couple ever sorted out? I would suggest that the analyst must have empathy for the patient's experience of the analyst's interpersonal impact (i.e., the analyst's countertransference) on the patient before going on to analyze the patient's resistance to acknowledging his or her contribution to the analytic relationship (i.e., the patient's transference). I would also suggest that in the analyst's private self-analysis of countertransference, the analyst must first have empathy for the analyst's need to maintain a self-syntonic sense of self in the face of the patient's negative transference before going on to analyze the analyst's own resistance to acknowledging self-dystonic aspects that have been evoked by the patient's unflattering characterization of the analyst.

The state of the analyst's mind is not autonomously regulated by the analyst alone but is rather intersubjectively regulated, with the patient exerting a regulatory influence. The patient is always in part a selfobject to the analyst who regulates the analyst's self-states. This regulation is effected through the analyst's perception (conscious and unconscious) of how the patient reflects explicitly as well as implicitly the analyst's selfhood. The analyst, especially the analyst attuned to the patient's transference, is always imagining how he or she is seen through the eyes of the patient. Though the analyst may harbor the illusion that his or her sense of self is relatively independent of how he or she imagines the patient is viewing the analyst and that the analyst's construction of the patient's perception of him or her (i.e., transference) is only factual information with no effect on the analyst's state of mind, it can be noted that the patient's perceptions of the analyst are always either validating or invalidating the analyst's own self-assessment. If the patient sees the analyst as the analyst sees him- or herself, then the analyst's self-syntonic self-assessment is validated and probably taken for granted, unless the analyst had some reason to suspect some sort of mutual collusion to avoid discerning self-dystonic elements in the analyst's personality. If the patient sees the analyst in a manner discrepant from the manner in which the analyst sees him- or herself, then the analyst's self-syntonic image is challenged. The analyst may either discredit the patient's perception of him/her or wonder whether perhaps the patient is observing some self-dystonic element in the analyst's personality of which the analyst was unaware. Thus the patient's perceptions of the analyst will either support or challenge the analyst's own self-syntonic view.

Countertransference will reflect how the analyst feels about the patient's either confirming or disconfirming the analyst's self-syntonic sense of self, which, just like the patient's self-syntonic self, entails the repudiation of self-dystonic elements. To the extent that the analyst's self-syntonic sense of self is narrowly constructed along unidimensional lines, it will prove to be relatively more prone to destabilization from self-dystonic feedback than a self-syntonic sense of self, which is flexibly organized along multidimensional lines. Thus, countertransference is going to be shaped by the nature of the analyst's level of characterological flexibility. The more rigid or brittle the character structure, the more the analyst may need to discredit perceptions that the patient has of the analyst that are self-dystonic.

The manifest countertransference of which the analyst is

aware will reflect in part a defensive repudiation of self-dystonic elements of the patient's transference. Regardless of the level of the analyst's characterological flexibility, repudiation of self-dystonic elements of the patient's transference is a normative process, as the self-syntonic sense of self, no matter how broadly constructed, is maintained on the basis of the repudiation of self-dystonic elements. In addition, as has been often noted in the literature on countertransference, the more severe the patient's pathology, the more likely the patient is going to perceive the analyst in a manner highly discrepant from the manner in which the analyst likes to think of him- or herself. For example, a paranoid patient in a negative transference is unlikely to serve as a selfobject who will reliably mirror the analyst's normal sense of herself. It may be difficult for the analyst to maintain a normal sense of herself if she is seen as an evil being who should be imminently assaulted and destroyed in a sadistic manner.

The question arises as to just how it is that the analyst can ever process transferences that reflect self-dystonic elements of the analyst's personality. Racker (1968) discussed the problem of the analyst's resistance to the countertransference resulting in a counterresistance that parallels the patient's resistance to the analytic process. For a patient's perception of the analyst's personality to be self-dystonic, it does not matter whether that trait is "really" present in the analyst's personality but is operating unconsciously or whether the patient is largely projecting a trait onto the analyst that the analyst does not actually possess. Either way, it is dystonic from the syntonic sense of self and therefore threatening. Who can say whether we are more disturbed by characterological assessments that are in effect false, unfair, and slanderous accusations or by assessments that are accurate appraisals fairly reflecting facets of our personality that we have been attempting to repudiate? It is exceedingly difficult to maintain a view of oneself that no one else shares, that is vociferously challenged by others, or that is not validated by someone who knows us well.

Minority opinions, especially a minority of one, usually need to be buttressed by a fair share of self-assurance in order to be maintained, whether or not that minority opinion is ultimately proven true or false in the end. Conversely, majority opinions are considerably easier to maintain even if eventually proven inaccurate. Consensual validation tends to supersede the autonomous reality testing of the individual, as in the phenomenon of mass hysteria. Nevertheless, regardless of the relative accuracy or inaccuracy of the patient's perceptions of the analyst, the analyst's natural role responsiveness (Sandler 1976) to the patient's role expectations makes it likely that the analyst does in at least some subtle way act in a manner congruent with the patient's perception of him or her.

The analyst's role responsiveness gives rise to what has been called "induced countertransference." Racker (1968) noted two types of induced countertransference: concordant and complementary, depending on whether the analyst identifies with the patient's self or the patient's objects. Concordant countertransference arises when the analyst identifies with the patient's point of view. Complementary countertransference arises when the analyst identifies with the point of view of the patient's internalized objects. Since the patient is always identified with his or her internalized objects and may also engage in role reversals in the therapeutic relationship, it is probably somewhat of an artificial dichotomy to assume that a clear-cut differentiation exists between the point of view of the self and the point of view of the other.

Countertransference, like transference, could be classified as either self-syntonic or self-dystonic. Self-syntonic countertransference has ready access to awareness, whereas self-dystonic countertransference tends to be repudiated. The relative degree to which countertransference derives from the analyst's defensive need to maintain a stable self-syntonic sense of self versus an accurate reading of the patient's personality as divined through the analyst's role responsiveness does not really matter, as the analyst's countertransference is always an intersubjective phenomenon that can only artificially be divided into its component parts. Nevertheless, even if countertransference could be divided up in that manner, it is unnecessary to do so, as all that needs to be articulated and expanded on is the patient's perception of the situation. The arduous task for the analyst in attempting to become aware of and acknowledge self-dystonic counter-transference is not to figure out whether he or she "really" possesses the trait the patient ascribes to the analyst but to pose to him- or herself the hypothetical question that if he or she did possess that trait, why would it be so difficult to admit it? That question may lead to self-empathy and perhaps to patient empathy if the patient is struggling with an analogous issue.

The analyst must approach countertransference by working from surface to depth and by balancing self-empathy with self-analysis. The analyst has a legitimate need to maintain a cohesive self-syntonic sense of self with positive self-esteem. The analyst must have empathy for this need because the patient is unlikely to prove a reliable selfobject. The analyst will have to assimilate innumerable narcissistic injuries and selfobject failures that the patient wittingly and unwittingly inflicts on the analyst in subtle and not so subtle ways. To some extent the analyst cannot take all this person-ally and must affirm the self in the face of the patient's invalidation. The analyst is in fact a role model for the patient in terms of how one maintains dignity and self-respect in the face of personal attack. Yet on the other hand, the analyst must question and analyze the countertransference for what it reveals about repudiated self-dystonic elements of the analyst's as well as the patient's personalities. After all, the countertransference is a compromise formation that serves multiple and conflicting functions; it affirms some aspects of the analyst's self while repudiating others, and it reveals certain aspects of the patient's self while concealing others.

The analyst must learn to tolerate the relativity of the self, that to each patient and with each patient he or she is to some extent a different person, no matter what connecting thread of self-sameness characterizes his or her personal style of being a clinician. To evade the relativity of the self, one could choose to prioritize a statistically normative sense of self that reflects the manner in which "most" patients (i.e., the average patient) seem to see the analyst. Or, one could choose to prioritize a specialized sense of self that reflects the flattering portrait derived from the perception of those patients who think highly of the analyst at the conclusion of their analyses and decide that such patients have achieved a more realistic perception of the analyst reflecting the analyst's "real" self. An analyst who imagined him- or herself brutally honest and open to entertaining all manner of self-dystonic perceptions might prioritize the most critical and unflattering portraits as plausibly reflecting at least some aspect of his or her "real" self. Another option would be to decide that one's analytic self is like a marionette on a string, the string being pulled by patients' transferences, and is therefore not one's "real" self at all but simply a professional role that one assumes—a role prereflectively molded to the particular role requirements of each patient.

This is not to say that the analyst is some sort of "as if" personality who does not possess a stable sense of identity but rather that the analyst, like the actor, is engaged in a profession that requires considerable role flexibility, not so much at the level of behavior but at the level of fantasy and feeling. To process countertransference, the analyst, like an actor, must rise to the professional challenge of assuming a role that seems to be out of character. Can a man play a woman, can a heterosexual play a homosexual, can a young person play an old person, can a nice person play a despicable person, can a jaded person play an innocent person, and so on? To process self-dystonic elements, the analyst must be able to identify with these roles at least in fantasy while refraining from acting such roles out overtly, though it may be that in some subtle form in keeping with an overtly professional demeanor these trial identifications are enacted in the intersubjective field.

Once the analyst surmounts his or her defensive repudiation of self-dystonic role assignments and assumes a self-syntonic trial identification with that role assignment in fantasy, it may be possible to use that role awareness diagnostically as a reflection of some aspect of the patient's personality. The crucial diagnostic question at this point in evaluating one's role responsiveness is whether the role relationship being enacted is self-syntonic or self-dystonic for the patient. If the role relationship is self-dystonic for the patient, then the diagnostic question is what role relationship is self-syntonic at this point in time and would be accessible to the patient's awareness. It may constitute a form of premature interpretation for the analyst to interpret the self-dystonic role relationship that has been divined through the analyst's reading of his or her induced countertransference if that interpretation bypassed the prerequisite analysis of the self-affirmative function of the self-syntonic role relationship that the patient has formed with the analyst. Interpretation of the self-dystonic that derives from the analyst's reading of his or her induced countertransference is likely to strike the patient as oracular because it seems so discrepant from the patient's self-syntonic self-experience. What is obvious, although perhaps taken for granted, is what is self-syntonic, and what is obscure, although perhaps unsettling, is what is self-dystonic.

Racker (1968), who processed transference–countertransference dynamics within the framework of Kleinian theory, seemed to bypass the issue of working from surface to depth in his clinical work, as do most Kleinian analysts. The example discussed here is an interesting one, because it is one in which Racker attempted to demonstrate how one could utilize countertransference to avoid making premature interpretations in working from surface to depth. As we shall see, Racker's conception of surface corresponded to something that I would still consider relatively deep. For this reason, Kleinian analysts have often felt it is an unfair criticism that they do not work from surface to depth, even though they openly acknowledge their belief that it is important to interpret at the level of greatest unconscious anxiety in the transference as soon as possible. Ironically, whereas Racker saw only what is "deep" in the patient's transference, he seemed to see only what is "surface" (i.e., self-syntonic) in his own countertransference. And it would seem that in this case example if Racker had analyzed what was self-dystonic in his countertransference, he may have been able to have had greater empathy for what was surface in his patient's experience of him in the transference.

The patient (Racker 1968, pp. 154–160), a physician, suffered chiefly from an intense emotional inhibition and a "disconnexion" in all his object relationships. He began a session by saying that he felt completely disconnected from the analyst. He spoke with great difficulty, as though he was overcoming a great resistance, yet always in an unchanging tone of voice. The patient recounted how in a conversation with another physician, he sharply criticized analysts for their passivity (they give little and cure little), high fees, and tendency to dominate their patients. The analyst recognized that although these accusations were couched in general terms, they alluded to the analyst, who was aware of feeling "slight" irritation in regard to the implicit accusation.

Racker hypothesized that the patient was projecting his own passive, exploitative, domineering, and selfish tendencies onto the analyst, whom he then attacked for being that way. This served as a defense against the patient's own accusatory superego. Racker believed it would be premature to interpret this "deeper situation." He suggested that the patient's complaint "has even at the surface still further meanings" (p. 155) such as rebellion, provocation, and vengeance, perhaps in the service of seeking punishment as well as controlling and subjugating the analyst. Here is an example of formulations that Racker would consider surface phenomena but that I would consider deep in the sense that I would suspect that the patient would deny that he was a provocative person trying to control the analyst while seeking punishment.

Racker utilized his countertransference in order to ascertain which of these interpretations was the appropriate response to the transference situation at the moment. The analyst recognized that he felt a "little" anxious and angry at the aggression he suffered from the patient. Perhaps the analyst's anxiety and anger paralleled the patient's inner conflict. The sense of disconnection and depression the patient experienced may have resulted from his guilt about his aggressive attacks on the analyst for which he should be punished. The analyst interpreted the patient's disconnection in these terms in order to alleviate superego anxiety. The patient confirmed that he had felt anxious voicing these complaints about the analyst but stated, "What am I to do with that?" The analyst was annoyed by these words. Yet Racker, having recognized his own anger at the patient, realized that it was important not to fall into the role of the patient's critical superego and counter the patient's accusation with a counteraccusation.

The patient admitted some connection but then denied it. Racker hypothesized that if the patient admitted connection, the patient would fall into intense dependence and be indebted to the analyst. The analyst interpreted the patient's fear of dependence. The patient's depression lifted, and the analyst took this sign of progress as an implicit admission that the analysis was of use. It emerged that a few days before, a mutual friend of the patient and the analyst told the patient that the analyst was going away on holiday and that the patient's next session would be his last. It turned out that this information was false. It became apparent that the analyst was important to the patient, but the patient was forging a protest against all analysts as an expression of as well as a defense against being abandoned by his analyst.

The strength of Racker's approach was that he utilized his own sense of anxiety and annoyance at having been implicitly accused of being passive, selfish, domineering, and ineffectual to recognize the emergence of superego anxiety in the transference. Recognizing the revival of a persecutory bad object, Racker, in containing his anger, tried not to give in to the temptation to interpret in a manner that would be experienced as retaliatory or punitive. Seeing past the accusatory superego transference, Racker was able to have empathy for the fact that the patient generated distance in the relationship out of fears of dependence. The interpretation of these fears of dependence brought to light the patient's mistaken expectation that the analyst was going away on holiday without telling him about it until the last session.

Though the worst of the patient's implicit criticisms of Racker—that Racker would not inform him of going away on holiday until the last session—was proven unfounded, the rest of the patient's criticisms (i.e., that the analyst was too passive, charges too much, and is domineering) were not addressed at least in their surface-level meanings. These accusations were appreciated as essentially displacements of the patient's genuine concerns and in the service of the defensive repudiation and projection of the patient's own despised self due to superego condemnation. Racker wondered why the patient felt disconnected from the analyst. Yet if the patient felt that his legitimate and consciously recognized desire for a more active, cheaper, and less domineering analyst were not appreciated, it was no wonder that he might have felt disconnected. The patient did seem to feel guilty about making such complaints, but maybe that was not solely because the complaints were unfounded unconscious projections of his own greedy self but in addition because at a more surface level he may have felt that he should defer to the analyst's authority and comply with the analyst's manner of conducting the treatment.

Racker made a point of noting that in response to the patient's implicit criticism, he was only slightly irritated and a little anxious, implicitly suggesting a self-syntonic sense of self that was not seriously threatened by challenges to his professional competence. At a self-dystonic level, the analyst's anger, annoyance, and anxiety in relation to the patient's accusations may have reflected some repudiated doubt on the analyst's part that the patient's implicit complaints about the treatment could be well founded. Evidently Racker was sufficiently sure of his basic technique, at least at a conscious level, so that he did not consider the possibility that he could be too passive, charge too much, or be too domineering. He did not consider the possibility that with this particular patient there could be any need to calibrate his technical stance to achieve a better working alliance given the magnitude of the patient's emotional "disconnection."

In the unfolding narrative, it is certainly dramatized as a moment of truth when it emerges that one of the patient's hidden complaints was unquestionably unfounded. Though Racker did not openly retaliate, neither did he take the patient's accusations seriously and explore them at face value as though they could possibly have been true. What would it mean to the patient for Racker to be a more active, less domineering, and cheaper analyst? It might have been Racker's persistent focus on the deeper rather than the more surface reading of the patient's complaints that the patient experienced as a form of interpretive domination.

Since the patient was a physician, perhaps he would have liked a more collegial relation with Racker than he felt Racker provided. Perhaps the patient felt that doctors should treat each other more equally, collaboratively, and with professional courtesy when it comes to fees. The patient as a physician may have felt humiliated in assuming the dependent patient role with someone with whom he felt he should have been on equal terms as a colleague. In retaliation, the patient put down all analysts. Though the desire to relate to Racker as a colleague could certainly have reflected a defense against deeper levels of involvement in the analysis, Racker did not seem to recognize the thwarted wish for greater respect in the patient's complaint.

The physician's complaint could certainly have touched on what may have been a repudiated sore point for Racker as a psychoanalyst—the difficulty psychoanalysis has had in obtaining respect and legitimacy in the medical community on par with other medical specialties. Presumably the patient's physician colleague, to whom the patient complained, commiserated with the patient's complaints about psychoanalysts rather than rebutted them. Evidently Racker practiced in part in a small community in which he and his patient had a friend in common. The patient's complaint could have stirred up issues in regard to the patient possibly tarnishing Racker's reputation in the professional community if his physician patient were to continue to bad-mouth his analyst to his physician colleagues. One might reasonably feel more than "slightly" irritated and a "little" anxious in relation to a hostile and mean-spirited patient who may have been discrediting the analyst to his potential sources of future referrals.

The patient felt slighted by Racker's analytic stance and retaliated by implicitly attacking Racker's authority. Racker,

despite consciously not wanting to retaliate, perhaps defended his authority and kept the patient in his place in
interpreting his fear of depending on the analyst. Racker did
not inquire how the patient imagined Racker might have felt
in hearing that the patient complained to his physician
colleagues that all analysts are too passive, charge too much,
and are too domineering. Of course, a self psychologist
listening to this material would have looked for the trigger of
the patient's narcissistic rage and tried to have empathy for
the slight that the analyst's technical stance may have
evoked. The thwarted need for a collegial relationship might
have been appreciated as the revival of a narcissistic patient's
need for a twinship transference that would have been
allowed to unfold rather than be rebuffed through insistent
interpretation of its defensive function in warding off underlying envy and hostility of the analyst, of which the patient
was guilt-ridden. The self psychologist might have appreciated that the patient's twinship transference could have been
experienced in the analyst's countertransference as a threat to
the analyst's sense of authority and proper professional
boundaries.

The analyst's role in the therapeutic situation is not solely
one in which the analyst processes the patient's role inductions. Such a view of the analyst denies the analyst's self-
agency—that the analyst acts on the patient in a manner that
encourages the patient to respond in a particular manner. The
analytic situation itself, independent of the analyst's personality or technical approach, is a powerful form of role induction (i.e., the lack of reciprocity of self-disclosure, the rule of
free association, the frequency of sessions, the duration of
treatment, the use of the couch, the introspective focus, and
so on).

Analytic technique reflects a method of regulating the
intensity and quality of the role induction to which the
analyst subjects the patient. Abstinence in frustrating the
patient tends to evoke a more hostile/dependent relationship
than alliance building, which treats the patient as an appren-
tice analyst, a role that may not be particularly infantilizing or
frustrating but that nevertheless remains a subordinate

role. Defense analysis tends to foster an adversarial relationship in which the patient may have to assume a defeated role, whereas a self-affirmative approach encourages the patient to assume a role in which he or she becomes more dependent on audience approval, support, and encouragement. Active transference interpretation encourages the patient to assume a role in which the analyst is a vitally important omnipresent object in relation to whom the patient is unfailingly and anxiously oriented, whereas a silently holding or containing approach in which the analyst allows the patient to take him or her for granted encourages the patient to become reliant on the analyst for maintaining a basic sense of security. Every technical approach fosters a particular role relationship between analyst and patient, usually some variation on the theme of a superior–subordinate role relationship. Although there is always an ongoing process of mutual influence between the members of the therapeutic dyad, it is mutual influence within an asymmetrical if not inherently hierarchical role relationship, which is not to say that role reversals or attempts at equality might not occur.

Possibly one of the reasons that differences in analytic technique become such a topic of controversy is that there is some underlying appreciation that each technical approach is fostering a particular sort of role relationship with the patient that is purportedly of greater therapeutic value than the role relationship fostered by another technical approach. The concept of technical neutrality has obscured the fact that the analyst is always overtly as well as covertly exerting considerable interactional pressure on the patient to assume a particular role relationship. Out of fear of exploiting the transferential relationship in acknowledging the analyst's suggestive influence, there is a denial that the analyst is indeed exerting a very calculating and strategic sort of interpersonal pressure on the patient. Although induced countertransference has been widely considered as well as the analyst's neurotic difficulties in processing induced countertransference, there is little acknowledgment of the fact that the analyst is engaged in an intentional though preconscious act of getting the patient to assume a particular role in relation to him or her and that the analyst applies all his or her powers of strategic thought and nonverbal influence to achieve this goal. The reason that Alexander and French's (1946) approach to the corrective emotional experience has been so actively repudiated is that they openly advocated that the analyst strategically assume a role to counter the patient's transference.

The analyst always has an interpersonal agenda for the patient, despite claims to the contrary, and employs state-of-the-art interpersonal skills to achieve this agenda, for better or for worse. To deny this state of affairs is to deny the analyst's self-agency in relation to the patient and to treat the analyst as a purely reactive being like a marionette on a string. The analyst's unique personality exerts interpersonal pressure on the patient to assume a certain sort of role responsiveness. Each analyst is going to bring certain gender role expectations, age role expectations, ethnic and racial role expectations, class role expectations, intellectual role expectations, and characterological role expectations to the therapeutic situation that will intermesh with the patient's expectations on these dimensions, raising the issue of goodness of fit for each analytic dyad. Of course, the analyst's personality is going to influence the choice of technical approach as well as provide the basis for his or her individualistic application or misapplication of a particular technical tradition. Yet despite the analyst's unique personality, the analyst's theoretical belief system, which is likely to be shared in part by many analysts of a similar orientation, has a major influence on the course of the analysis.

There is a temptation when utilizing countertransference diagnostically to become a naive realist who views countertransference as something unspoiled by the imposition of one's own theoretical assumptions. When countertransference is processed through the lens of a naive realism, the analyst might experience a sense of direct access to the patient's subjective universe, as though any bias deriving from the analyst's preconceived notions had been transcended. This is an illusion, for countertransference, like empathy, is a creative construction as much as it is a fact of the analysis that may be discovered and objectively analyzed for its diagnostic utility. Since countertransference is experienced as an emotion, it seems something more immediate, more like "raw" data that have not yet had the time to be filtered through the lens of the analyst's theoretical biases. I would suggest that countertransference is inseparable from our preconceptions, for our preconceptions prereflectively influence how we will feel about something. Countertransference reflects how the analyst feels about the patient in the light of the analyst's theoretical preconceptions. In this sense, countertransference reflects the analyst's prereflective characterization of the patient. Self-disclosure of the countertransference, be it explicitly or implicitly, is invariably experienced by the patient as a form of character analysis that either confirms or challenges what is self-syntonic. Thus the analyst must possess empathy for the patient's experience of the analyst's countertransference as an expression of the analyst's implicit characterization of the patient.

Here we begin to see that the dynamic tension between the intrapsychic and the interpersonal relates to the dynamic tension between empathy and analysis. The intrapsychic reflects the patient's relationship with his or her self. The interpersonal reflects the patient's relationships with others. From an intrapsychic perspective, the patient's relationship with the analyst is an externalization of the patient's relationship with his or her self. The problem for treatment is to analyze the patient's resistance to realizing that the transference is not *only* about the analyst but is *also* about an externalization of the patient's own intrapsychic conflicts. From an interpersonal perspective, the patient's relationship with the analyst is shaped by the analyst's unique personality, technical orientation, and countertransference. The patient's contribution to the relationship cannot be understood without empathy for the unique interpersonal impact of the analyst on the patient. Thus empathy for the unique interpersonal context of the patient's transference must precede analysis of the patient's resistance to recognizing its individualistic intrapsychic meanings.

Even a contemporary interpersonal analyst such as Ehrenberg (1992) may not always see how countertransference is invariably processed through the lens of the analyst's preconceived theoretical notions. Without empathy for the interpersonal impact of the analyst's preconceptions, the analyst is prone to seeing the countertransference as reflecting more about the patient's intrapsychic dynamics than it does about the analyst's own organizing principles. Ehrenberg (1992, pp. 105–107) provided an example of her method of constructively utilizing her countertransference response to the patient. The patient was a woman with whom Ehrenberg found it difficult to stop yawning. The patient indicated that she was hurt and angered by the yawning. Ehrenberg noted that since she was not always this way with the patient, it was important to consider what was happening between them now. The analyst also inquired if it felt familiar in some way. It seemed to Ehrenberg that it was very similar to experiences the patient had described in relation to her mother.

The patient associated that she had difficulty keeping her mother's attention. She could only be with her mother on her mother's terms. If she was too boring, she would lose her mother's attention. To remedy the situation, she had to "invent a self" to engage her mother. As an adult she would fake orgasms and pretend to enjoy sex when she did not. At this point the patient began to cry, saying that she was afraid her "real self" was "no good" and that she did not want to find out. As the analyst became engaged and was no longer yawning, the patient commented that the analyst's responsiveness was not out of compliance with her demand for full attention or out of conformity to the role of analyst but because it was genuinely felt. It became apparent to both parties that the analyst's yawning had been in response to the patient's effort to play a role, whereas when the patient was being genuine, the analyst really did respond. Ehrenberg acknowledged that at the time she did not explore whether the patient's role playing was in response to some aspect of the analyst's unconscious participation.

Some months later, the patient discussed how inadequate she felt professionally. Although it was difficult to admit, she felt that it was great progress not to have to pretend otherwise. Though she felt exposed, it was a relief to be so open. She realized that her pretenses resulted in feelings of inadequacy and isolation. The strength of Ehrenberg's approach was that in not trying to hide or deny her countertransferential response, it enabled access to deeply felt aspects of the patient's relationship with her mother. The analyst's openness and willingness to explore collaboratively the meaning of the incident seemed to be an extremely meaningful occurrence to the patient. The patient was able to transcend a role that she experienced as restrictive and isolating and developed the sense of trust and freedom to be open with aspects of herself about which she felt quite vulnerable and exposed.

Yet in a subtle way the material was organized by the patient as well as by the analyst according to certain preconceptions about the nature of the patient's self. It was assumed that there were role-playing selves that were false and hid genuine selves that were real. The self that was "invented" to please mother so she would not be bored was the self that bored the analyst. And it was assumed by both of them that any self that was playing a role rather than being genuine was intrinsically boring to anyone who was not taken in by the pretense, so that it was natural that the analyst would be bored. It was also assumed that the self that was isolated, inadequate, and exposed was a genuine self that would naturally engage the analyst's attention.

If one listened to this material with different preconceptions about the self, one could imagine other interpretive possibilities. If it was assumed that all selves involve an element of role playing, since selves are in part based on identification with the expectations and role example of others in addition to one's own spontaneous inclinations, then it would be appreciated that a false dichotomy had been established between a false role-playing self that was boring and an engaging real self that was hurt and vulnerable. If one envisioned the possibility that the overtly role-playing self had real elements and that the covertly isolated and inadequate self had false elements, then one could see a different sort of enactment, a repetition of a subservient relation to the mother in which the patient continued to define herself primarily in terms of her success at gaining the attention of mother/analyst despite the apparent breakthrough of exposing her sense of vulnerability to the analyst.

In reviewing the interpersonal sequence, we can see that the material is open to multiple, contradictory, and equally plausible interpretations. The patient was being her usual self as an analytic patient, the analyst was bored and yawned, the patient protested, the analyst encouraged the patient to look for analogies in past experiences, the patient provided such analogies, the patient burst into tears at her sense of inadequacy, this display of shameful inadequacy succeeded in engaging the analyst, and the patient was relieved to be able to be openly vulnerable in front of the analyst. How do we know that her tearful display of inadequacy was any more genuine than her faked orgasms? How do we know that she was not adopting the role of a hurt little girl to placate an analyst who she felt has treated her rudely in yawning in response to her just being her usual self?

Maybe her initial but treated-in-passing protest at the analyst's yawning was a genuine act of self-assertion in the face of conventionally rude behavior, to which she would have politely acquiesced in the past. Perhaps the analyst's inquiry that the patient search her past for analogous experiences was experienced as a dismissal of the legitimacy of her current complaint about the analyst's rudeness. Perhaps the patient responded to the dismissal characteristically through crestfallen acquiescence, which succeeds in regaining the analyst's attention, becoming a paradigm for their future transactions. The patient continued to prereflectively define herself largely in terms of her success in engaging the attention of others, as though her intrinsic value was defined by how interesting others find her. What was bypassed is the question of how interesting and engaging the patient found an analyst who yawned rather than listened attentively. Perhaps a bored analyst was a boring person with whom to work.

Ehrenberg made a point of noting that she did not interpret to the patient, "I am yawning because you are boring me" but rather asked, "Why is this happening now, because this is not my usual reaction?" Yet it is quite likely that the analyst's yawn as a nonverbal communication was plausibly experienced by the patient as expressing exactly that sentiment: "I am yawning because you are boring." For this reason, the patient protested as any self-assertive person might do. The analyst's yawn was in effect implicit character analysis that characterized the patient as a boring person, an unflattering characterization to which the patient took offense. In this context, Ehrenberg's interpretation would seem a disclaimer of her nonverbal character analysis to the effect of saying, "Don't be offended by my yawning because I'm not usually this way, and it is probably not my problem alone anyhow but something going on between us, of which you must assume at least partial responsibility." Interestingly, the patient went on to assume full responsibility in tearfully acknowledging her inauthenticity, and Ehrenberg was left completely off the hook for having done something conventionally considered rude.

If the surface-level self-syntonic sense of self to which the analyst responded with a yawn was appreciated affirmatively as possessing some genuine elements, a different treatment approach may have been adopted. When the patient protested and complained about the analyst's yawning, one might have empathized with what it was like to be treated by the analyst in a conventionally rude manner and explored how the patient experienced and dealt with conventionally rude treatment in the past. Perhaps it would have emerged that rude treatment has evoked neurotic self-doubt about her intrinsic interest to others. Perhaps because of such self-doubt she never even entertained the question of how interesting others were to her since she always had to prove her intrinsic interest to them first. Maybe she grew up with a bored and boring mother, whose unresponsiveness the patient attributed to her own lack of intrinsic interest. To work from the surface would be to assume that the patient was being herself, that she was not being intrinsically boring, and that therefore the analyst's yawn could have been an unappreciative response to what was intrinsically interesting material. The repetition was of a bored and boring mother's lackluster response to her child just being her ordinary, everyday self rather than the enactment of a role-playing invented self that pleased her mother but not her analyst, who intuitively saw through the pretense in responding with boredom.

The type of analytic material that an analyst finds boring or fascinating in many respects depends on the analyst's theoretical preconceptions. Ehrenberg made the material interesting to herself in pursuing the assumption that her boredom had been induced as part of a repetitive enactment. A self psychologist might have made the same material interesting in assuming that the patient had formed a mirroring transference in which the analyst was expected to do no more than listen appreciatively to the creations of the patient's "invented self" or to the daily updates and weekly progress reports of her ordinary, everyday self. The analyst's boredom is not a "fact" of the analysis that has been discovered but a creative construction based on preconceptions about what constitutes interesting material.

Ehrenberg treated it as significant that her boredom was not her typical reaction to the patient, as though this were evidence that her boredom was more in the nature of a role induction than a characteristic difficulty in becoming engaged with this particular patient or a characterological problem of her own in which she is frequently bored with others. Yet how do we know that her boredom had not been present silently for some time but repudiated and only at this point in the treatment had emerged into awareness? Perhaps the novelty and freshness of the material had been gradually wearing off, and the analyst was only now beginning to find the material stale and repetitive because it did not fit her preconceptions of how an interesting analysis would unfold. And even if Ehrenberg usually finds her patients fascinating, it still probably says something about Ehrenberg's own personality if one were to look at the common features of those infrequent instances when she is bored with her patients. The frequency or infrequency of a countertransference reaction does not make it any more or less a product of induced countertransference or the analyst's personality. All countertransference, regardless of the frequency, is a seamless blend of what the patient evokes and how the analyst processes that evocation through his or her characteristic preconceptions.

According to Weiss and Sampson (1986), the patient unconsciously carries out a plan in the therapeutic situation to test pathogenic beliefs in relation to the analyst. If the analyst successfully assesses the patient's unconscious plan and makes plan-compatible interpretations, the analysis is facilitated. The patient sets the stage unconsciously to test the analyst to assess whether the patient's grim beliefs about the analyst are true. The implication for technique is that if the analyst accurately evaluates the patient's unconscious plan and recognizes the nature of the patient's unconscious test as it is staged in the analysis, then the analyst would be able to behave intentionally and strategically in a manner designed to pass the patient's unconscious test. Was Ehrenberg's patient's test to see whether her hurt and vulnerable self could be exposed and accepted, or was it to discover whether she could protest the analyst's conventionally rude behavior and have the legitimacy of her complaint be recognized? Perhaps the patient was testing her in both respects simultaneously and thus establishing a no-win situation for the analyst in order to test the analyst's ability to extricate herself from a double bind.

In addition to the analyst's conscious assessment of the patient's unconscious plan, there is an unconscious transference–countertransference dynamic centered around a process of intersubjective negotiations in the service of passing unconscious tests. The analyst's unconscious countertransference may include certain unconscious tests that the patient is expected to pass, so that patient and analyst are constantly testing each other at an unconscious level. Perhaps Ehrenberg had a need to test the patient to discover whether the patient can still accept her as an analyst when Ehrenberg felt that she had become a bored and boring analyst with nothing interesting to say in response to the patient's current productions. The patient passed the test in reaching out to Ehrenberg through a variety of strategies to wake her from her state

of boredom rather than abandon Ehrenberg to her disen-
gaged state of mind in politely disregarding the yawn as
though she had not noticed. The failure of either party to pass
the other's unconscious test could lead to therapeutic stalemate as each party's repudiated self-dystonic elements are
confirmed, thereby destabilizing the consciously maintained
self-syntonic sense of self.

What is useful in the concept of selfobject transference in
terms of countertransference is that one can think in terms of
selfobject countertransference. An interactive view of countertransference makes it apparent that the patient is a regu-
lator of the analyst's self-states. The patient is never a neutral,
objective presence to the analyst but rather is always validating some of the analyst's self-experiences while invalidating others. The analyst experiences the patient as a
self-regulatory other through the filtering lens of the analyst's
own preconceived notions. This view of countertransference
makes it clear that whatever role the patient may be inducing
the analyst to assume is always processed through the filter of
the analyst's own selfobject needs and preconceived notions.
How the analyst utilizes his or her own countertransference
will depend on the preconceived notions the analyst employs
in his or her self-analysis of countertransference responses to
the patient.

The strength of the object relations approach to utilizing
the transference is that it recognizes that countertransference
may reflect repudiated self-dystonic elements of the patient's
personality. For this reason it may be of use diagnostically.
Yet the object relations approach tends to minimize the extent
to which the analyst's theoretical preconceptions shape how
countertransference is understood. Instead, countertransference is processed through the lens of a naive realism that
denies that countertransference reflects the analyst's characterization of the patient and is in effect an implicit form of
character analysis that may either flatter or offend the patient's narcissism. The analyst must first have empathy for
the patient's experience of the analyst's countertransference
as an expression of the analyst's own preconceptions before
going on to analyze the patient's resistance to acknowledging

the patient's own contribution to the analyst's countertransference. Otherwise, the patient is made entirely responsible for the analyst's feelings.

The analyst's countertransference to the patient is in a sense a transference to what the analyst has evoked in the patient. The analyst's interpretive framework and interactive style evoke a response in the patient to which the analyst's countertransference is a counterresponse. The analyst's choice of interpretive framework and interactional style is thus a choice of the sort of general transference–countertransference paradigms the analyst, consciously or unconsciously, hopes to evoke in the analytic situation and work through. Though countertransference does provide information about the patient, it provides just as much information about the analyst as it does about the patient. When the analyst's induced countertransference and role responsiveness are used as diagnostic tools without an appreciation of the role that the analyst's own preconceptions play in processing countertransference and in arriving at a formulation of what the countertransference says about the patient, the analyst may develop the pretense of being something of an oracle, oblivious to the possibility of having evoked from the patient what it is that the analyst is claiming to have been induced by the patient.

In returning to the case of Joe, it may be useful to consider the countertransference of the therapist as well as the supervisor in terms of self-syntonic and self-dystonic aspects. Many of the supervisee's "mistakes" could be seen as reflections of the supervisee's preconceived notions about how one works analytically. The supervisee assumed that to work analytically one must quickly get the patient to own unconscious resistances to treatment (i.e., arriving late, avoiding introspection, asking questions, etc.) and unconscious transferences (i.e., fear of depending on the therapist and consequent need for distance). These preconceptions led to premature interpretations in light of my preconceptions about treatment. Ideas like working from surface to depth, making the self-syntonic self-dystonic, establishing a therapeutic alliance, repairing ruptures to the alliance, and analyzing issues from multiple perspectives (i.e., different sides of a conflict) proved to be useful organizing principles for a beginning psychotherapist. Theoretical preconceptions tend to be largely preconscious and self-syntonic, constituting a countertransference that the therapist enacts as an interactional style and to which the patient's subjective universe will be assimilated. Hopefully, the therapist finished supervision with somewhat more refined preconceptions than when she initiated supervision.

At the self-dystonic level were the therapist's attempts to avoid being seen as either an infantilizing mother or a critical father and instead be seen as a supportive, autonomy-enhancing presence in the patient's life, which was a more self-syntonic role for the therapist. As a sort of parallel process in the supervision, my self-dystonic countertransference was that as a supervisor who was leading the supervisee in the direction of what I saw as a more effective way of proceeding, I was being an infantilizing mother who was showing the therapist the right way to do things while sparing her the consequences of her mistakes as well as an overly critical father who was pointing out all her premature interpretations. To what extent the countertransference is induced by the patient or is a reflection of the supervisee's as well as the supervisor's character structure is a question that cannot be answered in any clear-cut and ambiguity-free manner. If the treatment or the supervision were characterized mainly by the enactment of the self-dystonic countertransference, the patient as well as the supervisee would not have been helped by the experience, if not traumatized. If the self-dystonic countertransferences were never evoked or addressed, the treatment as well as the supervision would have remained superficial and falsely supportive.

Another aspect of the self-dystonic countertransference relates to role reversals in the relationship. When Joe treated the therapist with false reassurance as his mother treated him, it was both seductive and oppressive. The therapist did not like to think of herself as someone who might just go along with a superficial supportive relationship, given her self-syntonic investment in being an analytic clinician who does deep work with patients. In addition, the therapist did not like to feel incompetent when Joe put her on the spot with questions as he felt his father had exacerbated his performance anxiety by putting him on the spot. As a beginning therapist, she needed to establish some rudimentary sense of efficacy in her work. Likewise in the parallel process, as the supervisor I had to resist the temptation to be a falsely reassuring supervisor who would receive false reassurance in return from the supervisee as a means of covering over insecurities about my competence.

There is always some ambiguity as to which are the therapist's or the supervisor's "real" qualities, the self-syntonic or the self-dystonic ones? Is the self-syntonic view of self as an essentially supportive and facilitative therapist or supervisor the accurate self-perception, or is the self-dystonic view of being either an essentially infantilizing/critical or an infantilized/incompetent therapist or supervisor the accurate self-perception? Again, the question cannot be answered in an either/or manner. As the patient's character reflects conflicting and contradictory aspects, so does the supervisee's as well as the supervisor's character structure. I would suggest that in understanding one's own countertransference, one should also work from surface to depth with respect for one's own need to maintain a positively toned and cohesive sense of self while acknowledging the ubiquitous presence of conflicting and repudiated self-dystonic elements regardless of the years of personal analysis.

Curiously, most of the times that the therapist tried to interpret Joe's latent negative transference, he responded with a disclaimer that indeed they had a good working relationship, implying that the therapist was being overly sensitive or taking things too personally. Although this attitude in part reflected Joe's own resistance to acknowledging his underlying anxieties in the transference through identification with a falsely reassuring mother, it also reflected Joe's perception of the therapist's insecurity about not being seen as helpful. Joe responded with reassurance to bolster the therapist's sense of being seen as a helpful person. Though the therapist did not completely trust such reassurance as Joe had not trusted his mother's, it nevertheless did lower the therapist's anxiety that she needed to make something happen immediately. Thus reassurance serves adaptive self-regulatory as well as defensive functions. Similarly in the supervision, the therapist's increasing or diminishing sense of efficacy in the treatment served as feedback to me as to how helpful I was being.

The concept of countertransference requires that when one is empathizing with the patient's experience of the transference, there is some recognition that transference does not arise in a vacuum and has some basis in reality, some basis in the therapist's countertransference. And in empathizing with one's own countertransference, it is important to remember that there is not simply one unidimensional countertransference but that the countertransference is multidimensional, reflecting self-syntonic as well as self-dystonic aspects. Countertransference reflects a blend of the therapist's personality and style of being a therapist as well as the patient's role inductions. It may be a paradox to be tolerated that there is no unambiguous way of separating the two contributions from each other.

II

Relational Character Analysis

8

Impression Management and the Need to Be Seen as Normal

One of the challenges of character analysis is the patient's resistance to making the self-syntonic self-dystonic. Perhaps the most surface-level resistance to character analysis is the patient's assumption that the self-syntonic sense of self is a psychologically normal sense of self. To suggest otherwise is to imply that the patient is abnormal, evoking feelings of shame and humiliation. As a consequence, the patient resists character analysis in order to defend against being made to feel abnormal. A dialectical balance must be achieved between empathizing with the patient's need to experience the self as normal while analyzing the patient's defenses against being seen as abnormal, defenses that constitute a resistance to recognition of self-dystonic aspects of the personality. Empathy for the patient's need to be seen as normal must proceed yet be counterbalanced by the interpretation of the defensive function of needing to be seen as normal. As we shall see, such a balance is difficult to achieve, easily lost, and never unambiguously achieved. The dynamically balanced approach of today often turns out in retrospect to be the inherently skewed approach of yesterday that has neglected something that currently seems essential.

Psychoanalysis has gone far in demonstrating the fallacy of the concept of psychological normality. The original medical model of mental illness attempted to make a sharp distinction between a diseased mind and a healthy mind. Freud demonstrated that it was illusory to think of discrete qualitative differences between abnormal psychology and general psychology. The same basic principles of mental functioning apply to the normal as well as the psychopathological. If there is a difference between the mentally ill and the mentally healthy, it is a matter of degree or intensity rather than quality. Since unconscious conflict and compromise give rise to normal as well as deviant behavior, Freud had no difficulty with thinking of everyone as more or less neurotic. No one could claim title to being a mentally healthy, mature, or normal person. All adults were seen as saddled with persisting infantilisms, since the unconscious mind was conceived of as a childish mentality that had never grown up and never would. As a consequence of this outlook, the practitioners of psychoanalysis had to acknowledge their own neuroses, accept the role of a mentally ill patient, and enter into a personal analysis themselves.

The introduction of the cultural point of view into psychoanalysis alerted the psychoanalytic community to the cultural relativism of the concept of psychological normality. Cultural values define what shall be deemed normal or abnormal, mentally healthy or sick, mature or immature. Conceptions of psychological normality may reflect an arbitrary social convention rather than some universal fact of human nature that would prove valid across different cultures and different historic periods. If there is no such thing as psychological normality, there are then only varying degrees of adaptation or maladaptation to a particular social milieu. Whether it is good or bad to adapt to a particular culture with its particular biases and prejudices is a moral judgment relative to one's value system.

Kohut (1977) further critiqued the concept of psychological normality in questioning the residual mental health maturity ethic embodied in traditional psychoanalytic thought. Freud tended to substitute a developmental model for a medical model so that individuals could be assessed in terms of how far they had progressed in their psychological development. Freud assumed that individuals progressed from the pleasure principle to the reality principle, from subjectivity to objectivity, from dependence to independence, and from narcissism to object love. Freud viewed these dimensions of personality functioning as unfolding in a sequential developmental line in which earlier modes of functioning were progressively overlaid, suppressed, and superseded by later modes of functioning.

Perhaps these dimensions of personality functioning might be better thought of as polarities that resonate in dynamic balance, with each pole possessing its own distinctive line of development. The pleasure-seeking, subjective, dependent, and narcissistic dimension of the personality is not necessarily an immature, sick, or abnormal aspect of the self, but it could also reasonably be construed as a spontaneous, alive, vital, imaginative, creative, passionate, and intensely involved arena of self-experience. The continued evolution of this aspect of the personality is essential to a life experienced as rich and worth living. In contrast, the reality-seeking, objective, independent, and object-related aspect of the personality is not necessarily the healthy, normal, and mature aspect of the self. Rather, it can reasonably be construed as serving a function, a function that may be under- or overdeveloped, in the adaptation of the person to a communal existence, with its realistic expectations and limitations. The subjective, dependent, and narcissistic aspect of the self stands in a dialectic with the objective, independent, and object-related aspect of the self. It is a reflection of personal bias to favor one side over the other, a bias that a Kleinian might understand as a reflection of splitting.

The psychoanalytic deconstruction of the concept of psychological normality serves as a means of countering the apparently ubiquitous human tendency to construct standards of psychological normalcy by which to compare, measure, and evaluate oneself and others. To some degree everyone seems to possess a need to be seen as normal and experiences a distressing sense of abnormality when that need is not fulfilled. To experience the self as normal is to imagine that one is like everybody else and is in some sense a relatively ordinary, average, and conventional sort of person. To be normal is to fit in and be socially accepted by one's peer group in meeting the group's criteria for group membership. To experience the self as abnormal is to experience the self as different in a socially unacceptable manner. To be abnormal is to be socially deviant and perhaps to be doomed to a life as a social outcast.

In a culture that stresses the uniqueness of the individual, the need to be seen as normal has often been understood as reflecting a defensive position. In being mindlessly conformist in molding the self to a group norm, an excessively compliant and accommodating false self is erected, which hides and protects a wounded though vital center of individual initiative. The study of narcissism seemed to suggest that it would have to be a narcissistic injury to be thought of as "only" ordinary and average when there is clearly such a vital wish to be seen as a unique, special, or outstanding individual in one's own right. From the perspective of injured narcissism, the desire to be seen as normal would seem to be a defensive reaction-formation against the desire to be seen as special and unique. Overidentification with external appearances and disidentification with personal subjectivity is assumed to reflect a manner of protecting and preserving from traumatic violation some latent sense of distinct personhood. To some extent psychoanalysis, given its individualistic orientation, has lacked empathy for the patient's need to be seen as normal and has tended to treat that need as primarily a defense to be analyzed, a defense that obscures and denies deeper material.

Kohut (1971) expanded the concept of narcissism beyond the study of grandiosity to understand the narcissistic dimension of idealizing others as well as the narcissistic dimension of viewing others as being like the self. In idealizing others, one can bask in the reflected glory of someone truly special and unique even if one is not so special and unique oneself. In viewing others as one's alter ego or twin, there is a sense of being like someone else and therefore not alone or different. The need to be seen as normal appears to reflect an extension of alter-ego or twinship needs. One needs to be more than like just one other person who is like the self, but one needs to be like everybody else as well. The locus of selfobject experiencing is not so much a singular person but an imaginary group of similar people who define a group norm as a requirement for group membership. From this frame of reference, the need to be seen as normal is not necessarily a defensive position but rather a reflection of a need for group membership as a means of bolstering a sense of being a normal person. Whether or not the need to be seen as normal is understood as a defensive retreat from a dread of individuality or as a legitimate selfobject need for group membership is not a question that must be answered in an either/or manner. Perhaps a dynamic balance must be struck between experiencing the self as distinctive and unique and experiencing the self as an accepted member of a community of like-minded others.

The need to be seen as normal by the analyst is ubiquitous in the treatment situation. After all, the analyst as the assumed mental health expert and perhaps seen as a role model of mental health is imbued with the authority to grant the patient a sense of psychological normality, a "clean bill of mental health," so to speak. By virtue of his or her training, education, accreditation, experience, and reputation, the analyst is assumed to be a more or less adequate advocate of the normative standards of mental health established by the mental health community, which is empowered by the status that society affords a presumably scientifically based enterprise. Through the analyst as a representative individual, the patient experiences an implicit sense of connection to the larger group of which the analyst is an accepted part. It is the larger community of mental health professionals that establishes the accepted standards of psychological health, maturity, and normality in contemporary secular society. In an age of increasing dissemination of psychological knowledge to the public through a variety of media, there is an increasing public acceptance of the mental health establishment as a standard setter. Even those who indignantly claim that mental health professionals are crazier than everybody else are nevertheless being reactive to an image of the mental health professional as an all-powerful though malevolent authority figure. It is in this larger social context that individual treatment transpires.

Selfobject failure in the treatment situation means that the patient will experience the analyst as making the patient feel painfully abnormal. Selfobject success means that the patient experiences the analyst as supporting if not enhancing the sense of psychological normality. Since selfobject failure is an inevitable and necessary aspect of the treatment, the patient must gradually learn to assimilate the sense of abnormality, of being seen as unacceptably different from others, so that to be seen as abnormal is no longer experienced as a traumatic event. Working through this process so as to promote the development of transmuting internalizations is a gradual and painstaking process, since patients will have developed a variety of characterological adaptations in order to protect themselves from experiencing a traumatic sense of psychological abnormality.

Perhaps one of the most difficult-to-treat adaptations is what McDougall (1985) referred to as *normopathic* and Bollas (1987) as *normotic illness*. McDougall described the normopathic individual as someone who has achieved a robotlike adaptation to the demands of external reality and seems to possess no psychological problems in the sense of any distressing symptomatology. Normopaths seem to possess little imagination or affect. They deal with situations in a pragmatic manner. Their thinking is concrete, and they seem incapable of empathizing with other people's inner realities. McDougall suggested a link between normopathy and alexithymia, the inability to find words for feelings. Bollas defined a normotic person as someone who is abnormally normal. There is an attempt to erase personal subjectivity in favor of conceiving the self as a thing in the material world. According to Bollas, normotic individuals have a manner of transforming language so that their communication is deprived of all personal meaning. The person is enabled to vaporize conflict and as a consequence appear perfectly normal.

McDougall and Bollas, in their use of the terms *normopathic* and *normotic*, appear to be making an ironic statement to the effect that the need to be seen as normal reflects an excessively conformist mentality aimed at erasing the sense of individuality and that it is perhaps abnormality, illness, and immaturity that frame the uniqueness of the individual. If psychopathology reflects a creative process that expresses one's individuality, then normality constitutes an accommodative process that masks one's individuality. This ironic detachment from the patient's unfailing identification with normality appears to arise from the analyst's frustration in being able to deepen the analytic process with such patients. The normopathic individual challenges the analyst's faith in the analytic process. Yet the normopathic patient may begin to feel abnormal if he or she senses the analyst's frustration. The analyst implicitly conveys that a normal analytic patient develops a capacity for free association, introspection, and intense transference, which the analyst would find fascinating; whereas in contrast the normopathic patient remains unimaginative, reality bound, and uninvolved, which the analyst would find tedious and boring.

Bollas (1987, pp. 148–151) presented the case of Tom to exemplify a person with normotic illness. It illustrates what happens when the patient's appearance of normality is treated as primarily defensive in lieu of appreciating its self-affirmative function. Tom was an adolescent whom Bollas interviewed in front of the members of a psychiatry department in a large hospital. After a disappointment in school, he had attempted suicide but recovered quickly and was discharged, only to make another serious suicide attempt within a few days. Bollas interviewed him during his second hospitalization. Tom presented himself as a handsome, athletic, wholesome-looking lad, neatly dressed in stylish clothes. He opened the meeting with a humorous comment about the rather unusual nature of the event.

Tom behaved during the interview as if nothing was at all unusual in his immediate history. After 5 minutes of chat, Bollas interpreted that he must be in great pain or else he would not have attempted to kill himself. He politely rebuffed Bollas with an "OK," as though Bollas had not meant what he had said. Tom did acknowledge feeling socially isolated since he had moved to his new school. Yet when Bollas would try to discuss the deeper meaning of the move, Tom would refer to one of his father's remarks, such as "It will all turn out for the best" or "If you want to get ahead in life, you have to get on with life." Tom's family was characterized as normotic like him, a family who never discussed things at a deeper level and in terms of appearances appeared ideal.

Bollas felt he was confronted with a mentality that admitted of no inquiry or reflection. Once Bollas felt that it was useless to question him further, he began to disclose his own childhood conflicts and experiences. Bollas interpreted that Tom seemed to be more like one of his father's 50-year-old colleagues than a 16-year-old. Maybe he was trying to live up to some impossible standard that made him feel furious and incompetent, and if this was his fate, he may as well do himself in. Tom displayed some interest, anxiety, and uncertainty but remained composed and polite. Bollas saw Tom's breakdown as a refusal to live within normotic culture.

If Tom's overtly normotic character was seen as expressing affirmative as well as defensive functions (i.e., denying his suicidal despair), other interpretive possibilities may have been envisioned. Here was Tom put on display in a psychiatric hospital as an unusual case, a situation in which he was clearly being seen as abnormal. To show himself in public as an essentially "normal" person who was polite, intelligent, and good-humored could be understood as a quiet assertion of his human dignity. Tom could feel that suicide is a personal choice that is nobody's business but his own, and therefore he was being treated in a demeaning manner, being locked up and examined as an unusual specimen. To admit deep personal feeling in public could be experienced as allowing one's right of privacy to be violated. Perhaps interpretations along these lines may have evoked a different reaction. Bollas probably did not think of these interpretations since he considered the patient's normotic behavior primarily in terms of its defensive function.

Since the patient's need to be seen as normal is ubiquitous, though not always focal in the treatment situation, the analyst could be construed as functioning as a normalizing selfobject. The normalizing selfobject functions to reflect that the person is indeed a normal, average, conventional person who is just like everybody else. When Bollas was suggesting that Tom was like a 50-year-old man, he probably would have been experienced by Tom as suggesting that he was the opposite of a normal adolescent, an observation that would likely have added to Tom's feelings of abnormality. When Sullivan (1953) suggested that we are all more simply human than otherwise, he seemed to be highlighting the common-alities between people as a means of avoiding the stigmati-zation and scapegoating that may occur when someone is seen as different or unique. The normalizing selfobject pro-tects the person from the shame of stigmatization and the fear of being scapegoated in affirming the person's fundamental humanity. Like the Amish who believe that to be truly human one should be "plain," the normalizing selfobject affirms that to be truly human one should be just like everybody else. Being normal serves an adaptive function. It provides the security and comfort of belonging while relieving the fear of being shamed or persecuted for not fitting in. Perhaps it is normal to be somewhat normopathic.

Given that standards of normality are relative to social convention, different social standards will inculcate different styles of being normal. It is at the level of the public sense of self that a person attempts to accommodate to the social conventions of the culture in which the person is embedded. The person employs what Goffman (1959) referred to as the "arts of impression management" in order to present the self to others in a manner that is socially acceptable. The public sense of self is attuned to audience response, which functions as a normalizing selfobject, guiding the person to calibrate the self-presentation toward a seamless fit with social expecta-tion.

In the psychoanalytic situation, the public sense of self was initially conceived as a resistance to treatment. Freud recog-nized the transferential authority that society grants the physician, so that patients are predisposed to submit to the unusual procedures of psychoanalysis. Nevertheless, many aspects of analysis are contrary to and violate social convention, so that patients resist the analytic process in order to avoid the dread of being found socially deviant. Discussing one's sexual fantasies with a stranger, openly criticizing or lusting after one's doctor, talking about one's private life without mutuality of self-disclosure, and so on, constitute some of the unconventional aspects of the psychoanalytic dialogue in comparison to ordinary social discourse. Aspects of the principle of abstinence such as not answering questions, not giving advice, engaging in prolonged silence, and lacking certain common social courtesies could be seen as conventionally rude or impolite. The patient is expected to leave social etiquette outside of the consulting room and engage in all manner of behavior that would be considered ill mannered and offensive by conventional standards, such as openly speaking in graphic terms of incestuous, adulterous, homicidal, suicidal, grandiose, and self-abasing desires and fantasies.

Freud established the fundamental rule of psychoanalysis, free association, as a paradox. He instructed his patients to say everything that came to mind without self-censorship, knowing full well that they would prove incapable of complying with that instruction despite their agreement to make the attempt. Resistance was initially conceived as the patient's resistance to free association, and resistance analysis was initially conceived as interpreting the patient's self-censorship in order to allow the patient's associations to emerge more freely. It becomes apparent, though, that self-censorship is not a purely intrapsychic affair, as it is in part motivated by an interpersonal anxiety, the patient's concern with audience (i.e., the analyst's) reaction to the patient's self-presentation. The patient censors those associations that are imagined would create an unfavorable presentation of self in the eyes of the analyst. Thus resistance to free association is always a transference resistance, a fear of the analyst's response to one's free associations.

The patient can never leave concern with social etiquette outside of the consulting room, for the need to make a normal presentation of self is ubiquitous. What the patient soon learns is that psychoanalytic conventions are different in some respects from everyday conventions, so that the patient begins to assume a presentation of self that accommodates to the analyst's presumed expectations. The patient's reading of the analyst's expectations will to some extent be precisely attuned to the analyst's individuality as it is revealed in the analyst's conduct and to some extent be based on the patient's characteristic manner of making a good impression.

Given that the patient's public sense of self reflects a characteristic manner of attempting to make a good impression, one aspect of character analysis must then be to analyze the patient's characteristic manner of attempting to be and be seen as a normal person. Each character type must possess a distinctive style of self-presentation designed to make an impression of normality. Though no one possesses a pure character type, for the notion of character type is an abstract ideal that does not exist in reality, for the sake of illustration it may be interesting to examine the characteristic presentation of self as normal for the various character types. (For a more comprehensive analysis of the various character types in terms of a theory of multiple selves in conflict and compromise, see Josephs 1992.)

For example, the obsessive-compulsive character has traditionally been conceived as someone who is overtly compliant but covertly defiant. Because of unconscious guilt over sadistic fantasies, the obsessive-compulsive is unaware of being covertly defiant. Compliance as a character trait arises as a reaction-formation that repudiates unconscious sadism. Though compliance may be overt from the observer's point of view, the obsessive-compulsive does not necessarily conceive of the self-presentation as compliant. To be compliant implies a deviation from normality, an excessively accommodating attitude of which one might be somewhat ashamed. Thus, the obsessive-compulsive does not consider the self-presentation as compliant. Instead, the self-presentation is construed as conscientious and responsible. To be responsible and conscientious is not to be compliant but rather to be the way any normal, healthy, mature person should be, nothing of which to boast yet nothing of which to be embarrassed. If the analyst responds to the obsessive-compulsive as a compliant person rather than a responsible and conscientious person, the obsessive-compulsive will feel misperceived and misunderstood. The analyst fails as a normalizing selfobject who should be affirming what a normal person the patient is in being so responsible and conscientious. Instead, the analyst is experienced as a perfectionistic authority figure who is faulting the patient for not being an entirely responsible person in being ingratiating and obsequious instead.

The patient's need to be seen as normal thus constitutes the most surface-level resistance to the unfolding of the analytic process. Resistance analysis then must begin with an exploration of the patient's need to be seen and style of being seen as normal. As discussed previously, the affirmative, identity-maintaining function of resistance needs to be interpreted prior to the interpretation of its defensive, anxiety-avoiding function with which it is counterbalanced. To interpret the affirmative function of the obsessive-compulsive's self-presentation, the analyst might say, "It is important to you that others (or "I" if a transference interpretation) see you as a responsible person, and you feel misunderstood when you are not seen that way." Such an interpretation affirms that being responsible is an integral component of the patient's sense of identity. The defensive function of presenting the self as responsible could be interpreted along the lines of: "Since it is important to see yourself as a mature person who is responsible and conscientious, it is difficult to admit to yourself that you may become overly accommodating when you are afraid that others won't like you if you're not." This approach to character analysis could aptly be described as empathic character analysis since it analyzes character resistances in a manner that is respectful of the patient's sense of identity as a conscientious and responsible person.

The hysterical character has traditionally been seen as someone who is overtly innocent but covertly seductive. Overt innocence constitutes a reaction-formation against covert seductiveness that needs to be repudiated because of its incestuous implications. Though others might view the hysteric as cultivating a facade of innocence, the hysteric does not view the self-presentation in that light. To be innocent implies that one is naive, immature, not quite responsible for oneself, and not to be taken as a serious adult. The hysteric is offended by the implication of being thought innocent. Instead, the hysteric conceives the presentation of self as only being an ordinarily nice, friendly, and sociable person. If the hysteric felt that the analyst perceived the hysteric's self-presentation as innocent and naive rather than genuinely and maturely sociable, the hysteric would experience the analyst as a stern and distant authority figure who does not think of the patient as a serious or adultlike person. To interpret the affirmative function of the hysteric's self-presentation, the analyst might simply say, "You take pride in being a friendly person." To interpret the defensive function of the hysteric's pride in being friendly, the analyst might say, "Because you pride yourself on being friendly, it is difficult to admit to yourself that your friendliness might be taken as seductive or childlike. It's embarrassing to be seen that way when you want to be taken seriously."

The depressive-masochistic character has traditionally been conceived as someone who is overtly depressed but covertly reproachful. Depression has been understood as anger turned inward, anger being repudiated because of unconscious guilt. Yet the depressed person does not necessarily construe the self-presentation as depressed. To be depressed implies an element of irrational self-blame and unhappiness. It suggests that realistically one's depressive response is not completely justified by the situation, that one is overreacting. Freud (1917) originally differentiated mourning from melancholia on the basis of what he believed were rational and irrational responses to the experience of loss. In contrast, the depressive-masochistic character believes that the presentation of a suffering self is an entirely realistic and rational response to the current life situation and that any normal person would react the same way in the same situation. The depressive-masochist resents the innuendo that a normal person would not be as sensitive in the same situation. The depressive-masochist views the self-presentation of suffering as simply being an open, honest, and sincere person who will not hide suffering with a superficial false self. If the analyst were to imply that the patient's suffering was a neurotic rather than a healthy response to a painful life situation, the patient would experience the analyst as a cold, insensitive person who does not have genuine empathy for human suffering. To interpret the depressive-masochist's self-presentation affirmatively, one might say, "Given that you are trying to cope with a difficult life situation in as open and honest a manner as you can, it is important that others (or "I") take your feelings and your situation seriously." To interpret the defensive function of the depressive-masochist's self-presentation, one might say, "Given how important it is for others to take your feelings seriously, it is upsetting to admit that you might make yourself miserable and be your own worst enemy."

When the defensive function of the patient's self-presentation is interpreted, it constitutes a manner of making a self-syntonic character trait self-dystonic so that it can be subjected to deeper analysis. It is the patient's need to be seen as normal that constitutes the resistance to making the self-syntonic self-dystonic. The obsessive-compulsive must acknowledge that self-syntonic conscientiousness may entail self-dystonic compliance, the hysteric must acknowledge that self-syntonic friendliness may entail self-dystonic innocence and naiveté, and the depressive-masochist must acknowledge that self-syntonic common unhappiness may entail self-dystonic neurotic misery. The patient will, of course, argue that the self-presentation is indeed normal and that the analyst's pathologizing point of view is indeed a misconstrual, if not an attempt at character assassination. The analyst need not argue the point, for regardless of the question of the authenticity of the patient's presentation of self as normal, the analyst could pose the question of how the patient developed into such a normal person in the first place. The developmental history of the patient's particular style of being normal can be documented. How did the obsessive-compulsive develop into such a responsible person — in identification with responsible parents, in fear of authoritarian parents, in counteridentification with irresponsible parents? How did the hysteric become such a friendly person—to appease grumpy parents, to cheer up depressed parents, to be like outgoing parents? How did the depressive-masochist become such an unhappy person—growing up devalued, growing up abandoned, growing up neglected? The normal sense of self is experienced as the healthy adaptive response to the normative familial atmosphere in which one grew up. Thus to interpret the patient's normal self-presentation as the natural adaptive response to the family environment in which one was raised is to interpret that aspect of the self in an affirmative manner.

The patient is not necessarily able to articulate verbally the presentation of self as normal, though the patient is certainly emotionally reactive to the analyst's apparent misconstrual of the self-presentation when the analyst fails as a normalizing selfobject. The patient's presentation of self as normal tends to operate at a prereflective level, a silent and unformulated attempt to seamlessly fit into one's social surround. Thus the analyst's verbal formulation of the patient's public sense of self creates a more articulated and defined representation of one aspect of one's character structure that had never before been self-consciously delineated. Simply affirming the patient's normal sense of self and tracing its adaptive function across the patient's developmental history will have a therapeutic effect in and of itself in strengthening the patient's sense of self. Nevertheless, it is a limited therapeutic result that does not by itself allow the patient to integrate self-dystonic elements of the personality into a more complex and comprehensive structural unity. Yet it prepares the patient to tolerate the kind of analytic work that addresses self-dystonic elements.

In attempting to make the self-syntonic self-dystonic, it is inevitable that the patient will experience the analyst as attempting to make the patient feel abnormal. The patient argues that the self-presentation is indeed normal and that the analyst is painting an unfair and unflattering portrait of the patient. The analyst may then empathize with the patient's experience of the analyst in the negative transference prior to any attempt to interpret the defensive function of the negative transference as a resistance to acknowledging a self-dystonic trait. The obsessive-compulsive feels that the analyst is making an accusation that the patient is not "really" responsible; the hysteric feels that the analyst is making an accusation that the patient is not "genuinely" friendly; the depressive-masochist feels that the analyst is making the accusation that the patient has no "legitimate" reason to be unhappy.

Of course, the analyst should not attempt to invalidate the patient's experience of the analyst in the negative transference but rather should try to tolerate and empathize with that negative transference, even if the analyst feels unfairly accused by the patient of being unjustly accusatory of the patient. The analyst may attempt to empathize with what it is like for the patient to work with an analyst who seems to be unfairly critical of the patient and who fails to appreciate the patient's positive assets. To interpret the defensive function of the negative transference (i.e,. the negative transference as evidence of the patient's resistance to a correct interpretation) would be experienced as dismissive, as one more instance of the analyst being unfairly critical and intolerant of the patient's criticism of the analyst. It may seem to the patient that the analyst can "dish it out" but that the analyst "can't take it."

When the analyst is tolerant of the negative transference without having to deflect it by interpreting its defensive function, the patient may begin to address the possibility of not coming across to the analyst in a manner consistent with the impression the patient hopes to make. Since it is likely that this sort of discrepancy is not a unique event in the patient's life but a characteristic form of misunderstanding that occurs with others, that possesses a developmental history, the analyst may facilitate the exploration of the history of this characteristic sort of intersubjective disjunction. The patient tends to forgive the analyst's apparent misconstrual when it becomes apparent that the analyst is simply one in a long line of significant others who have misconstrued the patient. The obsessive-compulsive begins to accept the fact of characteristically coming across to others as compliant; the hysteric begins to accept the fact of characteristically coming across to others as innocent and naive; the depressive-masochist begins to accept the fact of characteristically coming across to others as complaining. If one is characteristically seen in that light by others, then maybe one really is that way but has difficulty admitting it because it is not quite as flattering a portrait of oneself as one had fancied.

To tolerate making the self-syntonic self-dystonic requires a form of empathy, of being able to recognize the difference between the impression one hopes to make and how one actually comes across to others. The patient must be able to decenter the self from an exclusively egocentric construal of self in order to take the other's perspective in viewing the self. To recognize the self-dystonic requires the ability to look at the self objectively, as an object from the other person's point of view. The more severe the character disorder, the more difficult it is for the patient to accomplish such a task. In addition, the more severe the character disorder is, the greater the distance is between the impression the person hopes to make and the way the person comes across. For the severely character disordered patient, to accept that the way one comes across to others is indeed a valid representation of the self is to accept a rather unflattering, unlovable picture of oneself.

The narcissistic character has traditionally been seen as someone who is overtly grandiose while feeling covertly inferior. Grandiosity is seen as compensatory to unconscious feelings of inferiority that are too shameful to acknowledge. Nevertheless, despite the fact that the narcissist's grandiosity is overt to others, it is not readily acknowledged, for that would mean admitting that one is an arrogant, superior, condescending, patronizing, and devaluing sort of person. Instead, the narcissist construes the self-presentation as simply being a secure, confident, self-satisfied, and happy person, the kind of person that any normal person is supposed to be. If others view the narcissist as grandiose, that viewpoint is summarily dismissed as a product of the uncon scious envy, competitiveness, and insecurity of others. The narcissist attempts to give little credence to the opinion of others as a means of not being sensitive to their opinions when those opinions prove unflattering.

We know from the work of Kohut (1971) that narcissistic characters are rarely successful in their attempt to remain oblivious to others' opinions. But in their defensive egocentrism, that is what they attempt to do in order to preserve their sense of normality. Though narcissists may be unconsciously dependent on the mirroring feedback of others, at a conscious level they experience themselves as counterdependent, as proud of their own high opinion of themselves independent of what others think. This creates an interpretive challenge for the analyst. The analyst is expected to mirror implicitly the patient's grandiosity without inadvertently implying that the patient's sense of self is based on a grandiose self-image rather than a healthy, realistic self-confidence as the patient imagines it is. If the analyst were to point out that the patient's self-confidence was based on grandiosity rather than a realistic self-assessment, the analyst would be seen as an envious spoiler who cannot be trusted.

The schizoid character has traditionally been viewed as someone who is overtly detached and withdrawn while covertly dependent and needy. Overt detachment constitutes a reaction-formation against intense merger wishes that are repudiated due to fears of engulfment. Despite being seen as detached and unrelated, the schizoid character does not construe the self-presentation as unrelated. To be detached and unrelated implies that one is a cold, uncaring, and indifferent person. The schizoid person feels wounded to be thought such a heartless person. Instead, the schizoid construes the self-presentation as being a gentle, polite, and nonthreatening person who is extra careful not to disturb others by being overly intrusive. To the schizoid, any normal person should display this sort of tact and sensitivity in dealing with others. If the analyst were to imply that the schizoid patient is unrelated rather than related in this especially sensitive way, the analyst would be experienced as an overly emotionally demanding person who is unreasonably rejecting. Though the schizoid patient is aware of being socially isolated and not close to anybody, in order to maintain a sense of normality, the schizoid patient imagines that not fitting in is no sign of social deviance, since the schizoid has no desire to fit into a neurotic society of overbearing, intrusive, and insensitive people. The schizoid imagines that in some other healthier society in which people were gentler and more polite, the schizoid would feel a sense of belonging and fitting in.

The paranoid character has been seen as someone who is overtly suspicious but covertly hostile. Overt mistrust and suspiciousness is thought to derive from the projection of one's own hatefulness and hostility onto others. The paranoid cannot acknowledge hating others, for that might entail acknowledging loving others; the paranoid is also ashamed of loving feelings, presumably homoerotic love especially. Yet it is well known that the paranoid character does not like to be seen as paranoid and is quite offended by that appellation. To be paranoid suggests that one's suspicions are unwarranted, so that one's reality testing is poor and that one is an unreasonably querulous person who is accusatory without just cause.

The paranoid construes the self-presentation as someone who is an ordinary person "just minding his or her own business" but who as a self-respecting person is unwilling to allow others to take unfair advantage of him or her. The paranoid hopes to be seen as someone who believes in a "live and let live" philosophy but who is secure enough to stand up for oneself if given reasonable provocation. The paranoid character believes that to be labeled as paranoid is a way that exploitative others might try to get the upper hand by dismissing and discounting one's legitimate grievances. If the analyst were to imply that the paranoid patient was paranoid, the patient would feel that here is an analyst who cannot be trusted with a confidence, as the analyst might use the patient's confidences against the patient in the future. The paranoid person has no desire to fit into a society of dishonest, disloyal, and scheming people. The paranoid character imagines that in some hypothetical world of trustworthy, honest, decent, forthright, and plain-speaking people, the paranoid would be a normal person who would belong.

The antisocial person has traditionally been seen as someone who is overtly exploitative while covertly dependent. Overt exploitation serves as a manner of being gratified in one's sense of entitlement to be taken care of without ever having to acknowledge that one needs to be taken care of in the first place. Dependent wishes are disavowed since there is a sense of humiliation in being needy. Overt exploitation is an unflattering character trait for obvious reasons, for the exploitative person is seen as lacking in morals and common human decency. Though the antisocial person is thought to lack a conscience, the antisocial person, nevertheless, takes offense at being thought immoral and indecent. The antisocial person views conventional morality as a "scam" that justifies the privileges of those in power while blaming the "have nots" for their own unhappy lot in life. If it is a "dog-eat-dog world," then why not be honest about it and take what one can get "by hook or by crook"? This philosophy of living strikes the antisocial person as more genuinely moral than conventional values, which hypocritically deny that life is about the survival of the fittest (i.e., the most ruthless and powerful). The antisocial person believes that people get what they deserve: if weakness is a moral failing and strength is a virtue, then it is only fit that the weak should suffer at the hands of the strong. Thus, below the hypocrisy of conventional morality, the antisocial person conceives the self-presentation as that of a normal person who is shorn of the pretenses of polite society. If the analyst cannot appreciate the normality of the patient's self-presentation, the analyst is experienced as either a fool or a liar.

It becomes apparent that with the more severe character disorders a seemingly impenetrable narcissistic attitude is established that insulates the normal sense of self from invalidating experiences. The invalidating other is immediately neutralized as a threat to self-stability through devaluation, detachment, dismissal, or domination. The sense of normality is maintained in establishing a fantasy world of like-minded people in which the person belongs, in contrast to the real world, which seems inhospitable. Higher-level character types tend to be invested in finding a manner of obtaining a normalizing response through accommodation to the expectations of the invalidating other. The obsessive-compulsive is bent on gaining approval, the hysteric is bent on being liked, and the depressive-masochistic is bent on gaining sympathy. There is a reluctance to give up the attachment to the invalidating other in the hopes that he or she might eventually come around. The more severe character disorders are just as likely to swiftly lacerate the connection rather than tolerate selfobject failure. This distinction echoes Freud's (1914a) distinction between the transference neuroses and the narcissistic neuroses. The former maintains a stable attachment in the face of frustration whereas the latter does not. Analysis of self-dystonic elements of the personality requires some capacity to remain related to the analyst despite the negative transference evoked in making the self-syntonic dystonic.

What Reich (1928) referred to as "character armor" can now be appreciated as a mode of relatedness to others in the service of maintaining a normal sense of self. The unobjectionable positive transference reflects a mode of engagement in which the analyst is experienced as a normalizing selfobject. The negative transference that is generated when the patient's character armor is analyzed, in making the self-syntonic dystonic, is a mode of relatedness in which the analyst is failing as a normalizing selfobject and the patient is engaging in compensatory and defensive activity in order to restore a sense of psychological normality. The analyst's empathy with the patient's experience of the analyst in the negative transference—that is, the patient's experience of selfobject failure—allows a new mode of relatedness to be established in which the patient can begin to tolerate the self-dystonic element of the personality as an acceptable and therefore normal aspect of the self. This acceptance is in part based on an identification with the analyst who nondefensively tolerated the patient's criticism of him or her for being less of a normally accepting and empathic analyst than the analyst is conventionally supposed to be.

At the time of selfobject failure, the analyst reflects in the negative transference an unacceptable aspect of the patient's self—either the patient's intolerant and judgmental self, which is identified with rejecting others, or the patient's despised and devalued self, which was identified as the object of that rejection. The obsessive-compulsive patient experiences the analyst in terms of perfectionistic standards, so that the analyst is experienced as being hypercritical and judgmental or as failing to uphold high standards. The hysterical patient experiences the analyst as either condemning the patient for being immature or as being inadequate and not to be taken seriously. The depressive-masochistic patient experiences the analyst as reproaching the patient for complaining or as being a cold, insensitive, and uncaring person who is essentially unlovable. The narcissistic patient experiences the analyst as either threatening and competitive or as weak and impotent. The schizoid patient experiences the analyst as either emotionally demanding and overintrusive or as pathetically fragile and easily wounded. The paranoid patient experiences the analyst as either a dangerous persecutor or as a contemptible person by virtue of being passive and submissive. The antisocial patient experiences the analyst as either a domineering aggressor or as a stupid, incompetent fool.

Selfobject failure leads to a return of the repressed in projected form. Unacceptable aspects of self begin to emerge into awareness as a result of the breakup of the normal sense of self, and in order to defend against awareness of those self-dystonic aspects they are projected onto the analyst. The patient, in repudiating the analyst, is then able to repudiate a self-dystonic aspect of self. The patient attempts to restore the normal self-syntonic sense of self in using the analyst as an "adversarial selfobject" (Wolf 1988). An adversarial selfobject shores up the sense of self by providing an object through which the self can define itself in contradistinction. Through defining the other as the opposite of the self and then opposing the suggestive influence of that opposite in defying it, the self becomes more clearly defined, articulated, and solidified. The patient solidifies the normal sense of self by saying in effect to the analyst, "I am clearly me and proud of

it, and you are clearly not me, and that is your misfortune."
To the extent that the patient is a precariously or rigidly
integrated person, character analysis will be a painstakingly
slow and tedious process. The patient will require extensive
and prolonged affirmation of the normal sense of self prior to
tolerating awareness of self-dystonic elements, and the patient may require a lengthy adversarial selfobject transference
in which the analyst is experienced as "containing" (Bion
1967) the patient's self-dystonic aspects.

Analysts have long recognized that patients are resistant to
recognizing their character styles. Hysterics do not like to
think of themselves as hysterical, and paranoids do not like to
think of themselves as paranoid. And it has long been
recognized that the reason for this state of affairs is that one's
character style tends to be ego-syntonic and that it is a
narcissistic injury that one resists when what is ego-syntonic
is made dystonic. Yet the intersubjective dimensions of how
this narcissistic resistance is worked through have rarely been
addressed in the literature on psychoanalytic technique. The
reason for this is that the problem has usually been conceived
in primarily intrapsychic terms. Psychoanalysts have tended
to assume that what is overt to the analyst—that the patient is
hysterical, paranoid, or narcissistic—should be overt to the
patient as well with a little confrontation and clarification, as
the major resistance to analysis is usually thought to be in the
recognition of primitive unconscious content rather than in
the acknowledgment of superficial but ego-syntonic character
traits.

Although analysts have been cognizant of what patients
are avoiding in opposing the attempt to make the ego-
syntonic dystonic, analysts have been less aware of what
patients are attempting to achieve. Their resistance serves to
maintain a normal sense of self as the patient defines it, a
self-definition that tends to be unformulated and of which the
analyst is often unaware for lack of appreciation of the fact
that the way in which the patient is overtly coming across to
the analyst may not correspond to the way in which the
patient hopes to present the self to the analyst. If the analyst
assumes a stance in which it is taken for granted that the

analyst possesses an objective perspective, then it is likely
that the analyst will fail to appreciate the discrepancy between the patient's view of his or her self-presentation and
the analyst's view of the patient's self-presentation. Thus the
manifest content (i.e., the patient's overt self-presentation)
does not appear in the same light to both parties in the
analytic encounter.

Traditionally, analysts assumed that the nature of latent or
unconscious content was a matter of debate and controversy
but that manifest content was obvious and could be taken for
granted. After all, the manifest content was a superficial layer
of the mind that people oblivious to unconscious content
were overly susceptible to taking at face value. But the
manifest content is not obvious. It only seems obvious to
those who are egocentric and oblivious to the fact that what
is overt, manifest, surface, or superficial can appear in a
different light to people who assume different observational
perspectives. Traditional analysts have tended to assume that
the only source of observational bias derived from defensive
distortions that are derivative of unconscious conflict. If one
had undergone an "analytic purification" oneself, then the
assumption was that one's analytic instrument no longer
possessed significant observational bias. Though it may be
true that after a training analysis there may be less observational bias due to unconscious conflict, observational biases
may still remain from other sources, such as being selectively
attuned to intrapsychic dimensions of treatment while remaining unattuned to the wider intersubjective dimension.
An understanding of the analyst's prereflective role as a
normalizing selfobject in relation to the patient's unformulated self-presentation allows for an appreciation of the
intersubjective dimensions of making what is self-syntonic
self-dystonic.

To make the discussion more concrete, I will present a case
report as an illustration. Since I view case reports as reflecting
primarily an application of the analyst's preferred story lines,
it provides a good means of illustrating the sort of clinical
process that can be generated utilizing a particular model. As
mentioned previously, I do not see case reports as a means of

providing factual evidence in the service of validating hypotheses. I believe the data of analysis are always open to multiple interpretations. In addition, short of presenting verbatim transcripts of an entire treatment, case reports cannot help but be a reflection of selective recall, selective presentation of events, and a particular style of writing with its unique rhetorical and dramatical devices.

I will present the treatment of a 34-year-old single man who was seen for over 8 years at two sessions weekly and whose character style could be described as largely a blend of obsessive-compulsive and schizoid issues. I will try to highlight in the presentation how coming to appreciate the nature of his self-presentation and need to be seen as normal was one important dimension of the analytic process. I also hope to convey to the reader a sense of what a dialectical approach looks like in clinical practice. I try to balance empathy for the patient's need to be seen as normal with analysis of the patient's resistance to recognizing any aspect of the self that is felt to be abnormal.

The patient, whom I will call Carl, was a 26-year-old accountant when I began working with him. His presenting problem was feeling depressed in realizing that a woman with whom he was quite infatuated was interested in him as only a platonic friend. Carl felt humiliated by this rejection, which proved to be severely damaging to his masculine self-esteem. Carl had never had a girlfriend, rarely dated, and had occasional sex with prostitutes. Alongside feelings of mortification at having been rejected, Carl maintained an active fantasy that he would win her love sooner or later if he just persevered.

Carl initially conceived of treatment as a course of short-term counseling, in which in a few months either I would enable him to get over his infatuation and move on with his life, or I would teach him the interpersonal skills to win his heart's desire. Once Carl recounted his presenting problems, he had little to say and expected me to provide him with answers or to direct the session with questions. After explaining to him the idea that he was free to discuss whatever came to mind, I realized that he felt only the more self-conscious in being unable to carry forward the dialogue spontaneously on his own initiative. In discussing Carl's difficulty in freely expressing himself, I learned that Carl had always been a fairly quiet person who was a better listener than a talker and that his reticence seemed to reflect an entrenched characterological inhibition that could only be resolved through considerable analysis. Carl reported that it took him over a year of intense ambivalence to finally decide to seek therapy. It seemed to me that we had barely begun treatment but that already Carl was experiencing the treatment as quite injurious to his narcissism, as he felt that his self-dystonic sense of passivity, shyness, timidity, and unmanliness were shamefully exposed.

With the idea of working from surface to depth, I tried to conceptualize Carl's self-syntonic self-presentation. Given his conception of psychotherapy, it seemed that his conception of a "normal" psychotherapy patient was someone who dutifully showed up for sessions, conscientiously described his problems, and patiently deferred to the therapist's authority and wisdom. Carl expected to be seen as a cooperative patient for acting in such a manner. To the extent that I did not engage him in the manner in which he felt most comfortable, I was not mirroring his normal self-syntonic sense of self. In contrast, my expectation that he speak openly and freely only highlighted his inadequacy to do what it became apparent to him a normal psychotherapy patient was expected to do, at least one in treatment with me.

I adjusted both my interpretive and interactive stance with him in order to bolster his sense of himself as a normally dutiful, conscientious person. I assumed a more actively facilitative stance in which Carl experienced me as an instructor who would give him guidance and to whom he would defer. Interpretively, I noted the importance to him of being a responsible person who is dutiful and conscientious. Such an interpretation met with ready agreement, and we proceeded to explore the implications of attempting to be such a person. Carl described how with potential girlfriends he assumed the role of loyal friend, and at work he assumed the role of the quietly competent worker who gets the job done without self-promotion. The result, though, of this style of engaging others was that he was typically taken for granted. Women he befriended did not respond romantically, and at work promotions were few and far between.

Growing up he had always been the responsible and well-behaved son and eldest brother of three without getting much recognition for his good conduct. His mother was described as a somewhat "queenly" and entitled person who put considerable emphasis on following rules of propriety. His mother expected him always to be the proper gentleman. His father was described as a casual, easygoing person who was somewhat henpecked by his wife, to whom he always deferred. Both parents expected him to defer to his mother's wishes and took for granted that he was a well-behaved child who did not need much attention. Carl envied his two younger brothers who seemed to monopolize parental attention and who did not seem to be held to as high standards of propriety as he was. Carl became rather withdrawn as a child but feigned a facade of everything being "OK," which both parents took at face value.

Enabling Carl to be a successfully dutiful and conscientious patient with me as well as affirmatively interpreting this aspect of his character style led to a marked improvement in his self-esteem, and he began to talk more freely in the sessions. I had given him a thematic focus that he could pursue on his own initiative. As we discussed his sense that no one appreciated what a good person he was, Carl began to articulate other underlying feelings that heretofore had been defended against and hidden by his dutiful self-presentation. Carl admitted resenting being so responsible without getting anything in return and that he felt a fool for continuing to act that way, knowing that he would be taken for granted. He despised himself for being so sensitive to the expectations of others and so eager to please. Thus Carl's private but hidden sense of himself began to emerge, his private resentment and self-contempt that he hid from others for fear of being seen as a person who was being responsible not of his own free will but begrudgingly and out of a need to ingratiate himself. His self-presentation as dutiful and conscientious began to feel self-dystonic, a manner of being that seemed a false self that hid more genuine feelings and attitudes.

After a year in treatment, a major shift took place in the transference and the way in which Carl presented himself to me. He began to express a wish to engage women in a different manner that was more initiating, more assertive, and more open about his sexual desires. As his infatuation with his platonic friend became a diminishing topic of discussion, he began to voice his interest in "sowing his wild oats." Carl saw himself as a "late bloomer" who needed to begin doing in his mid-twenties what he should have been doing in high school and college. In his relationship with me, Carl shifted from viewing me as an authority to whom he would defer to seeing me as "one of the guys" with whom he could engage in "man talk" regarding his sexual desires toward women. Concurrently he began to see himself as a patient in long-term treatment and started attending two sessions weekly.

The beginning phase of treatment could be understood as involving a partial working-through of a particular narcissistic trauma of childhood—that he always tried to please his parents and meet their expectations but that nothing he did could really evoke their enthusiastic attention. My initial interactive stance as relatively silent, nonintrusive, and waiting for him to take the lead was experienced as rejecting his attempt to engage me as a responsible person who would defer to my authority. His narcissistic vulnerability as a painfully shy and inhibited person was prematurely and traumatically exposed. Responding both interactively and interpretively to his self-presentation in a more affirmative manner quickly bolstered his sense of self and generated a productive working relationship. No sooner was the affirmative function of his responsible self-presentation interpreted than Carl began to interpret of his own independent volition its defensive function as a cover for resentment, fears of rejection, and self-contempt at being so eager to please and comply. As his responsible self-presentation became self-dystonic, he began to assimilate the narcissistic wound of not being as assertive a person as he would like to be.

Focusing on surface structure in one's thinking and clinical work does not mean that one need be oblivious to considerations of deep structure. In many ways I experienced Carl as an unconsciously withholding person who wished to be catered to without reciprocation. I felt that I was expected to be an especially hardworking therapist just to get him to stay in treatment and that there would be little recognition for my hard work. It seemed reasonable to assume that unconsciously he was identified with the entitled mother about whom he complained so that he unconsciously treated me as he had been treated while consciously feeling that I was the one who would expect his compliance without giving anything in return. Focusing on surface structure enabled me to decenter from my countertransference resentment of him as an overly demanding person who made me do all the work, a dynamic that reflected an unconscious deep structure that seemed premature to interpret. Certainly, it would have been unsettling to his masculine self-regard to interpret that he was acting like his "queenly" mother. (It did emerge later in treatment that as an adolescent he had dressed up as a ballerina for Halloween as a lark.)

The need to present the self as normal is not simply an issue of the beginning phase of treatment that is then overcome to go on to deeper issues. It is an ever-present dynamic through all phases of the treatment. During the second and third years of treatment, Carl focused on his desires to date women and make sexual conquests. After a brief honeymoon phase in which he believed therapy would relatively quickly cure his inhibitions, it became apparent that dates and sexual experiences were not forthcoming. Carl was often impatient and angry with himself and me for what he felt was his slow rate of progress. He often expressed the fantasy of terminating treatment, feeling imprisoned by therapy, and wanting to tell me off and defy me. He began to feel that I was an impediment to his sexual freedom and that he would make better progress if he quit and did it all on his own. In fact, Carl wished to prove that he did not need me and could solve his problems independently.

Notably, now that self-syntonic dutifulness had been changed into self-dystonic ingratiation and obsequiousness, Carl was highly critical of himself for being such a willing psychotherapy patient, whereas if he were a truly assertive person, he would just quit treatment. The earlier deferential relationship to me to which I needed to accommodate in order to allow him to feel comfortable enough to stay in treatment was now replaced by a defiant relationship, the logical conclusion of which was to get rid of me. His new self-syntonic sense of self demanded that he be a fully assertive, independent, and self-sufficient person and that if therapy had worked, he should be ready by now to go it alone. The surface-level self-syntonic sense of self is not a static phenomenon but rather a fluid and shifting one that changes with shifts in the transference.

Once again treatment appeared to be exposing a shameful inadequacy, his inability to get a date or have sex with women. I realized that in having assumed the role of mirror of his unfolding phallic narcissism, our relationship had also stimulated considerable performance anxiety. Whereas he wished to demonstrate his phallic prowess to me, instead I became a constant witness to his failure with women. If getting dates and having sex with women had become established in Carl's mind as the goals of treatment, then it became apparent that he was not living up to those goals. From a surface perspective, it was important for Carl to present himself to me as just a "normal guy." Instead, our sessions served to rub in the fact that he was not a "regular guy." He would prove to me that he was a "regular guy" by defying me and showing me that he could be successful with women on his own.

It emerged that growing up Carl had not felt like "one of the guys." He was always somewhat overweight and not good at sports. After puberty when he found himself pain-fully shy around women, he worried that perhaps he was homosexual even though he felt no sexual desire toward men. Carl did not feel his father was a "regular guy" either but a passive, henpecked husband whom his mother kept under her thumb. Carl expressed disappointment that he felt his father had not been a sufficient male role model. He viewed his mother as an emasculating woman to whom his father had abandoned him.

Carl's idea of a "normal guy" was someone who was highly adept at obtaining casual sex with women without strings attached. Someone who was not a "regular guy" was someone who was foolish enough to pay the price of commitment as the cost of having sex with a woman. Carl's fantasy of a normal male had a long developmental history. He still frequently indulged in latency age fantasies of being an adventurer or explorer out in some rugged wilderness in which he could be free, independent, and self-sufficient. His desk job made him feel like a Walter Mitty type of character. He also fantasized about being a playboy type in the James Bond tradition. In exploring his conception of a normally virile male, it began to become somewhat self-dystonic as it seemed the fantasy of an early adolescent that did not feel quite right for a 30-year-old whose "normal" friends were all getting married. I suggested the possibility that perhaps this view of masculinity might defend against underlying fears of intimacy with women. Carl responded to my interpretation of the defensive function of his view of "normal" male sexuality with a noncommittal attitude, suggesting that the interpretation was plausible but not compelling.

In the fourth year of treatment, Carl's negative transference evaporated when he developed a relationship with his first steady girlfriend that was an actively sexual relationship. Now he felt like a "regular guy" in my presence and granted me partial credit for his newfound success with women. I felt pleased that after 4 years of hard work, I had finally been given some credit for being a dutiful and conscientious therapist. The first year of the relationship was relatively conflict-free for Carl, as he seemed to be enjoying all the sexual gratification that he felt he had been missing out on for years. The relationship became problematic when his girlfriend began to express desires for a serious commitment that would lead to marriage. Carl did not view her as someone he wished to marry, but he was reluctant to break up with her for fear of returning to a lonely bachelor's life. He felt stuck in his ambivalence, unwilling to make a commitment and unwilling to end the relationship. Yet he felt guilty leading her on to keep the relationship going when he suspected that he would end it as soon as he felt sufficiently confident to begin dating again.

What was interesting in terms of our work together is that in the sixth and seventh years of treatment, Carl began to act more like a traditional analytic patient. He was able to free-associate, would work with his associations for lengthy periods of time without needing any intervention on my part, was aware of experiencing intrapsychic conflict, and began to recognize introspectively his own defensiveness. In our relationship, it was a point of pride that he could do it himself, and on occasion, when I was about to make an interpretation, he would interrupt me so that he could analyze the issue for himself. I believe his sense of self had become sufficiently resilient so that he could be a "good" patient without feeling that he was shamefully deferential and dependent and that he could be an assertive male without having to defy me to prove it.

In his relationship with his girlfriend, Carl felt split between two apparently irreconcilable ways of being himself. If he was a "regular guy," he should just end the relationship so that with his newfound sexual confidence he could get on with "sowing his wild oats" before finally settling down in some distant future. On the other hand, if he was really a mature and responsible adult, he should try to make the relationship work and overcome his fears of commitment. Thus his two self-syntonic senses of self were dystonic in relation to each other and left him in conflict and feeling hopelessly ambivalent. If he was normal by one standard of normality, he could not be normal by the other standard of normality.

In the transference, Carl often tried to position me to take one side or the other of the conflict. If I tried to analyze his fear of intimacy, he felt I was arguing that he should make the relationship work, and I was making him feel guilty for wanting out. If I tried to analyze his fears of ending the relationship and resuming dating, he felt I was arguing that he should end the relationship, and I was making him feel ashamed of not having the courage to tell her it was over. If I tried to analyze his ambivalence, he felt I was criticizing him for not being able to make a decision and get off the fence. If I tried to analyze his experience of me as critical or pushy, he felt criticized for not being sufficiently appreciative of my well-intentioned helpfulness. Treatment was once again exposing an underlying narcissistic vulnerability—that he felt paralyzed by ambivalence. Unsure whether he was a henpecked male like his father or an immature adolescent who was unwilling to assume adult responsibility, Carl felt either way it was an unflattering picture of someone unable to make an autonomous decision.

My analytic stance contributed to his sense of exposure. As he became more able to work like a traditional analytic patient and work with him began to feel less like pulling teeth, I tended to make more interpretations of conflict, as he seemed quite receptive to them. Yet Carl experienced interpretations of conflict as implicit demands to resolve conflict the moment it was exhibited to him. Thus I, like his girlfriend, seemed to be pressuring him to make a decision, making him feel guilty about disappointing us and ashamed in exposing his inability to "fish or cut bait." What seemed to be exposed and reexperienced was a sort of power struggle often engaged in with his mother, in which he was too guilt-ridden to be openly defiant, too proud to be compliant, and found a compromise in doing nothing but then felt shamed by his apparent impotence. In adjusting my stance in the direction of becoming more silent and noting his freedom to resolve his conflicts and make his decisions on his own timetable, Carl began to feel he could just "be" in treatment without having to "do."

At this point, it began to be possible to begin interpreting more meaningfully how this surface-level conflict may have been defending against a deeper conflict. Perhaps his conception of a normal male reflected an unconscious defense against as well as an indirect expression of his attraction to, hostility toward, and fear of closeness with a sexually alluring but domineering woman who might emasculate and enslave him. Perhaps his conception of a normally responsible adult reflected an unconscious defense against as well as an indirect expression of dependence on, submission to, and fear of abandonment by a seductive, domineering, and emasculating woman. In the transference as his male ally, I might fail him either by forcing him to leave a woman to whom he was quite attached and would be lost without or by forcing him to stay with a woman who might turn him into a eunuch. In sum, Carl was unconsciously conflicted between desires to remain in and escape from a relationship with his mother who was experienced as a seductive, domineering, and emasculating phallic woman while unconsciously conflicted between desires to identify and disidentify with his father who was experienced as a genuinely caring but castrated man who would ultimately fail him in his struggle with his mother.

As Carl experienced these conflicts in his relationship with his girlfriend as well as in his relationship with me, these interpretations of unconscious conflict were experienced as not only plausible but compelling as well. Carl began to recognize that he experienced his girlfriend and myself as domineering and controlling like his mother and that he was in a power struggle with us in order to extricate himself from that control. What was a more disturbing and guilt-ridden recognition was that he was unconsciously trying to win the power struggle by "turning the tables," by getting us "under his thumb." As he began to surmise his girlfriend's low self-esteem and masochism in sticking with him despite his refusal to make a commitment, Carl began to feel quite guilty about "taking advantage of her insecurity." Thus he began to see that he was inflicting the same trauma on his girlfriend that he felt his mother had inflicted on him and that in this respect he was like his entitled mother who expected others to do all the accommodation.

Interpretations of deep structure are by definition interpretations of what is highly self-dystonic. Unconscious characterological trends such as being sadistically emotionally withholding, masochistically subservient, needy of feminine nurturance, and fearful of emasculation by women were all dystonic in terms of Carl's seeing himself as either proudly independent and self-assertive or proudly dutiful and conscientious. What I hope to have illustrated in the current example is how an analysis can be done in terms of examining surface structure alone in all its intrapsychic and interactive complexity. I also hope to have demonstrated how a variety of incipient treatment impasses were resolved through an appreciation of how my interactive and interpretive styles were experienced as invalidating to Carl's surface-level self-syntonic sense of self. Such invalidation led to the reexperiencing of childhood narcissistic trauma in the transference that could be understood and worked through. Typically, as soon as the affirmative function of the self-syntonic sense of self was reestablished, its defensive function could be meaningfully interpreted, allowing for deeper analysis and greater characterological flexibility in not being so wedded to only a single, unidimensional manner of being a normal person. It was important for me to not be too wedded to any one interactive style. I moved through a variety of styles such as active facilitator, phallic mirror, conflict analyzer, and silent catalyst, as each style elicited a variety of positive and negative transferences that required analysis. I think this case example also highlights the utility of a model that conceptualizes character in terms of multiple selves in conflict and compromise, each self structure striving for validation and defending against invalidation.

9

Strategic Thought in the Analysis of Defense

Character analysis has traditionally been seen as virtually synonymous with defense analysis. Innovation in character analysis has often resulted from increased analytic rigor in the understanding and analysis of defense. I believe that a dialectical approach to defense analysis can allow for greater sophistication in the analysis of defense. If defense is appreciated from holistic as well as microscopic perspectives, as anxiety avoiding as well as identity affirming, and as being simultaneously intrapsychic as well as interpersonal, it can be analyzed with greater rigor. I hope to highlight that aspect of defense that reflects an overarching strategy of interpersonal engagement in the service of protecting the sense of self, for it is that aspect of defense that is minimized when defenses are looked at as primarily microscopic intrapsychic events that serve to allay anxiety.

Reich (1928) initiated a holistic approach to the analysis of defense when he focused resistance analysis on the problem of "character armor." Whereas concepts such as repression, denial, projection, displacement, and so on, referred to discrete defense mechanisms, the concept of character armor referred to the overall patterning of defenses. Characteristic attitudes, beliefs, values, ambitions, ideals, as well as any other aspect of what might be considered a personal style, can be used defensively as a means of remaining unaware of unconscious conflict. Fenichel (1941) criticized Reich's "layer" approach to character analysis since it led to conceiving the mind in an overly stratified way. Reich seemed to suggest that the outer layer, the patient's character armor, was analogous to an impenetrable stone wall beyond which lay the patient's infantile conflicts. One had to penetrate or shatter this stone wall in order for the patient to abreact repressed affect.

Fenichel (1941) distinguished between frozen and mobile defenses. Frozen defenses were analogous to Reich's character armor and reflected relatively fixed, rigid, and ego-syntonic character traits that were not easily amenable to analysis. In contrast, mobile defenses were fluid in their mode of operation, reflecting a momentary defensive move on the patient's part, and therefore more amenable to the patient's observing ego if the analyst were to attempt to demonstrate their operation to the patient. Mobile defenses also illustrated the fact that the mind is not as rigidly stratified as Reich portrayed it to be. Fenichel discovered that the distinction between resistance and content, drive and defense is not so clear-cut once it is realized that drives can serve defensive functions and that defenses can serve as a means of drive discharge. For example, a drive may serve as a defense when heterosexual promiscuity serves as a defense against latent homosexual impulses. A defense may serve as a means of drive discharge when the projection of one's hateful feelings onto another gives one a covert manner of venting one's aggression in being blaming and accusatory. And, of course, defenses do not defend against only the awareness of drive derivatives but also the awareness of other defenses. There are defenses against the awareness of defenses. For example, a person who is sexually repressed may not admit to being a repressed person. In projecting repudiated sexual desires onto others, the person could claim that others are oversexed in comparison to oneself who possesses a normal and healthy interest in sex, a level of sexual interest that could only be unfairly characterized as repressed. In this instance, projection serves as a defense against awareness of the utilization of repression, which serves as a defense against the awareness of forbidden sexual wishes.

The interchangeability of drive and defense and of one

defense for another defense means that what is surface and what is depth can be fluid and interchangeable. Thus, as in the case of borderline personality structure, a patient could be well aware of all manner of primitive sexual and aggressive fantasies as well as of primal scene experiences of childhood yet be totally unaware of possessing a defensive style, consciously thinking of oneself as though a particularly open and nondefensive person. Freud (1923) made it clear that the defensive operations of the ego could be just as unconscious and just as inaccessible to awareness as the most archaic infantile wish. Therefore, character armor cannot be thought of as a surface dimension in contradistinction to archaic affect and drive that is then a depth dimension in contradistinction. Rather, both character armor (i.e., defensive style) and drive possess surface and depth dimensions.

Brenner (1982) resolved this confusion about what is drive and what is defense in developing a functional definition of defense. All psychic events reflect compromise formations and as such serve multiple functions. Thus, all compromise formations possess a defensive component and a drive component as well as other components of compromise formations, such as superego components and affective components. Any behavior or psychic event may serve a defensive function. Sexual fantasy can serve a defensive function; conscience can serve a defensive function; even reality testing can serve a defensive function in denying one's most fantastic fears. Brenner defined a defensive function as any psychic activity that serves to diminish anxiety or depressive affect. He argued that one need not think in terms of discrete defense mechanisms that stand apart from the rest of the mental apparatus or that are specialized tools of the ego. Rather, ego functions are all-purpose. Be it reality testing, impulse control, or any other sort of cognitive operation, all ego functions can be used defensively as well as adaptively.

Resistance is ubiquitous and all-pervasive because there is no psychic activity that does not serve in part a defensive function. Thus, as Reich originally suggested, the personality as a whole (i.e., one's character style) can serve a defensive function. Yet, whereas Reich believed that underneath one's character armor lay the human being *au naturel*, it becomes apparent that we cannot demarcate some hidden inner self buried beneath layers of defensive attitudes. Though we may work from surface to depth in a manner analogous to peeling the layers of an onion, we never discover a solid core or a bedrock, only more layers to be peeled away ad infinitum.

Theorists such as Horney (1950), Winnicott (1960), and Guntrip (1969) appeared to treat what is surface as defensive, false, and inauthentic in contradistinction to what is deep as true, real, and authentic. This dichotomy, though not necessarily a false dichotomy, may nevertheless serve a defensive function: it may deny the possibility that how we appear to others (i.e., our self-presentation) is just as much a "real" self as any other aspect of the self, and it may deny the possibility that how we appear to ourselves in private inner fantasy, which is hidden from others, may in some manner be unreal, a highly selective construction that excludes many aspects of self that do not fit into the desired self-image being privately cultivated. Perhaps one's defensive style in both its surface and depth dimensions is one's real self.

The personality as a whole serves not only a defensive function but an identity-maintaining function as well. Thus, defenses should not be thought of as "not self" or "not me" processes that stand in contradistinction to the true self or one's "real" feelings. The self is an agent, engaging in defensive activity as an expression of and as a means of maintaining a sense of identity. One's defenses do not so much oppose the expression of who one "really" is but rather constitute one essential expression of who one is as a person. Defenses reflect personal values and ideals. For example, if one is quite an angry person but never admits to being angry, the essence or core of one's personality is not necessarily that at bottom one is an angry person. It might be equally, if not more, accurate to say that in essence, if one were to attempt to reduce a person to an essence, this person is someone who as a matter of principle will not admit to being angry. That principle could be said to be more reflective of the person's true self than the fact of the individual's chronic anger.

Psychoanalysts who still subscribe in some respects to an

abreactive or cathartic model of treatment tend to privilege affective experience as something basic, innate, primary, genuine, or authentic. Defenses are construed as a manner of blocking authentic affective experience, and it is in getting in touch with one's true feelings that the curative process transpires. This perspective, though, tends to ignore the defensive function of affect. Love can defend against hate, and hate can defend against love. Elation can defend against depression, and depression can defend against elation. Guilt can defend against shame, and shame can defend against guilt. That an affective state may serve a defensive function does not invalidate that state, or make it unreal, or imply that one should not empathize with that state for fear of colluding with a defensive attitude. It only implies that an affective state, like any other psychic phenomenon, can be subject to an analysis in terms of its multiple functions, and one of those functions is always a defensive function.

Not only can affect be used defensively, but so can developmental progressions. New or more effective ego functions that arise as an outcome of successful analytic work can also serve a defensive function. Paradoxically, ego development enables one to become a more complexly and well-defended person. A newly developed sense of independence and autonomy can bolster defenses against awareness of dependency needs; a newly developed trust in relying on others can serve as a defense against individual initiative; a newly developed capacity to articulate one's feelings verbally can serve as a means of intellectualizing feelings that had previously been acted out.

Defense analysis thus entails the interpretation of the defensive function of whatever psychic activity it is in which the patient is engaged. As discussed previously, although the defensive function is ubiquitous, the affirmative, identity-maintaining function of psychic activity is equally ubiquitous. Interpretation of the self-affirmative, identity-maintaining function of psychic activity tends to enhance self-stability. In contrast, defense interpretations tend to decrease self-stability in confronting the patient with self-dystonic elements of the personality. Thus, defense analysis always provokes the anxiety of identity loss and spoilage, of exposing the patient to the cognitive dissonance of recognizing that the patient is not quite the person the patient fancied him- or herself to be. This anxiety will then trigger increased defensiveness in the service of re-repressing the self-dystonic element that the defense interpretation has brought to the fore. Thus, defense analysis must eventually entail interpretation of the patient's defenses against the recognition of being defensive (i.e., resistance to the awareness of resistance).

Freud sometimes likened resistance analysis to a game of chess, an analogy that highlights the strategic thought involved in developing either a defensive or an offensive plan of action. Chess involves a battle of wits, of move and countermove, of being able to accurately anticipate the opponent's next move, of planning a countermove as a follow-up, and of possessing a broad repertoire of response options if the opponent were to move in an unexpected manner. Strategic thought is obviously a sophisticated ego function that requires accurate anticipation, contingency planning, the capability to envision multiple futures, the ability to see the world from the opponent's point of view in which one is seen as the adversary to be defeated, elements of gamesmanship such as bluffing and other forms of deception to throw one's opponent off the track, and the ability to think quickly on one's feet under pressure.

Although the primitive prototypes of psychological defense may be a sort of automatic, reflexive flight-or-fight-response or affect blunting to stimulus overload that do not require any higher-level cognitive operations, it is impossible to grasp how character style operates as a defensive style without looking at character style as a strategy of defense. A. Freud's (1936) reduction of a character style to its predominant mechanisms of defense neglects the element of strategic thinking in the genesis of defensive attitudes. To think of a hysteric as someone who predominantly defends the self through repression, to think of the paranoid as someone who predominantly defends the self through projection, or to think of the obsessive-compulsive as someone who uses several defenses such as reaction formation, regression, intellectualization, and rationalization does not actually tell us much about the particular defensive strategy of that particular character type. Defense mechanisms are better thought of as universally present defensive options that any character type could utilize in different situations of danger. Hysterics utilize reaction formation in thinking of their love as wholesome and pure rather than as dirty and self-serving. Obsessive-compulsives utilize projection in viewing others as being as dogmatic as their own superegos. Paranoids utilize repression in being as oblivious to their incestuous desires as any hysteric. It is the strategic patterning of defenses that distinguishes one character type from another.

Transference resistance reflects the interpersonal manifestation of defense in the treatment situation. Though the concept of defense developed as an intrapsychic concept—an unconscious manner of blocking anxiety-arousing psychic content from gaining access to consciousness—intrapsychic defense invariably manifests itself as a transference resistance, that is, as an interpersonal event. Thus, a defensive style is always manifested in an interpersonal style. An interpersonal style operates as a defensive style by engaging the social surround in a manner so as to support rather than destabilize intrapsychic defensive operations. The interpersonal destabilization of intrapsychic defense may lead to a failure of defense, a return of the repressed, and symptom formation. One avoids interpersonal situations that challenge defenses, and one seeks interpersonal situations that bolster defenses. A defensive style therefore requires a strategy of interpersonal engagement.

In sum, character style functions in one of its multiple functions as a defensive style. As a defensive style, it possesses both surface and depth dimensions, self-syntonic and self-dystonic aspects. A defensive style cannot be reduced to mechanisms of defense alone but must be understood in terms of a sophisticated strategy that entails complex and high-level cognitive operations. A defensive style can be thought of holistically in the same manner that a strategy may be said to reflect a distinct and coherent principle of organization—a game plan, so to speak. Though a principle of organization may be relatively fixed, its mode of implementation may be fluid and varied since a strategy must be responsive to multiple and sometimes unanticipated contingencies. Though the concept of defense is basically an intrapsychic concept defined by those psychic activities that function to attenuate anxiety and depressive affect, defensive activity manifests itself as an interpersonal style, as interpersonal events will either support or challenge defenses. Defensive style is thus reflected in a strategy of interpersonal engagement that possesses both surface and depth dimensions. And it should be kept in mind that, in any interpersonal event, what is surface to one observer might be depth to another observer and vice versa.

This view of psychological defense as a mostly unconscious strategy of interpersonal engagement in the service of warding off threats to the self-syntonic sense of identity is analogous in some respects to Weiss and Sampson's (1986) concept of the patient's unconscious plan for self-cure. They noted that Freud's (1923) theory of unconscious ego processes suggests that high level ego functions such as reality testing, planning, and anticipation may transpire unconsciously. Automatic and reflexive unconscious ego defense is only one small aspect of what the unconscious ego does. As a consequence of childhood experiences, certain pathogenic or grim beliefs are formed about what constitutes a situation of danger to be avoided. These situations of danger in the interpersonal world are not simply automatically avoided, but rather the unconscious ego develops a plan of action, a strategy to subject those grim beliefs to reality testing in order to discover whether they are true. Disconfirming pathogenic beliefs through an unconscious plan of action constitutes a form of self-cure. Thus, unconscious plans and strategies serve not only a defensive function—to avoid the materialization of a grim belief—but also an adaptive function—to subject grim beliefs to unconscious reality testing in order to disconfirm them and thus be free of them. Weiss and Sampson noted that in the treatment situation, the patient's unconscious plan manifests itself interpersonally as an unconscious test of the analyst, to assess whether the analyst will behave in a manner consistent with the patient's pathogenic beliefs.

Though to focus on the adaptive function of a patient's unconscious plan is an important emphasis, it should not be taken in lieu of a recognition that a patient's unconscious plan also possesses a defensive function. Even unconscious reality testing can serve a defensive function. There is a reason that the patient's plan is executed unconsciously rather than consciously, which is because the underlying plan is in some respects self-dystonic. For example, a patient is unconsciously frightened of depending on others for fear that they will prove unreliable. As a consequence, the patient unconsciously tests the analyst's reliability by acting out in a variety of ways and, in discovering that the analyst is reliable, settles into the treatment situation and stops acting out. Despite the analyst's having passed the patient's unconscious test, the patient does not admit to being dependent on the analyst or to having been unsure of the analyst's reliability in the first place. Instead, the patient overtly exhibits a newly enhanced sense of independence. The reason for this state of affairs is that a patient possesses not only an unconscious plan but also a conscious plan. In this case, the conscious plan was to become a more autonomous person. The conscious self-syntonic plan to become an autonomous person, so one need not worry so much about others' reliability, conflicts with the self-dystonic unconscious plan, which is to make sure that others are absolutely reliable because one is such a dependent person who would be lost without others' reliability. Paradoxically, it is the patient's unconscious faith in the analyst's reliability that allows the patient to sustain the illusion of autonomy prior to its having become a reality that can be sustained independent of the stable holding environment that the analyst provides.

Patients can be understood as possessing multiple plans— some conscious, some unconscious, some self-syntonic, some self-dystonic, conflicting in some respects and compatible in others, and each plan serving both defensive and adaptive functions. The unconscious plan of testing the analyst's reliability serves a defensive function in denying the patient's capacity for autonomous functioning, whereas the conscious plan of becoming more autonomous serves a defensive function in denying the patient's need for and mistrust of the reliability of others. In terms of a strategy of interpretation, one should interpret the adaptive function of a plan or a strategy prior to the interpretation of its defensive function with which it is counterbalanced.

Weiss and Sampson (1986, pp. 93–95) presented the case of Mr. B. to illustrate how inaccurate interpretations of the patient's unconscious plan hindered the patient from carrying out his plan. This case example illustrates the limitation of viewing behavior as either adaptive or defensive rather than as simultaneously adaptive as well as defensive. Perhaps unconscious plans are compromise formations serving multiple and conflicting functions. The patient misled the analyst into believing that he suffered from a "primary" homosexual attachment to the analyst, whereas in fact he suffered from unconscious worry about him. The homosexual attachment to the analyst was not the expression of a primary impulse but rather an attempt to placate the analyst, whom the patient unconsciously feared would be hurt, envious, and retaliatory if the patient were successful with women. The analyst's interpretations of the patient's apparent primary homosexuality made the patient "worse," worse in part defined by an intensification of the patient's homosexual attachment to the analyst (p. 94).

Mr. B. was a young man with an obsessive-compulsive character who aspired to be an architect. He sought treatment for his inhibitions in love and work. Mr. B. had been highly competitive with his father and three older brothers while growing up. He perceived them as highly competitive with him, envious of him, and vulnerable to his challenges. To test the analyst, the patient provided what could be called "multiple-choice tests." He would report enjoyable sexual relations with women but imply that he was struggling with strong homosexual impulses. In retrospect, it seemed that the patient was testing the analyst to see whether the analyst could tolerate his success with women, so that to focus on the patient's implicit homosexuality would be construed as failing the test. At the time, though, the analyst believed that the patient was unable to accept his repudiated homosexual desires and began to interpret along those lines.

When the analyst initially listened to the patient's success with women relatively silently, the patient became more outspoken about his relations with women. When the analyst began to interpret the patient's shame over his alluded-to homosexuality, the patient became depressed and anxious. The patient stopped dating women and provided corroborating memories from childhood that confirmed the analyst's ideas in regard to the patient's "primary" homosexuality. Yet over time the analyst became alarmed by the patient's growing inhibition and depression despite the patient's acknowledgment of his homosexual tendencies. After consultation with colleagues, the analyst began interpreting the patient's oedipal fears of competing with men by being successful with women. Mr. B. immediately began to do better and after 7 years of analysis did well in graduate school and made a satisfactory marriage.

It is interesting how the dynamics of the case were formulated in either/or ways. The patient's homosexuality was assumed to be either primary and defended against by secondary heterosexuality or secondary as a defense against primary heterosexuality. The patient was then testing the analyst in either one of two ways: testing the analyst to see whether the analyst could accept the patient's homosexuality or testing the analyst to see whether the analyst could tolerate the patient's heterosexuality. Why could it not be both simultaneously? It seems that the patient's surface-level self-syntonic sense of self was heterosexual, whereas there was a repudiated but alluded-to self-dystonic sense of self that was homosexual. It is therefore no surprise that the patient was destabilized by the interpretation of the repudiated self-dystonic homosexuality and stabilized by the implicit affirmation of the self-syntonic heterosexuality.

In being presented with a "multiple-choice test" for which the analyst assumed there was a correct answer (i.e., the accurate assessment of the patient's singular unconscious plan for self-cure), the analyst had been seduced into taking sides in a conflict that the patient had in regard to his sexual orientation. The analyst's either/or interpretive choices, deciding whether to highlight the defensive nature of the patient's heterosexuality or the defensive nature of the patient's homosexuality, entailed the analyst implicitly making a decision about sexual orientation for an obsessive patient who could not decide for himself. Part of the transference with an obsessive-compulsive patient would be looking to the analyst as an authority figure to whom to defer in resolving whatever issues have become embroiled in obsessive self-doubt and ambivalence.

Sexual orientation as a compromise formation can be seen as serving multiple functions, affirmative as well as defensive. The affirmative function of the patient's homosexual transference may have been to have a relationship with a man which is primarily loving rather than primarily competitive, as he had with his father and brothers. Yet the patient may have feared that his father, brothers, and analyst would have disdain and contempt for a homosexual man who would have been seen as unmanly by them, as unlike them. Thus to own his homosexuality may have been a depressing affair, if it meant the loss of the regard of the important men in his life. When the analyst returned to taking the side of heterosexuality, the patient was relieved that he was allowed to be a "normal heterosexual" male once again. The patient's competitiveness with his father and brothers suggested that he was also quite identified with them as male role models, so that there may have been unconscious fears of the consequences of disidentifying with them in choosing alternative male role models.

The important point here is that character structure can be thought of as a complex, sophisticated plan or strategy of interpersonal engagement that possesses self-syntonic and self-dystonic dimensions and that serves defensive, adaptive, and identity-affirming functions. The various character styles can be analyzed in terms of their defensive strategies of interpersonal engagement. For example, the obsessive-compulsive can be understood as utilizing self-control as an overarching strategy of defense as well as of interpersonal engagement. The basic idea is that as long as I remain adept at controlling myself, I will not fall in harm's way, because as long as I can control myself I am free of the control of others. This strategy possesses self-syntonic and self-dystonic elements. The self-syntonic element is that self-control is a virtue, a sign of maturity, of which one could be proud and that others should admire. The self-dystonic element is that self-control may in a certain interpersonal context reflect an emotionally withholding and ungiving attitude. Self-control serves a variety of defensive functions. It most especially wards off a fear of losing self-control, but it also deflects the control of others in being stubbornly self-controlled and offers a manner of controlling others indirectly by setting an example for others to follow. Since self-control serves as an all-purpose defensive strategy, it can be utilized to ward off any sort of anxiety, from castration anxiety to fears of oral impregnation.

Mr. B. may have experienced heterosexuality as compatible with self-syntonic self-control, whereas he may have equated homosexuality with a self-dystonic loss of control. Interpretation of the patient's homosexuality would have threatened the patient with fears of loss of control, as the patient would likely have experienced the analyst as taking sides in a conflict by implying that he should give in to his homosexual desires. The patient then defended himself through the intensification of his characterological "inhibition" (i.e., self-control) as a means of preserving an endangered but necessary sense of self-control. Conversely, implicit affirmation of his heterosexuality may have spared him the anxiety aroused by the threat of an out-of-control homosexual self-experience and assured him that he could continue to live a self-controlled heterosexual existence despite anxiety-ridden unconscious desires to do the exact opposite. Thus, given his obsessive-compulsive character, Mr. B.'s conflicts over sexual orientation may have in part expressed a conformity = controlled/nonconformity = impulsive conflict.

The hysteric employs an overarching strategy of defense and interpersonal engagement in which the basic principle is to make oneself desirable to others. The basic idea is that as long as others are attracted to me, I need not fear them. At the self-syntonic level, the idea is that being a friendly, likable person is a good way to get on with people and find a place in the world. At the self-dystonic level, the idea is that in seducing others before being seduced by others, I remain in a safer position. To always be an attractive and desirable object to others serves as an all-purpose defensive strategy that can defend against fears of initiative or fears of one's own sadism toward others. A defensive strategy should not be thought of as something that is erected to protect oneself against some particular anxiety from some particular source. Rather, it is akin to a philosophy of living that provides one with a generalized style of coping suitable to any conceivable contingency or situation of danger. A defensive strategy is like an all-purpose remedy. In this sense it reflects magical thinking and is in the nature of a superstition. A defensive strategy functions as a talisman, a secret charm that will avert evil and bring good luck.

The depressive-masochistic character utilizes an overarching strategy of defense in which looking to others for completion becomes a way of life. At a self-syntonic level, the idea is that as long as I look to others for sympathy, solace, and support and as long as I am successful in obtaining that result, all will be well in the world. At a self-dystonic level, the idea is that as long as I remain a submissive and suffering individual, I will avert all potential catastrophes.

The narcissistic character utilizes an overarching strategy of defense in which remaining a center of attention is the secret of maintaining a sense of psychological security. At a self-syntonic level, the idea is that as long as I present myself as a confident and secure individual, I will be treated with respect and need not worry about my status. At a self-dystonic level, the idea is that as long as I remain superior to others and can force them to recognize my superiority, I will not have to worry about anything in the world.

The schizoid character employs an overarching strategy of defense based on the idea of being self-sufficient. At a self-syntonic level, the idea is that it is admirable to be independent and self-sufficient, and as long as I display these admirable traits, I will be accepted by others. At a self-dystonic level, the idea is that as long as I do not need or depend on anybody, nobody can hurt me in any way, so I will refuse to warm up to anybody who tries to get close to me. We see that all defensive strategies serve to maintain an illusion of invulnerability.

The paranoid character employs the overarching strategy of defense that one should always remain in control of a situation. Whereas the obsessive-compulsive controls the self, the paranoid tries to control the situation. At a self-syntonic level, the idea is that if I just mind my own business and do my own thing, no one should bother me. At a self-dystonic level, the idea is that if I remain hypervigilant, keep others at a protective distance, and take immediate offensive action if anyone invades my personal space, I should remain safe and secure.

The antisocial character utilizes the overarching strategy of defense that in a "dog-eat-dog world" one should try to remain "top dog." At a self-syntonic level, the idea is that in a world in which everybody is trying to exploit and take advantage of everyone else, in order to fit in I should be and become like everybody else. At a self-dystonic level, the idea is that although not everybody is as ruthless or exploitative as I am, that is all for the better—I can get the upper hand over them and get my piece of the pie in a world in which there is not enough to go around.

Defensive strategies possess self-syntonic and self-dystonic aspects. The self-syntonic aspect reflects that aspect of the strategy that the person feels is admirable, that seems to demonstrate maturity, objectivity, and normality in adapting to the world. As such, it is a strategy that reflects well on who one is as a person and affirms one's basic values. The self-dystonic aspect reflects that aspect of the strategy of which one is ashamed or guilt-ridden. The self-dystonic aspect of the strategy strikes the person as self-serving, opportunistic, of low moral standards, and lacking in integrity, so that it is repudiated. The self-syntonic and the self-dystonic reflect different qualities of object relations. At the self-syntonic level, others are treated as individuals in their own right. Though one is entitled to assert one's own rights in relation to others, others are to be treated in a manner that seems fair and justifiable. The self-syntonic level reflects a sense of protecting oneself in which one plays by the socially accepted rules of engagement. At the self-dystonic level, others are treated as obstacles to be overcome rather than as persons. At the self-dystonic level, it is not how you play the game that counts but winning. Thus, at a self-dystonic level one does not play by the rules. Not only is this strategy hidden from others, but the intention to break the rules is hidden from oneself as well. If in order to gain a sense of security at others' expense, one depersonalizes others in treating them as though only inanimate obstacles without subjectivities of their own, it would seem to make one somewhat inhuman oneself.

The problem for defense analysis becomes immediately apparent. Patients will have relatively less difficulty owning their self-syntonic defensive strategies, as they seem to reflect a mature and reasonable style of coping; whereas patients will be resistant to acknowledging their self-dystonic defensive style, for it would suggest that the patient covertly influences and manipulates others in order to feel secure. Much work, though, can be accomplished at the level of analyzing the self-syntonic strategy of defense. The analyst could confront the patient with the ineffectiveness of his or her self-syntonic strategy of defense. The obsessive-compulsive could be confronted with the fact that dedication to self-control may entail an abdication of the freedom and pleasures of spontaneity. The hysteric could be confronted with the idea that the need to be everybody's friend may interfere with self-assertion. The depressive-masochist could be confronted with the fact that the need to gain sympathy may be at the expense of one's own autonomy. The drawbacks of each defensive style could be elucidated, as each defensive style reflects a limited worldview that may be valid in a particular context but is not universally valid in every conceivable situation as the patient would have it.

Though it is difficult for a patient to refute the logic of a debate that argues for the superiority of multiple perspectives over a more limited perspective, the patient will nevertheless attempt to resist the analyst's confrontation by attempting to make such a refutation. The analyst would have to win such a debate on logical grounds, which seems to be the method of Ellis's (1985) rational-emotive therapy as well as cognitive therapy of the personality disorders (Beck et. al. 1990). Yet such a debate masks the narcissistic injury that the patient may experience in discovering the maladaptive nature of a strategy that had previously been considered an especially fine strategy of adaptation. The patient's confidence in his or her own adaptive resources is undermined at the same time that the patient is impressed with the greater perspicacity of the analyst's worldview.

To the extent that the patient is capable of assimilating the analyst's higher level of integrated functioning and is motivated to identify with the analyst, the patient may adopt the analyst's broader perspective as an organizing framework. Loewald (1980) suggested that the therapeutic action of psychoanalysis derives from the patient's opportunity to develop an object relation with a person at a higher level of integrated functioning. Such a person can help the patient learn to see the world from a higher ground with a broader perspective. Nevertheless, the patient's confrontation with the narrowness of his or her own perspective in comparison to the analyst's broader vision is a narcissistic injury to be resisted to the degree that the patient is wedded to a relatively egocentric construal of relationships. No matter how much the patient wishes that the analyst would be no more than a narcissistic extension of the patient's self, the reality is that the analyst is an independent subjectivity with a separate perspective no matter what cultural or characterological common ground they may share. The analyst may, through an especially nonintrusive and nonimpinging interpersonal style, mute that element of separateness, allowing the patient the illusion that the analyst is an extension of self. Yet the patient cannot help but register the fact that the analyst's mind employs different principles of organization than the patient's mind.

The analyst may trace with the patient the historic development of the patient's self-syntonic defensive strategy. How did the schizoid learn to be so self-sufficient, the paranoid person develop so much respect for the value of personal space, the antisocial individual become so convinced that being dominant is all that counts, the narcissist become so invested in remaining a center of attention? When the patient begins to see that the self-syntonic defensive strategy was a perfect fit for the familial and cultural environment in which the patient grew up, then it becomes more palatable to accept the possibility that other interpersonal and cultural environments may require other strategies of adaptation and defense. Nevertheless, patients may resist this sort of historic analysis, as affirmative as it seems to be, because it too entails the assimilation of a narcissistic injury. To the extent that one's own family, culture, and value system have been construed as universal, normal, healthy, or perhaps superior, there will be a resistance to assimilating a point of view that challenges that universality, normality, and so on. The patient's narcissism through extension of the grandiose self, idealization, and twinship is extended to family, gender, race, religion, occupation, and so on. Thus, if the analyst were to challenge any of the assumptions (or should I say presumptions) of the groups with which the patient is identified, it is like questioning the patient him- or herself. For this reason, the "blame the family" approach, even with a family that tolerated incest or other forms of abuse, is dependent on the patient's disidentification with the perspective of the family of origin and identification with the analyst's critical perspective. Yet the patient, despite whatever overt disidentification with family values, is at least unconsciously identified with the family values that the analyst opposes. To the extent that family values are self-syntonic, the analyst's values and perspective may seem to be alien, lacking universality, abnormal, and narrow-minded. Despite the fact that an analyst's entitlement to practice is based on a belief in possessing a broader psychological perspective than the patient, patients often accuse analysts and analysts often accuse each other of being rigid and narrow-minded.

In challenging self-syntonic defensive attitudes in which

the patient is narcissistically invested, there is a characteristic sort of negative transference that is likely to be elicited. The patient—in feeling accused by the analyst of being narrow-minded, egocentric, constricted, rigid, maladaptive, self-defeating, and of confusing childhood realities with current realities, not seeing the forest for the trees, distorting reality due to overgeneralization, and so on—will probably feel that it is indeed the analyst who is imposing the analyst's reality on the patient, and that it is indeed the analyst who claims to possess an all-purpose system in which all patients can be pigeon-holed. So much of the current literature warning clinicians not to foist their own preconceptions on the unwitting patient and to instead listen with an unprejudiced openness to the patient's point of view seems to avoid the unpleasant fact that clinicians tend to hear primarily what their theoretical preconceptions allow them to hear. Patients are well aware of that fact and possess strong feelings in regard to how the analyst is going to assimilate their life story. Patients, though not as theoretically sophisticated as clinicians, nevertheless seek out a mental health professional because they know that that person possesses a specialized point of view that is not common knowledge and that the clinician will assimilate the patient's life story and problems in terms of this special point of view.

The patient is, of course, highly ambivalent about having his or her life story and identity reinterpreted in terms of the analyst's system of thought. On the positive side is the hope of cure, insight, empathy, and understanding. On the negative side is the fear of just what it is that a "good" analyst is not supposed to do with patients—that is, to be judgmental, prejudiced, rigid, narrow-minded, pigeon-holing, formulaic, stereotypic, authoritarian, and so on. The feared result of such analytic misconduct would be something along the lines of what Shengold (1989) has called "soul murder"—that the analyst will rob the patient of the patient's sense of identity by either malevolently or ineptly interpreting the patient's experience in terms of preconceived notions that are inappropriate to the patient's real experience. Analysts of all persuasions have been vulnerable to this accusation, an accusation that

particularly stings given that analysts have based their professional identity on the attempt to be the opposite.

Though it would be interesting to examine the dynamics of
the use of this accusation when analysts are making such an
accusation of each other, I think it is especially interesting to
look at the dynamics of those times in the clinical situation
when the patient makes some such accusation in response to
attempts at defense analysis. It would seem that it is at those
occasions when the analyst is challenging what seems to be a
self-syntonic defensive attitude that the patient tends to
experience the analyst as a coercive person who is trying to
force a patient to accept a point of view that would be in
violation of the patient's sense of identity. To submit to the
analyst at such a point would seem to be to act without
personal integrity, so that to resist the analyst at such a point
is to act with self-respect. Here, then, would be an example of
role reversal and turning the tables as a defense. When the
analyst interprets the patient's defensive attitude, the patient
turns it around to accuse the analyst of imposing a precon-
ception on the patient. In making such an accusation of the
analyst, the patient evades the anxiety-arousing implications
of the analyst's interpretation. Yet we know that patients
tend either to become incensed or submit begrudgingly when
the analyst follows up a defense interpretation with an
interpretation of the patient's defensive response to the
analyst's defense interpretation.

Once again Kohut's (1971) recommendation to empathize
with the patient's experience of the analyst's empathic failure
seems relevant. The issue is not so much whether the analyst
is "really" judgmental, although the analyst "really" possesses preconceptions. Nor is the issue whether the patient's
negative transference to the analyst as a judgmental person
possesses a kernel of truth or is primarily a defensive projection or displacement of some aspect of the patient's preexisting representational world. What is relevant is whether the
analyst can empathize with what it is like for a patient to work
with an analyst who seems to have been imposing his or her
own narrow-minded preconceptions on the patient. This
does not mean apologizing to the patient for an error of

technique or a countertransference-based misunderstanding. It means appreciating the patient's struggle to maintain the integrity of his or her own point of view in the face of the authority of the analyst who appears to possess a different point of view, one in which the patient does not seem to be seen in such a flattering light. It also means tolerating and containing the patient's counteraccusation that perhaps it is the analyst who possesses the egocentric point of view and who is incapable of grasping the patient's perspective without mauling and destroying it. The patient may then identify with the analyst's capacity to deal with what may be fair or unfair criticism to which the patient subjects the analyst. Initially, at least, the patient's criticism of the analyst seems warranted as it has been provoked by the analyst's confrontation, which the patient has construed as an unwarranted imposition of the analyst's biased perspective.

If interpreting self-syntonic defensive attitudes that are accessible to consciousness evokes so much resistance in their examination, how is it that self-dystonic defensive attitudes that are inaccessible to consciousness are ever addressed? If the obsessive-compulsive takes offense at the suggestion that perhaps self-control stifles spontaneity, then how is it that the obsessive-compulsive will ever admit to being unconsciously withholding and critical? If the schizoid character takes offense at the suggestion that self-sufficiency may get in the way of intimacy and closeness, then how will the schizoid ever admit to being unconsciously cold and rejecting toward others in order to keep them at a distance? If the depressive-masochist is offended at the idea that the need for sympathy may interfere with becoming more independent, then how is the depressive-masochist going to admit to being a clingy, submissive person who would rather accept abuse than abandonment? If the hysteric is offended that undue friendliness precludes self-assertiveness, then how is the hysteric ever going to admit to being unconsciously seductive as a means of exerting interpersonal influence?

The self-dystonic level, as a result of the failure of defense when self-syntonic defensive attitudes are challenged, tends to return from repression in projected form. The analyst is then experienced as employing the same self-dystonic defensive strategies that the patient unconsciously utilizes. When the analyst notes the rigidity of the obsessive-compulsive's self-control, the patient experiences the analyst as overly critical and emotionally withholding the praise that is the patient's due. When the analyst notes the hysteric's need to be friendly to everyone and liked by everyone, the analyst is experienced as seductive in trying to have an especially intimate relationship with the patient in which the patient relinquishes the friendly persona. When the analyst notes the schizoid patient's self-sufficiency, the schizoid patient feels that it is the analyst who will be aloof and distant if the patient were to warm up to the analyst. Thus, the analyst must be able to empathize with what it is like for the patient to work with an analyst who employs the same defensive strategies that the patient utilizes unconsciously (i.e., transference of unconscious defense). In the negative transference, the patient does not see the analyst as a generic "soul murderer" but as a particular kind of soul murderer—one who possesses a personal signature, a particular strategy of obliterating the individuality of the other. It is not enough to empathize with the fact that the analyst has failed or might fail the patient in some essential manner. The analyst must interpret the particular devious technique through which the attempt to annihilate the patient has been or might be made. The analyst experienced as narcissist must be superior to the patient but deny it; the analyst experienced as paranoid must attack the patient who violates the analyst's personal space and then justify it; the analyst experienced as depressive-masochist must expose the patient's sadism in letting the patient abuse the analyst and then act the martyr; the analyst experienced as hysteric must seduce the patient and then play innocent; and the analyst experienced as obsessive-compulsive must be emotionally withholding with the patient for the patient's own good.

So we see that a patient's strategy of defense manifests itself as a transference resistance. Gill (1982) delineated two types of transference resistance: (1) resistance to the awareness of transference and (2) resistance to the resolution of transference. Resistance to the awareness of transference essentially means resistance to the awareness of the latent transference, for there is always a manifest transference of which the patient is aware that is readily subject to verbal articulation and discussion. As Reich (1928) noted, a latent negative transference is stimulated as soon as the analysis begins to move beyond what is ego-syntonic. Thus the analyst's technique determines the extent to which the latent negative transference becomes manifest. To the extent that the analyst affirms the self-syntonic, the manifest positive transference will be strengthened and the latent negative transference weakened; and to the degree that the analyst challenges the self-syntonic and stimulates the self-dystonic, the positive transference will be weakened and the latent negative transference will become manifest as a conscious experience. Interpretations of resistance to the awareness of latent negative transference, in implicitly or explicitly challenging the self-syntonic manifest positive transference, cannot fail to make the latent negative transference manifest to the patient. In this sense, one might say that the negative transference is induced by the analyst's technique, as is the positive. Any analysis that either stimulates inadvertently or actively addresses self-dystonic elements of the patient's personality will have its share of manifest negative transference to be analyzed.

Resistance to the resolution of transference refers to the resolution of a manifest transference that the patient does not seem to move beyond. Since we see that defense analysis is invariably evocative of a manifest negative transference in stimulating self-dystonic elements of the personality, how is it that that negative transference is resolved? One cannot do character analysis without stimulating the patient's experience of the analyst as a sadist engaged in character assassination, employing exceptionally cunning and devious methods of destroying the patient's sense of identity. I would suggest that the affirmative function of the manifest negative transference needs to be addressed prior to the interpretation of its defensive function. To interpret the affirmative function of the manifest negative transference is to empathize with the patient's experience of the analyst in the negative transfer-ence. This means articulating the patient's sense of how the analyst has failed the patient as well as the patient's affirma-tive attempt to assert the sense of identity in the face of an analyst who appears to be undermining that sense of iden-tity. This interpersonal configuration constitutes an adversa-rial selfobject relation in which the patient asserts the sense of self against an adversary who is opposing that sense of self. This opposition to the analyst serves as a means of preserving a sense of self in the face of an annihilatory threat. It is only after the sense of self is stably defined in opposition to the analyst that the defensive function of the manifest negative transference may be addressed (i.e., that it serves to deny another sense of reality, that it defends against an underlying positive transference, or that it reflects an identification with the aggressor and as such constitutes a pathological enact-ment and repetition of the past in the present).

Spence (1987) noted that the psychoanalyst's task has been represented in an analogous manner to detective work in the tradition of Sherlock Holmes. The detective accumulates clues through which the criminal betrays him- or herself. The detective and the criminal are embroiled in a strategic battle of wits, the criminal attempting to get away with something and the detective attempting to apprehend the criminal. In con-trast to the game of chess, which is a morally neutral competition, the battle of wits in which detective and criminal are engaged is a battle between good and evil. The criminal has broken a rule, a taboo, and as a moral transgressor deserves to be punished, though the criminal will attempt to evade that punishment. The detective upholds the moral order in exposing the identity of the criminal. Freud (1916) believed that the clues the criminal leaves behind for the detective to discover are left due to unconscious guilt. Freud believed that many criminals unconsciously desire to be caught and punished for their misdeeds.

A self-dystonic defensive strategy is one that is felt to be morally reprehensible. It is felt not to be a legitimate manner of defending oneself—like hitting below the belt in a boxing match. It is a defensive strategy that breaks the socially acceptable rules of resolving interpersonal conflict. It is a strategy that gives one an unfair advantage in dealing with others. As a consequence, the pangs of conscience object to such a strategy of defense and repudiate it to the extent one needs to think of oneself as a basically decent, fair-minded, good, and moral person whose actions are justifiable on ethical grounds. As mentioned previously, even antisocial characters need to convince themselves that exploitative and criminal conduct is morally justified, and employ quite a bit of tortured reasoning to rationalize their misconduct. Through an act of self-deception, one continues to engage unconsciously in a morally unacceptable strategy of defense while consciously continuing to think of oneself as a fundamentally decent person.

The self-deception is not foolproof, due to the person's unconscious sense of guilt and need for punishment. The person's unconscious superego cannot allow the person to engage in a morally reprehensible defensive strategy without consequence. An unconscious strategy then must be devised to ward off superego anxiety. The superego must be bribed or corrupted in order to be convinced to look the other way. To the degree the integrity of the superego is compromised, the strategy of self-deception proves successful. This intrapsychic conflict is externalized in the treatment situation as an interpersonal conflict. The analyst as a superego figure is experienced as a detective attempting to expose a criminal who is deviously attempting to get away with something. The patient, experiencing the self in the role of criminal, both wishes and fears being exposed, caught, and punished. The ambivalent patient yields clues in order to be caught but then conceals clues in order to remain hidden.

In unconsciously employing a self-dystonic strategy of defense in the treatment situation, the patient is relating to the analyst as an adversary. And whereas the analyst is an adversary who is supposed to play by the rules, the patient as criminal may not. Unconsciously, the patient may try to gain an unfair advantage over the analyst in attempting to deceive, mislead, sabotage, or deviously outwit the analyst—a fifth columnist who is overtly a friend but covertly a foe. Unconsciously, the patient feels guilty about mistreating the analyst but then rationalizes such treatment. The analyst is seen as receiving the sort of treatment that the analyst deserves to receive. The more effective the patient's unconscious strategy of defense is in defeating the analyst, the greater the unconscious sense of guilt becomes in achieving an ill-gotten victory. Defeating the analyst is a pyrrhic victory, for unconsciously it proves that the patient is irredeemable (i.e., unanalyzable). Overall, the patient must choose between the lesser of two evils: to defeat the analyst through deception or to allow oneself to be caught by the analyst and face the consequences. It is more the patient's readiness to be apprehended than the analyst's clever detective work that allows a patient's unconscious strategy of defense to be acknowledged. Perhaps the patient's unconscious sense of guilt does not lead so much to a negative therapeutic reaction, reflecting an unconscious need for punishment, as it leads to expiation and atonement, with the analyst as a witness to the patient's confession. The patient's unconscious sense of guilt is then a motive that may in certain respects support the analysis, as the analytic cure is experienced as a form of reparation for one's misdeeds.

Just as the analyst is not supposed to be a character assassin who reduces the patient to a stereotype, neither is the analyst supposed to be a prosecutor for the defense who is out to prove the patient's guilt beyond a shadow of a doubt. Yet I would suggest that the attempt to analyze self-dystonic defensive strategies evokes just such a negative transference. The patient experiences the analyst as a skeptic who never takes what the patient says at face value. The patient feels that his or her honesty, integrity, accuracy, and decency are suspect, as though the patient were a person with something to hide and who would fool the analyst with an act of deception. Feeling unfairly prosecuted and judged by the analyst, the patient must defend the self by questioning the analyst's moral authority. The patient implicitly accuses the analyst of being moralistic, judgmental, authoritarian, self-righteous, morally pompous, punitive, condemning, and prosecutorial—just the opposite of what a good analyst is supposed to be.

In analyzing self-dystonic strategies of defense, the negative transference for which the patient requires empathy is to understand what it feels like to work with an analyst who is felt to be detective, prosecutor, judge, and jury. What is it like to work with an analyst who is accumulating evidence in order to make a case against the patient? What is it like to work with an analyst who calls into question one's honesty, integrity, and intentions? What is it like to be seen as someone who cannot be trusted by virtue of being seen as defensive, deceptive, evasive, covertly hostile, secretly manipulative, and unwilling to be responsible or be held accountable for the consequences of one's actions? So much of the prescribed analytic attitude is designed to avoid being seen by the patient in such a light, given how predisposed patients tend to be to regarding the analyst so once the analyst attempts to analyze the patient's unconscious defensiveness.

The patient establishes an adversarial selfobject transference with the analyst in conceiving the self as a defendant on the witness stand at a trial in which the patient is falsely accused. In defending oneself against a prosecutorial analyst, the patient is seeking moral vindication and exoneration. The patient defends the integrity of the self against the analyst's slanderous attack. To maintain one's self-respect in the face of libelous accusations and charges is no easy feat. The analyst as prosecutor is seen as possessing a distinctive strategy or technique for winning the case against the patient. As always, the analyst is feared to be a formidable adversary. The analyst as an obsessive-compulsive catches the patient in logical inconsistencies; the analyst as a hysteric is shocked by the patient's indiscretions; the analyst as a depressive-masochist grieves for the plight of those victimized by the patient; the analyst as a narcissist looks down on the patient as an inferior specimen; the analyst as a paranoid has contempt for the patient's hypocrisy and pretense, and so on. The patient feels prosecuted and judged in a manner analo-

gous to the way in which the patient unconsciously prose-
cutes and judges him- or herself.

The affirmative function of such superego transferences is
addressed in recognizing the patient's self-assertion of innocence in the face of the analyst's prosecution. The defensive
function of such superego transferences is addressed in
noting that the analyst seems to blame the patient in a
manner that is not dissimilar to the patient's own self-blame.
When analysis is construed as analogous to courtroom
drama, it highlights the element of strategic thought in the
attempt to build a case point by point or to refute a case point
by point. Analysis can then be seen as unfolding as a dialectic
of point and counterpoint. The elements of skillful debating—
the use of rhetoric, sophistry, narrative coherence, and logical
argument in the process of establishing a successful defense—
speak to an extremely complex and sophisticated level of ego
functioning. The verdict of guilt or innocence depends on
which side can tell the most convincing story to a jury whose
sense of logical coherence as well as human sympathy must
be engaged.

Traditionally, it had been assumed that the ego-syntonic
could be made ego-dystonic with the formation of an observing ego. The patient could identify with the analyst's
scientific attitude, that is, the analyst's presumed objectivity,
and learn to observe oneself as would a dispassionate observer. If a patient possessed an observing ego, then it would
be possible for the patient in the process of introspection to
observe defensiveness and self-deception. As previously
noted, a problem with this theory of personality change is
that the patient's observing ego is not the analyst's most
reliable ally in the analysis, since such a split in the patient's
ego can serve a defensive as well as adaptive function.
Possessing an observing ego does not solve the problem of
defensively motivated observational bias. The observing ego
always possesses an observational bias in that self-
observation is always conducted in a characteristic manner.
Obsessive-compulsive individuals observe themselves with
fine attention to trivial details, and hysterics observe themselves impressionistically. Only schizoid characters attempt

to observe themselves in a manner that aims to be detached, dispassionate, and objective, as a scientist might.

It is probably incorrect to say that a patient has not developed an observing ego, for it is in the nature of personality organization to observe oneself on the basis of an identification with how one has been observed by others. When we say that a patient lacks an observing ego, it probably refers to a patient who in the act of self-observation sees a person who is average, conventional, and normal—in other words, a nondescript generic human being. Observing nothing out of the ordinary, there seems nothing of note to say about oneself. It is not that such a patient does not possess an observing ego but rather that such a person observes the self in a naive, innocent, and nondiscriminating manner. When an analyst attempts to help a patient develop an observing ego, it is to enable the patient to learn to employ a different style of self-observation, one that is more skeptical and does not take things at face value. The patient is encouraged to identify with the analyst's Socratic method of investigation.

A skeptical observing ego that never takes anything at face value and is always on the lookout for hidden meanings behind surface pretenses is akin to a paranoid style of observation. Perhaps the problem is not to help the patient develop an observing ego, for all patients already possess one; and perhaps the problem is not to help the patient develop an observing ego that is free of observational bias, for one can only observe oneself through a particular lens or filter. The problem may be to enable the patient to deploy multiple rather than singular observational styles. Patients will possess a characteristic self-syntonic style of self-observation through which the patient observes a familiar self that has been seen many times before and may be taken for granted. All other styles of self-observation are dystonic to this familiar style and generate an image of oneself that is unfamiliar and strange, which may be repudiated as "not me."

To see oneself as someone who can be unconsciously defensive and engaged in self-deception requires an ability to look at oneself from multiple perspectives and styles of self-observation. Self-dystonic elements of the personality are revealed when one can look at oneself through a novel style of self-observation. If an obsessive-compulsive could observe the self impressionistically as a hysteric does, then the obsessive-compulsive would see that despite being so conscientious in attending to small details, the overall impression is of being fault finding and hypercritical. If a hysteric could observe the self in fine detail as the obsessive-compulsive does, the hysteric might notice a person who despite attempting to create an overall impression of being genuinely friendly could be seen as superficial in treating everyone indiscriminately in the same friendly manner without making any fine distinctions between individuals. The more styles of self-observation one is capable of deploying, the greater the number of self-dystonic aspects of self can be recognized. We possess as many sides of ourselves as we possess styles of self-observation: each style of self-observation reveals a different aspect of self. To observe self-deception, it helps to assume a skeptical and ironic style of self-observation in which one does not take the self-syntonic view of self too seriously or at face value.

To the extent a new style of self-observation reveals an aspect of self that is strange, unfamiliar, and unflattering in comparison to the familiar view of self, that style of self-observation will be resisted and rejected as self-dystonic. In the analytic situation, the analyst will be experienced as empathic to the degree the analyst views the patient in the same manner in which the patient views him- or herself. To the degree that the analyst departs from this self-syntonic view, the analyst will be experienced as unempathic, at least until a time in which the patient comes to identify with the analyst's view of the patient. Thus, the analyst as a mirror of the patient often reflects back to the patient an image that is unfamiliar and strange—unflattering if the analyst is doing defense analysis and flattering if the analyst is attempting to be especially affirmative and validating. Thus interpretations of affirmative functions tend to flatter patients' narcissism and pave the way for interpretations of defensive functions that tend to be unflattering and injure patients' narcissism.

Analysis requires that the patient learn to tolerate the relativity of self. After all, the patient is seeking personality change and hopes to be at least a somewhat different person after analysis than before, despite whatever thread of continuity remains the same.

I will present a case illustration in which I hope to illustrate how unconscious psychological defense is organized holistically and reflects a defensive strategy of interpersonal engagement that in the analytic situation unconsciously tests the analyst. This unconscious strategy is self-dystonic, and therefore the patient resists its exposure. I hope to demonstrate a dialectical way of working both with the patient's defensiveness and the patient's negative transference in which I am alternately empathic and challenging. Ironically, this is a case in which the patient often experienced my questioning of his self-criticism and self-blame as unempathic rather than as reassuring.

The patient, whom I will call Peter, was 32 years old, married, and had been in treatment once and twice weekly for the past 4 years. Peter came for treatment having suffered from mild-to-moderate-level depression for most of his life. He displayed a predominantly obsessive-compulsive character style with underlying depressive-masochistic trends. The current source of his depression was the sense that careerwise he was in a rut. A music major in college, he had originally hoped to have a career as a musician. After graduating college, he made little headway as a musician because of depression, low self-esteem, and lack of initiative. After getting married in his mid-twenties, Peter decided he needed a responsible job and a steady income, so he switched to a job in sales in which he did well but was not enthusiastic. He often did not get along with authority figures at work, tending to be covertly provocative and antagonistic.

Peter appeared to have established a hostile/dependent relationship with his wife. He viewed his wife as a nurturing, caring person to whom he was quite attached yet also viewed her as insecure and needy. Peter often found himself treating her in a contemptuous and fault-finding way, not infrequently snapping at her in an irritable manner followed by feelings of guilt and remorse. He also found himself troubled by adulterous fantasies that he feared he might enact. Prior to marriage, Peter had had girlfriends and sexual experiences, but for the most part he construed himself as unsuccessful with the women whom he saw as the most desirable and difficult to obtain, of which he did not consider his wife one. Peter felt that his wife needed him more than he needed her, and one of her insecurities was that if Peter ever found his self-confidence, he would leave her. Nevertheless, Peter felt highly committed to the marriage and believed that his marital problems were more an issue of his own inner conflicts than a problem in his choice of a mate.

In the treatment situation, Peter quickly recruited me as an ally in his desire to make a career change from sales to music. Within the first year of treatment, he switched jobs to a sales job with an easier schedule and was able to find an evening job as a musician. He felt he was off and running and attributed his progress to the effectiveness of his treatment with me. His depression was significantly alleviated and his self-esteem was improved. It emerged that Peter was a talented musician growing up but that his parents never praised his musical talent. When he was practicing and his father was reading the newspaper, his father would tease him about making a lot of noise. Both parents seemed to feel that praise would lead to an inflated ego, so they both treated Peter in a manner designed to remind him constantly not to develop excessive pride. His father felt it was a waste of money to spend college tuition on becoming a musician.

What was also salient in Peter's discussion of his childhood was the fact that he was adopted in the first year of life, as was his older brother. Peter attributed his chronic depression to a lifelong sense of the loss of the mother who raised him during the first 6 months of his life. He felt that his adoptive parents had always loved him in a conditional manner. His parents were described as people who above all wanted him to follow their rules and believed that he should feel lucky and grateful to have been adopted by them. Peter always possessed a sense that perhaps his parents would send him back to the orphanage from which he came if he ever refused to follow their stringent rules of conduct. In contrast to Peter, his elder brother was a defiant rule breaker who became a delinquent adolescent and eventually an alcoholic adult. He was disowned by the parents, who finally became fed up with him after years of futile power struggles. Peter had a poor relationship with his brother, who he felt had mercilessly teased and bullied him growing up, leaving him with an impotent rage.

As the honeymoon phase of the first year of treatment began to dissipate, Peter's depression began to return during the second year of treatment as he began to feel that he had gone only so far and was stuck going any farther. He was bored with his new sales job and also felt that his evening job as a musician was a dead-end, uncreative endeavor, working with amateurs. The nature of the transference relationship began to change subtly. Whereas during the first year I was experienced as an encouraging mirror of his potential as a creative musician, during the second year I became a constant reminder of his failure to live up to his potential as a musician. Peter was not averse to being reminded of his failure, as he believed that constant confrontation with his failings would provide a good incentive to overcome his procrastination and laziness. Nevertheless, I felt I had been seduced into a role in which I would be seen as browbeating him for failing to take initiative and that he would masochistically submit to my admonishments.

Believing that I had unwittingly taken sides in an unconscious conflict in becoming the mirror of his musical aspirations, I felt that that stance had become an implicit message to the effect that the life he was currently living was somehow unacceptable and unworthy. The mirroring stance seemed to mirror his self-criticisms to the effect that as someone who failed to live up to his musical potential, he was a miserable failure as a person. I then attempted to analyze what I believed to be his excessive self-criticism for being an underachiever as a musician, which Peter then took as my believing that the only reason I thought he should accept himself for who he is is that I did not really believe him capable of establishing a successful career as a full-time musician. Thus I was making him even more depressed than he was already.

A similar transference dynamic emerged in his discussions of his adulterous fantasies. Peter believed that having adulterous fantasies was a sign of immaturity, and he hoped that treatment would alleviate him of such thoughts. To the extent adulterous fantasies continued to be experienced as intruding themselves on his consciousness against his will, Peter continued to criticize himself for a lack of progress in that regard, which depressed him. When I attempted to analyze his self-criticism for having fantasies that he had no apparent intention of acting on, Peter felt that I was encouraging him to indulge in such fantasies and that indulgence was only one step from action. He stated, "Why bother fantasizing about something if you're not going to do it?" I became the representative of the wish that he should cheat on his wife rather than the person who was supposed to be holding him back from that possibility.

My role, from his perspective, was not to be neutral but to be an ally who would enable him to advance his musical career while preventing him from cheating on his wife. To the extent his musical career did not advance and to the extent he still felt tempted to cheat on his wife, I was not helping him. To the extent I addressed his self-criticism for not advancing musically and for continuing to entertain adulterous fantasies, I was seen as an unsupportive person who did not have confidence that he could achieve his goals. It became clear that Peter had a conscious self-syntonic plan for how treatment was supposed to help him. He felt that with a therapist who believed in his ability to achieve professionally and remain faithful maritally, he would be able to achieve his goals. To the extent I enacted this role, Peter felt I was supportive, but then he beat up on himself for being unable to achieve his goals even with my support. Then it seemed he had only his own laziness to blame. To the extent I addressed his beating up on himself, Peter felt I was relinquishing my role as supporter of his aspirations and encouraging him to settle for less, to be a run-of-the-mill salesman who cheats on his wife.

It became apparent that in the treatment, Peter was reexperiencing a trauma to his narcissism. Peter was never much impressed with his father, whom he tended to see as a rather pathetic figure. His father was described as a petty bourgeois person who lived a narrow, boring, and conventional life. Peter saw his father as a rather dense person who tended to be grumpy, irritable, and fussy and whose dignity was easily threatened and offended. His father, like himself, had many times been reduced to an impotent rage by his brother's rebelliousness. He took himself quite seriously and was intolerant of any sign of irreverence or disrespect from his sons. Whenever Peter felt he was following in his father's footsteps, he became quite depressed and ashamed to think that he would live a lackluster and unimpressive life like his father's. Peter's goal was to live a life unlike his father's, to have a career that was creative and enjoyable and to be in a marriage about which he felt enthusiastic and completely gratified. Anything less than achieving these goals meant he was a pathetic loser like his father.

Growing up Peter felt treated by his parents as someone who was quite ordinary and unexceptional, who would never do anything special with his life, and whose fantasies of doing something special were the sign of an inflated ego that needed to be cut down to size. His dream from a young age was to prove them wrong by doing something special with his life. To the extent his life was turning out to be ordinary and conventional, Peter felt disgraced and humiliated. It was inconceivable to accept himself as an ordinary person. To the extent I seemed to be suggesting that he should accept himself as he is, I was, just like his parents, trying to get him to tone down his inflated ego and be content following in his father's footsteps.

What perplexed me was what was holding him back from making the life changes he claimed he wanted. Initially I might have believed that with a facilitating environment he would have been off and running. The beginning of the treatment seemed to suggest that with the help of a mirroring selfobject, his self-esteem would be bolstered sufficiently to pursue his goals. It seemed that some kind of unconscious inhibition was holding him back as he seemed stuck in an orgy of moral masochism. Of course, my attempts to explore the unconscious roots of his moral masochism were experienced as my being unsupportive and undermining of his self-syntonic plan for self-improvement. I had the feeling that he would have liked me to become a sort of drill sergeant who would browbeat and cajole him into doing what he felt he should be doing and that anything less on my part was felt as insufficiently supportive. As Peter began to think about starting a family and buying a home with a mortgage, any sort of significant career change began to seem increasingly unfeasible for financial reasons. It started to seem like a no-win situation for both of us in which it seemed too late to change careers, but neither could he ever accept himself for living a conventional life that did not live up to his creative potentials.

In the fourth year of treatment, an incident occurred that began to reveal the nature of an unconscious dynamic in our relationship. Peter rarely canceled sessions but canceled one at the last minute in order to drive his wife to the doctor as she was not feeling well. My cancellation policy was that I charged for late cancellations but would offer a makeup session if scheduling permitted. The next session after the missed session, we discussed scheduling a makeup session. When I did not have any available times that were convenient for Peter, he seemed annoyed. I noted that it seemed that he wished I would not charge for the missed session because he did not want to come for a makeup session at an inconvenient time or pay for a session that would not be made up. Peter replied testily that he knew the rules, that he would attend a makeup session at an inconvenient time, and that he did not want to waste any more of his session time discussing scheduling. I asked him how he felt about me wasting his session time. He said that he thought that when it came to scheduling, I was officious and stuffy. After discussing what it was like for him to work with a therapist whom he experienced as officious and stuffy, he asked me whether I saw myself as officious and stuffy. I asked him what it would mean to him whether I said I was or I was not such a person. He said that if I said I was not officious and stuffy, it would mean that I was not honest with myself and that if I admitted I was officious and stuffy, it would mean that I was honest. I then suggested that he was not so concerned about whether I agreed with his assessment of my officiousness, since he was confident that I actually was officious, but that he wished to figure out whether I was honest and trustworthy and was asking me a sort of trick question to ferret out my true nature.

This interpretation brought tears to Peter's eyes. He reported that he wanted to know whether I really cared about him as a person or was just interested in his money. He felt that if I bent the rules for him, that would demonstrate I really cared. He reported a memory that when he was in college and living at home and needed a ride from his parents, they would give him a ride but would make him pay the same price as they thought it would have cost to take a taxi. I attempted to empathize with his feeling that I, like his parents, did not love him for himself but merely tolerated him when he played by the rules and rejected him when he did not. I went on to interpret how he saw a willingness to bend the rules as a sign of love.

The next session Peter came in to tell me that he was planning to terminate treatment. He stated that during the last session I had had the perfect opportunity to tell him explicitly that I cared about him and that when I missed that opportunity, it was proof to him that I did not care about him. I interpreted that he was now planning on rejecting me by terminating as punishment for my rejection of him in not telling him explicitly that I cared about him. In addition, I questioned his assumption that my refraining from explicit self-disclosure meant that I did not care about him. He asked what other reason I could possibly have for not answering his question. I responded that his question put me on the spot. If I answered in the negative, that would only confirm what he suspected already; that if I answered in the affirmative, he would not have believed me anyhow since he would have

succeeded in coercing me to say what he wanted to hear just
to avoid his anger and retaliation. Peter then recalled a similar
strategy of entrapment that he had employed with his mother
in which he would always ask her for a glass of orange juice
at times he believed were inconvenient for her as tests of her
love. If she refused to give him the orange juice, he sulked;
but when she gave him the orange juice, she often did it
begrudgingly so that he never felt she really cared about him.
Like his parents, I am the overly rule-bound person who only
cares about him conditionally, as long as he does things my
way. Yet at an unconscious level there is also a reversal of
roles—Peter will threaten me with abandonment (i.e., termination) for not conforming to his way of doing things just as
he felt threatened with abandonment for not conforming to
his parents' expectations.

A later session revealing a similar dynamic involved Peter
recounting an interesting dialogue that he had with one of his
best friends. The friend began sharing his adulterous fantasies with Peter in the hopes of engaging Peter in a dialogue in
which two faithful and monogamous husbands could com-
miserate about their sexual longings and frustrations. Curiously, though, Peter would not admit to his friend of entertaining such fantasies as his friend, who had already
confessed his, started trying to pry Peter's fantasies out of
him. Finally, Peter blurted out that he was attracted to his
friend's sister, to which his friend responded with shock and
indignation and said that he did not want to discuss it any
further. Peter then responded defensively that he was only
sharing his fantasies under duress because his friend pres-
sured him. As Peter recounted this incident to me, he was
quite amused.

In listening to this vignette and finding myself identifying
with his friend, I interpreted how with his friend and with me
Peter often presented himself as a sexually innocent person in
comparison to whom anyone else who admitted actually
enjoying prurient sexual fantasies seemed dirty-minded. Yet
then he would say something shocking to demonstrate that
not only was the other more prurient than him but more
prudish as well. Peter could then contend that whatever he

said that seemed outlandish if not perverse was evoked in him by the other person so that he was still essentially innocent. Peter was adept at exposing others as prurient prudes and thereby unmasking others as pretentious hypocrites who are both more prudish and more perverse than they care to admit to themselves or others. Peter then recalled a memory in which after he was toilet trained, his mother thought that Peter was making faces as though he had to go to the bathroom, but Peter denied it. Shortly thereafter it was discovered that Peter had made a bowel movement in his pajamas, and his mother was quite annoyed. Peter acted as though it were an innocent accident and that his mother's annoyance was proof of her intolerance, as anyone can make an innocent mistake.

At a self-syntonic surface level, Peter presented himself to others and himself as an essentially innocent person working diligently to live up to high standards of career achievement and moral conduct. To the extent he failed to live up to these standards, Peter took full responsibility and only blamed himself. In the service of living up to these standards of which he fell short, he would willingly submit himself to a regimen of self-improvement such as psychotherapy. If others responded to him as a provocative or passive-aggressive person, Peter felt shocked, hurt, and indignant, as though others were unappreciative like his parents of what a considerate, hardworking, and talented person he was. Thus Peter repeatedly reexperienced a trauma to his narcissism for which he sought reassurance and comfort.

At an unconscious level, though, Peter appeared to be constantly testing others through a very clever sort of inter-personal entrapment. Peter would constantly test others to see how they would respond to minor violations of rules and standards of social propriety. If others made a big deal about what he felt were minor violations, he would have exposed their latent authoritarianism and believed that they cared more about following the rules than about him. If others did not seem to mind minor violations of the rules, Peter would continue to test their sincerity by continuing to break the rules in various minor ways. In this manner, Peter could be experienced as unconsciously provocative, tending to irritate others and eventually getting under their skin. Even when others were apparently accepting and tolerant of minor violations, Peter could imply that they had become indulgent and lax and were therefore not doing their job. Thus Peter put others in a no-win situation: if they responded to Peter's violations of minor rules, they were being petty, but if they did not respond to these violations, they were being careless.

The unconscious test, though, did not have so much to do with complying with or defying the rules as it had to do with finding out whether others really cared about him as a person. By engaging others in petty power struggles over rules, Peter was defending against the fear that no one really loved him for himself and that he would be abandoned if he did not play by others' rules. To the extent others stuck by him despite being a difficult person who constantly tested the rules, Peter was reassured that he was loved for being himself no matter how much he irritated and annoyed others in attempting to expose their pettiness, prudery, hypocrisy, and hidden perversity. In this unconscious testing of others, Peter was in effect being an emotionally withholding and intolerant person like his parents, who would withhold his emotional acceptance of others until they passed his arduous test, not once but repeatedly in endless forms and guises. Like his parents, Peter was a person for whom it was difficult to prove oneself good enough to be worthy of his spontaneous and enthusiastic approval.

As I attempted to interpret this level, which was self-dystonic, Peter had a dual reaction of shame and pleasure. On the one hand, Peter was quite amused by these interpretations since they exposed a side of him that seemed like a mischievous, naughty little boy who took pleasure in teasing and fooling others and who felt quite potent in so doing. On the other hand, Peter felt ashamed that he seemed more invested in playing this covertly sadistic game than in getting on with his life and felt vulnerable in realizing how insecure he was in needing constant reassurance that he was loved and would not be abandoned. Unconsciously, Peter felt like an orphan who had to ingratiate himself so that he would not be sent back to the orphanage. He resented ingratiating himself and felt humiliated by it. So instead, he only pretended to ingratiate himself on a manifest level while covertly defying the rules to assert his autonomy and make others prove to him that he did not have to follow the rules to be accepted. As this dynamic was elucidated in the transference, our relationship became freer and more playful as an alliance began to develop between myself and his mischievous trickster self. In addition, in a less overt way Peter began to feel that I had empathy for what it was like for him as an adopted child with a dread of abandonment who tried to act as though he was just a normal kid trying to grow up to be a normal and successful person.

In summary, Peter's more overt defiance/compliance conflict with authority served as a defense against an underlying fear of a traumatic abandonment. To the extent the transference–countertransference relationship remained embroiled in conflicts with authority, the underlying fear of abandonment remained untouched. Peter engaged others so cleverly in power struggles over rules and standards of propriety, finding fault if they were overly strict yet finding fault if they were overly lax as he maintained a stance of his own essential innocence, that it was not easy to extricate oneself from this form of engagement with Peter. It was in gradually discerning this unconscious defensive strategy of interpersonal engagement through which Peter continually tested me, that the seeming therapeutic stalemate began to be worked through. Of course, to expose this strategy was to challenge Peter's self-syntonic innocence in confronting him with his unconscious and self-dystonic sense of being a trickster who made a fool of others as well as his unconscious sense of being an abandoned orphan who would never grow up to be a normal and successful person. In making the self-syntonic self-dystonic, I was often experienced as an unsupportive, fault-finding, officious, and stuffy person who was less than helpful and genuinely caring. Yet in working through this negative transference, we were able to achieve a more playful relationship in which performance pressure was significantly alleviated.

10

Personal Idiom and the Principle of Identity Maintenance

As character analysis proceeds past the patient's surface-level self-presentation, it reaches what I would call an intermediate level of depth, the level of the patient's private sense of self. This is the aspect of the self of which the patient is aware (i.e., it is often preconscious rather than unconscious) but that is hidden from others for fear of rejection. This is the aspect of the self that the patient experiences as precious, vulnerable, and fragile and therefore must be carefully guarded. It is an aspect of the self that the patient experiences as a vital inner core that may be endangered if exposed to external reality. Thus the patient often resists being open about this aspect of the self in analysis.

If the private sense of self is construed as a compromise formation serving multiple functions, identity affirming as well as defensive, then it must be approached with a balance of empathy and analysis. On the one hand, the analyst must be experienced as having empathy for what the patient experiences as an exquisitely sensitive aspect of self that should be treated with "kid gloves." To do otherwise is experienced as an outrageous violation, as "soul murder." Yet to take the patient's sense of preciousness, fragility, and vulnerability at face value as though it were sacrosanct (i.e., to analyze it would be sacrilegious) may be to collude with a defensive attitude on the patient's part. Maybe it is part of the patient's masochism to construe the self as fragile, maybe it is part of the patient's grandiosity to construe the self as infinitely precious, maybe it is part of the patient's omnipotent control to make others a slave to the patient's vulnerability, and maybe it is part of the patient's paranoia to assume that others are out to violate the patient's inner core. Thus empathy for the sacrosanct nature of the patient's private sense of self must proceed yet be counterbalanced by interpretation of the defensive function of needing to construe the private sense of self as sacrosanct.

Although the psychoanalytic vision of human nature would seem to imply that to be defensive and self-deceiving is as much a human essence as any other aspect of personality functioning, the recognition of the extent of human defensiveness led to the postulation of aspects of the personality that are nondefensive—aspects that can be understood as basic, fundamental, primal, and irreducible. The topographic (i.e., surface–depth) approach to the mind suggested that the surface of the mind was a defensive superstructure that covered over and concealed a depth dimension that reflected a human essence. For Freud (1937a) the sexual and aggressive instincts constituted a biological bedrock and as such represented an authentic core of human nature. Reich (1928) conceptualized the surface as a "character armor" surrounding and repressing a wholesome and natural instinctual being that needed to be liberated. Winnicott (1960) conceptualized the surface as a false self that concealed a deep inner true self. According to Winnicott, the true self is based on the somato-affective vitality of the body and reflects a distinctive personal idiom. The true self represents the innate core of the sense of individuality that will unfold over the course of maturation. Bollas (1989) suggested that Winnicott's true self contained a "destiny drive" that is bent on actualizing the latent creative potential embodied in the distinctive personal idiom of one's true self.

Though psychoanalysts have vociferously debated the essence of human nature (i.e., whether it is essentially sexual, aggressive, narcissistic, object related, and so on), there seems to be agreement that human nature contains some innate biological essence that is obscured by a defensive superstructure. The whole point of defense analysis is to bring to the surface this hidden, suppressed essence of human nature and in so doing set in motion a curative process. Much of psychoanalysis reflects a modernist view of the self, positing a unique inner self that is biologically grounded and struggling to affirm its existence despite the inhospitality of the modern world. Erikson (1959) spoke of the sense of identity to grasp that sense of distinctive personhood that provides a sense of personal continuity over time and in different situations. Lichtenstein (1977) posited a principle of identity maintenance as the superordinate organizer of the personality that supersedes both the pleasure principle and the reality principle. He conceptualized the sense of identity as analogous to a musical theme that, though distinctive, could nevertheless be played out in creative variation. Kohut (1977) spoke of nuclear ambitions and nuclear ideals that organize and direct the development of the sense of self.

Sullivan (1953) suggested that the sense of personal individuality was a culturally derived illusion. According to Sullivan, there is no unitary "I" or "me" but rather as many self-identities as social roles that we assume. We assume as many different social roles as there are different social situations in which we find ourselves. Mitchell (1991) stated that "we are all composites of overlapping, multiple organizations and perspectives, and our experience is smoothed over by an illusory sense of continuity" (p. 128). Stolorow and Atwood (1991) posited, "Our view is that the concept of an isolated, individual mind is a theoretical fiction or myth that reifies the subjective experience of psychological distinctness" (p. 193). These theorists reflect a postmodernist view of the self in which there is no essential biologically grounded self apart from culture and that all aspects of self are social constructions. The self is relative to culture rather than fixed by biology.

Despite the fact that the felt cohesiveness and continuity of the self may be demonstrated to be illusory, it can be appreciated as a necessary illusion that exerts an adaptive organizational influence on personality functioning. Winnicott (1971) made a case for the adaptive import of illusion in psychological functioning. Illusion serves as a creative bridge between subjective and objective senses of reality. The capacity for illusion is what makes life feel meaningful, worthwhile, and real. From a postmodernist point of view, the illusion of a whole and essential self reflects the ideology of individualism that characterizes Western society in general and American society in particular. Thus to adapt to an individualistic culture requires a firmly separate and autonomous sense of possessing a unique self.

The illusory sense of an essential inner self or sense of identity can be appreciated as a compromise formation, and as a compromise formation it can serve multiple functions, adaptive as well as defensive. As an adaptive function, the sense of identity, as Lichtenstein (1977) suggested, serves as the superordinate organizer of personality functioning that supersedes other organizational principles. The sense of identity enables one to function as an integrated unit and in an organized fashion. The sense of identity provides one with a coherent set of purposes and goals that guide and structure the cast of one's life. The defensive function of illusions about oneself, especially illusions of one's essential uniqueness and individuality, is to repudiate aspects of the self that are not so special or unique. The sense of identity reflects a dialectical tension. The affirmation of a unique and distinct sense of individuality requires a negation: to say that "this in particular is me" requires saying that "this in particular is not me." The sense of identity is based on differentiation, identification and disidentification, being like something and being unlike something else. What one is like then stands in polar opposition to and in contradistinction to what one is unlike. If one defines oneself as a conscientious person, then one is also defining oneself in contrast to those who are irresponsible. Irresponsibility then becomes a "not me" element of the personality that would need to be repudiated. The unconscious can then be understood as all those aspects of the personality that prove incompatible with the sense of identity by virtue of standing in polar opposition to it.

Fast (1984) discussed how gender identity develops on the basis of differentiation and repudiation. Originally the child is psychologically undifferentiated in terms of male and female. For the undifferentiated child, everyone is a generic human being, all capable of bearing babies and all capable of growing penises or breasts. Gradually, the child learns that one is either male or female with each sex's distinctive anatomy, sexual capacity, reproductive function, and socially derived gender role. On making this differentiation between male and female in terms of both biological and social differences, the child identifies with one or the other role and disidentifies with the opposite role, which must be repudiated. The conscious sense of identity as either male or female then stands in contradistinction to an unconscious sense of being identified with the opposite sex. Goldner (1991) noted that the coherence, consistency, and continuity granted by a sense of identity may prove constricted, limited, inflexible, and conformist as when the sense of identity is based on rigid sex role stereotypes. To the degree that the sense of identity is established on the basis of a narrow or unidimensional self-definition, it may prove to be more confining than enabling of personality development and enrichment. Perhaps a balance must be struck between role flexibility and identity diffusion.

The sense of identity as an illusory sense of self is a private sense of self. As a precious illusion about oneself, it must be maintained as a relative secret hidden from others, who may attempt to relieve one of one's illusions. Since external reality is a source of disillusionment, the illusory sense of self must be sequestered from exposure to external reality, especially protected from the debunking and deflating attitudes of skeptical others. The illusory sense of self tends to be cultivated in private fantasy and daydreams in which omnipotent control can be exerted. In one's private daydreams, one's nuclear ambitions and ideals can meet with the longed-for happy ending toward which one might strive in real life, with no guarantee of ultimate success. This sacred domain of privacy in which others are forbidden to trespass must not only be protected from the disillusioning impingements of

external reality but from the equally disillusioning impingements from the unconscious that are always threatening to
return from repression. How can one maintain a private
sense of self as chaste and innocent in the face of sexual and
aggressive wishes, and how can one maintain a private sense
of oneself as independent and self-sufficient in the face of
wishes for nurturance and dependence?

Disillusionment in one's privately cultivated sense of self
entails the threat of identity spoilage and loss. Defensive and
compensatory strategies will be initiated in order to maintain
the illusion on which the sense of identity is based. Protection
of the private sense of self in which illusions of individuality
and distinctiveness are cultivated is the origin of defensive
attitudes. To lose these illusions about oneself is to lose one's
sense of identity. Thus fear of disillusionment is the equivalent of fear of identity loss. The anticipation of identity
spoilage or loss functions as a signal anxiety that triggers
defensive and compensatory strategies in the service of
sustaining the illusion on which the sense of identity is based.
Analysis, in its attempt to bring what is deep to the surface—
and especially defense analysis, in its attempt to confront
self-deceptions—constitutes a threat to the sense of identity.
Freud was well aware that psychoanalysis was a threat to the
narcissism of humanity in dethroning consciousness as the
seat of human intentionality and agency in demonstrating the
power of the unconscious to determine human conduct.
Freud prided himself on being an iconoclast who would
debunk humankind of its illusions through objective observation and rational analysis. Yet from a contemporary perspective we can appreciate that Freud's sense of identity as
the detached, dispassionate, and objective observer of the
human condition reflects an illusion through which Freud
denied the relativity and the subjectivity of his own self-
identity as a scientist.

Winnicott (1963) suggested that the illusion on which the
sense of selfhood is based must never be exposed to external
reality, for to do so would be a sacrilegious act equivalent to
soul murder.

> I suggest that in health there is a core to the personality that corresponds to the true self. . . . I suggest that this core never communicates with the world of perceived objects, and that the individual person knows that it must never be communicated with or be influenced by external reality. . . . [E]ach individual is an isolate, permanently non-communicating, permanently unknown, in fact unfound. . . . At the centre of each person is an incommunicado element, and this is sacred and most worthy of preservation. . . . I would say that traumatic experiences that lead to the organization of primitive defences belong to the threat to the isolated core, the threat of its being found, altered, communicated with. . . . Rape, and being eaten by cannibals, these are mere bagatelles as compared with the violation of the self's core. . . . For me this would be the sin against the self. We can understand the hatred people have of psycho-analysis which has penetrated a long way into the human personality, and which provides a threat to the human individual in his need to be secretly isolated. [p. 187]

Winnicott (1963, pp. 186–187) provided an example of a 17-year-old girl's need to maintain the privacy of her secret self. The case illustrates the importance of being sensitive to a patient's need for privacy and of seeing the need for privacy in a self-affirmative light. However, it also illustrates the liability of not considering the defensive function of the patient's desire for privacy as perhaps a defensive retreat from a thwarted wish to have one's creative productions celebrated by an appreciative audience.

The patient's mother worried that she might become schizophrenic because of a family history, whereas Winnicott saw her as in the middle of the usual doldrums and dilemmas of adolescence. The patient discussed the glorious irresponsibility of childhood: "You see a cat and you are with it; it's a subject, not an object." Winnicott said, "It's as if you are living in a world of subjective objects." She said, "That's a good way of putting it. That's why I write poetry. That's the sort of thing that's the foundation of poetry." She added, "Of course, it's only an idle theory of mine, but that's how it seems and this explains why it's men who write poetry more than girls. With girls so much gets caught up in looking after children or having babies and then the imaginative life and the irresponsibility goes over to the children."

The patient had kept a diary when she was 12 and 14. Currently she was writing poetry but was not interested in publishing her poems or showing them to anyone. She was not interested in whether the poems were good or whether others thought the poems were good. She was fond of each of her poems for a little while and then lost interest in it. In this brief vignette, Winnicott quickly developed rapport with the patient through his empathy with and respect for the patient's private world of creative imagination, on which he had no wish to intrude. Clearly the patient in the privacy of her diary and poetry was working through developmental issues of adolescence, and any violation of this right of privacy could have derailed a necessary developmental process. Given a mother who worried that her daughter may have been schizophrenic, respect for the patient's right of privacy seemed all the more essential.

Yet Winnicott did not entertain the possibility that her need for privacy may have been a compromise formation serving multiple functions. Perhaps her need to keep her poetry to herself without seeking an audience may have had something to do with her ideas that men write poetry more than girls because girls grow up to have and look after children and can therefore as adults only experience imagination vicariously through their children. Mothers, in contrast, have the grim responsibility of worrying about whether their imaginative children will grow up to be schizophrenic. No wonder the patient was in the adolescent doldrums if this was her conception of what adult life had in store.

The patient clearly enjoyed having Winnicott as an appreciative audience to whom to air her theories, theories that she characterized as "idle." After all, who was the patient as a "girl" to presume that her theories would be taken seriously in the world of adult "men"? If the patient experienced writing poetry as a transgression of traditional gender role expectations to which she felt expected to conform, then it might be expected that she might have had some defensive need to hide her creativity in order to disguise what may seem to her an audacious appropriation of a traditionally masculine prerogative. Mitchell (1993) noted that "the self-conscious designation or coronation of one version of self as the true self brings with it an inauthentic foreclosing of experience and an arbitrary claim made both on oneself and others" (p. 134). For Mitchell, what is true or authentic in self-experience is a social construction rather than something inherent or innate in the individual. Was Winnicott's patient "truly" a private poet who wrote only for herself, or was she perhaps "really" a poet secretly in search of an audience who would celebrate her work, or was she "authentically and genuinely" both sorts of poets simultaneously? Maybe in an unappreciative world she wrote for herself as her only appreciative audience and in a genuinely appreciative world she would have happily written for others as well.

Though it is true that the private illusion of individual selfhood needs to be hidden from others who might deflate that illusion and thereby undermine the sense of identity, Kohut (1971) suggested that the core of an individual's selfhood craves recognition, affirmation, and indeed joyful celebration. For Kohut, the self comes into being through mirroring, through being seen and reflected by others. Thus, Winnicott's fear of the deleterious effects of communication and the resultant need for a sacred domain of privacy seems to downplay the traumatic effects of an absence of communication—what Kohut would call a failure of mirroring. Winnicott seemed to have implied that only the false self was based on identification, whereas the true self reflected the person *au naturel*, unspoilt by human contact. Nevertheless, if the sense of self is based on an identification with the other's view of one's self, there could be no self-experience that is not an intrinsically social (i.e., intersubjective) experience. Though certain abilities, predispositions, and temperaments may be innately determined (e.g., musical talent), it is not until such abilities, predispositions, and temperaments are given social definition that such innate factors can become a biological basis for a sense of identity (e.g., to think of oneself as a gifted musician).

The capacity to develop a sense of identity is probably "hardwired." Stern (1985) discovered an infant is capable of intersubjectivity beginning somewhere between the seventh and ninth months of life. At this point, the infant discovers that others possess separate minds with independent points of view and intentions. Once the infant is capable of recognizing the parent's point of view, especially the parent's view of the infant, the infant may begin to identify with that point of view and make it his or her own.

Lichtenstein (1977) suggested that the sense of identity is imprinted on the infant during certain critical periods of development. The infant is granted an identity theme by the parents, largely unconsciously, and it is this identity theme that will color the developing individual's existence. Lichtenstein noted that an identity theme is not so much like an architectural blueprint that would strictly determine one's ultimate structure but rather like a musical theme that could be played out in creative variation. Whatever one's innate talents, it is the parents who grant the child a name, a cultural heritage, a social status, and most importantly the facilitating environment in which innate talents can be actualized and given personal significance.

The private illusion of unique individuality thus requires recognition and affirmation for its maintenance and development, yet it must be hidden from others in order to protect its integrity. As Winnicott noted, it is an exquisitely vulnerable illusion. There are a number of reasons for the precariousness of the sense of identity. First, as the sense of identity is based on an identification with how significant others see us, then it becomes apparent that different people see us in different lights and that even the same person may see us differently in different situations or in different states of mind. The relativity of the self is a fact of life with which one is confronted at an early age. If one's mother sees a needy baby at one moment and a cute adorable child at another, if one's father sees a chip off the old block one moment and a crybaby the next, and if one's sibling sees a rival one moment and a twin the next, then which one of those self-identities is real? Who am "I"?

The child's narcissism requires that the most flattering role relationships will be declared to reflect the "real me" and the least flattering role relationships will be declared to be "not me." Thus, as both Winnicott and Kohut noted, the child's sense of self is based on the illusion of infantile omnipotence. Role relationships that gratify the child's grandiosity and narcissistic need to idealize the parents will constitute the role relationships on which the sense of identity will be based. Role relationships that are injurious to the child's narcissism will be repudiated yet survive unconsciously, and they may return from repression and destabilize the more narcissistically gratifying sense of self that is maintained preconsciously and prereflectively. Thus, the privately maintained illusion of individuality is endangered in a variety of ways. As it is based in part on infantile omnipotence, exposure to external reality may be deflating. As it requires mirroring for its maintenance, failure of mirroring may lead to a fragmentation of the sense of self. As it is based on the repudiation of aspects of self that seem contradictory and incompatible with a particular sense of identity, that sense of identity is threatened whenever defenses fail and there is a return of repressed aspects of the self. As the sense of identity reflects an ideal sense of self, of who one is meant to be and become, any attempt at objective self-evaluation runs the risk of revealing that who one actually experiences oneself to be is indeed a far cry from who one is ideally supposed to be.

Each character type can be understood as possessing a distinctive private sense of self in which an illusory sense of identity is cultivated and protected from spoilage and loss. The obsessive-compulsive character privately cultivates the identity theme of being a morally and intellectually superior being who takes pride in self-containment and self-control. A recognized life of productivity and achievement validates this identity theme. The hysterical character privately cultivates an identity theme of being a romantic idealist. A life filled with passionate and blissful love relationships satisfies this identity theme. The depressive-masochistic character privately cultivates the identity theme of being a saint or martyr. A life dedicated to appreciated altruistic endeavors satisfies

this identity theme. The narcissistic character privately cultivates the identity theme of being an exceptionally attractive,
powerful, and successful person who stands above others in
status and prestige. A life spent being an admired center of
attention and adulation satisfies this identity theme. The
paranoid character privately cultivates the identity theme of
being a courageous and morally superior lone rebel. A life
spent winning the fight against injustice and gaining vindication satisfies this identity theme. The schizoid character
privately cultivates the identity theme of being a self-
sufficient and ironic observer of the absurdities of life. A life
spent in creative solitude satisfies that identity theme. The
antisocial character privately cultivates the identity theme of
being a top dog in a dog-eat-dog world. A life spent successfully exploiting others satisfies this identity theme.

Though an identity theme reflects a mission in life, the
actualization of which is the purpose of one's existence, an
identity theme also entails a constriction to the breadth and
depth of the personality. An identity theme provides a focus
that excludes other focuses, an exclusion that may contain a
tragic element. The obsessive-compulsive whose life is dedicated exclusively to work and achievement may never experience the joys of play, spontaneity, and abandon to one's
passions. As a consequence, life may become a burdensome,
never-ending chore. The hysteric whose life is dedicated to
romantic love may never come to feel like a responsible and
autonomous adult. A life dedicated to romance can turn into
a life filled with seduction, betrayal, and abandonment. The
depressive-masochist whose life is dedicated to selfless and
altruistic pursuits may never experience a sense of a right to
a life of one's own. As a consequence, one ends up feeling
taken for granted and exploited. The narcissist whose life is
dedicated to being a center of attention may never experience
a sense of belonging and community. Never feeling a part of
something greater than the self leads to a sense of the
meaninglessness of life. The paranoid whose life is dedicated
to being a rebel never has the experience of trusting friend-
ships with others. Despite the quest for recognition through
vindication, the paranoid remains alienated from others. The

schizoid whose life is dedicated to self-sufficiency never becomes attached to others. As a consequence a life is spent warding off feelings of loneliness. The antisocial character whose life is dedicated to successfully exploiting others never gets to enjoy that success, living in constant fear of getting caught and retribution.

Invalidation of the identity theme leads to experiences of identity spoilage and loss. When the obsessive-compulsive discovers that she is not a morally and intellectually superior person who is expertly self-controlled, she feels herself to be a humiliated failure with a pathetic weakness of willpower. When the hysteric discovers that romantic aspirations are but pipe dreams, he feels unlovable, unattractive, and worthless. When the depressive-masochist discovers that she is not a saint, she feels undeserving, pitiable, and hopeless. When the narcissist discovers that he is not an exceptional person, he feels contemptible, foolish, and ridiculous. When the paranoid person discovers that she is not a triumphant avenger of injustice, she feels a deserving object of scorn and abuse. When the schizoid discovers that he is not self-sufficient, he feels like a social deviant and outcast who is exquisitely fragile. When the antisocial person fails to be top dog, she feels like a lowly loser who is a "have not" in a world of "haves."

Identity themes reflect impossible dreams to the extent they are based on infantile omnipotence. As identity themes represent human hubris, there is a tragic inevitability in their ultimate disillusionment. Despite being doomed to pursue an identity theme that can never be fully actualized, neither can a person relinquish an identity theme, for one cannot function without the illusion of being a unique individual. Resistance to character change is essentially resistance to changing the core of one's sense of identity. The drive toward self-actualization, the need to maintain and enhance the coherency, continuity, consistency, and stability of the self constitutes the essential resistance of the personality to structural change. According to Lichtenstein (1977), the principle of identity maintenance supersedes both the pleasure principle and the reality principle. No matter how unpleasurable, anxiety laden, self-defeating, and maladaptive the pursuit of an identity theme may be, it will be pursued to the bitter end nonetheless. Thus, we are all like Cervantes's Don Quixote, driven to materialize an impossible dream no matter how naive or foolish it may seem to others.

This paradoxical state of affairs—that the privately cultivated illusion of individuality serves both adaptive and defensive functions simultaneously—creates some interesting problems in terms of character analysis. If the analyst interprets the defensive function of the illusion of personal individuality, the analyst does not merely inflict a passing narcissistic injury but is undermining the patient's sense of identity, with the result that resistance to change is intensified in the service of preserving the coherency, continuity, and stability of the self. If the analyst interprets the affirmative function of the illusion of individuality, the analyst may be supporting a constricted and limiting self-definition that seems to be the source of the patient's neurotic suffering. Should the patient be encouraged to accept him- or herself as is or attempt to change and become a somewhat different person? And what if who the patient is is someone who cannot accept him- or herself for who he or she is?

Prior to the question of how the analyst should relate to and interpret the patient's experience of a core self is the question of how it is that the analyst makes contact with the patient's experience of a core self. After all, the experience of a core self is a private experience that is hidden from others in fear of their invalidation of that aspect of self. It is the public sense of self that the patient puts forward as that aspect of the self that the patient assumes would be socially acceptable to others. The preconscious sense of self is established as a dialectic: "Though outwardly I am a normal person like everybody else, privately I am special and unique, if not exceptional." The analyst is expected to overtly mirror the patient's outward sense of normality while covertly mirroring the patient's private sense of unique individuality. The private sense of self is a sort of hallowed ground that the analyst is expected to respect without impingement, intrusion, or violation. To the extent the analyst is felt to be trespassing on this sacred domain of privacy without permission, the analyst is experienced as a disrespectful intruder who must be driven away.

There are a variety of ways in which the analyst could be inadvertently or advertently intrusive. To fail to covertly mirror the private sense of self may force the patient to seek mirroring more overtly in a manner that makes the patient feel shamefully exposed. The particularly silent, nongratifying, and abstinent analyst is likely to evoke that response. To mirror the private sense of self too overtly may lead to a sense of exposure, as such mirroring is too much like flattery that embarrasses the patient. The analyst is openly gratifying a need that the patient never admitted having or asked to have gratified. The analyst who is overzealous in being supportive and affirmative is likely to embarrass the patient in overstimulating and exposing the patient's hidden grandiosity. To treat the public sense of self as a defensive superstructure and interpret the private sense of self that it conceals may feel like a defiling psychic rape. The analyst who overzealously interprets the latent transference cannot tolerate the patient's distance, superficiality, formality, or apparent uninvolvement in the transference and has a need to quickly make contact with the patient's core sense of self.

If the analyst either explicitly or implicitly conveys that the patient's private illusion of individuality is based on immature, naive, egocentric, or unrealistic notions that do not merit respect as the self-identity of a mature adult, then the patient's private sense of self is deflated, resulting in a traumatic disillusionment with oneself. The analyst who is too wedded to a developmental model of personality change is going to be ever assessing the patient's progress in attaining so-called higher and more mature levels of development. Such an analyst will be bound by what Kohut (1977) referred to as a "mental health maturity ethic." If the analyst either explicitly or implicitly conveys that the private sense of self serves as a self-deceptive illusion that conceals a less reputable aspect of the self that has been disavowed, the patient is confronted with a negative anti-identity that undermines all that the patient ever believed and hoped him- or herself to be. The analyst who is zealously committed to the search for the truth and as such is driven to expose hypocrisy will be intolerant of the patient's self-deceptions. For these reasons the patient is judicious and exercises discretion in exposing the private sense of self to the analyst.

The implication for technique is that the analyst should be content to covertly mirror the patient's private sense of self while patiently waiting for him or her to share that aspect of the self when ready. The patient is ready when the patient sufficiently trusts the analyst to affirm rather than invalidate the private sense of self. The private sense of self, at least initially, is best addressed by providing an ambience, a holding environment or an atmosphere of safety, that ensures what Winnicott (1960) referred to as a "continuity of going-on-being." In terms of the private sense of self, a facilitating atmosphere is established in communicating an attitude or worldview that seems promising for the actualization of the privately maintained identity theme. The obsessive-compulsive must feel that the analyst is one who respects and believes in hard work and achievement. The hysteric must feel that the analyst is someone who values and appreciates romantic love. The depressive-masochist must feel that the analyst is someone who appreciates altruism and self-sacrifice. The narcissist must feel that the analyst is someone who recognizes the importance of status and prestige. The paranoid must feel that the analyst is someone who believes that the world should be a fair and just place. The schizoid must feel that the analyst is someone who can appreciate the ironic absurdities of life. The antisocial person must feel that the analyst is someone who understands that life is based on the survival of the fittest.

It is the sense of being a "soul mate" with the analyst, of sharing a common worldview, that allows the patient to trust the analyst sufficiently to begin to share the private sense of self. The response to the patient's sharing of the private sense of self is simply acknowledgment, as it is an affirmative experience for the patient when the analyst makes contact with and recognizes the patient's experience of a core sense of self.

Though the therapeutic goal is to make contact with and

affirm the patient's experience of a core self, such a goal is never achieved in some nonconflictual manner through the provision of a wholesome atmosphere, for the patient must constantly test the analyst's reliability and authenticity. The patient views the analyst as possessing a public self that conceals a private sense of self. The patient does not trust the analyst's professional self-presentation, for it seems to constitute an obfuscating facade through which the analyst can hide genuine feelings and attitudes toward the patient. The analyst's self-disclosure does not offer much reassurance, since the patient is well aware that any self-disclosure the analyst makes is likely to be highly selective, perhaps drawing attention away from the way the analyst "really" feels. Over time the patient must assess the analyst's authenticity in a variety of subtle and not so subtle ways. The patient may attempt to surprise the analyst and catch the analyst with his or her guard down. The patient may provoke the analyst in a variety of ways to see what the analyst is like under duress. And the patient may attempt to wear the analyst down and try the analyst's patience to test the durability of the analyst's commitment.

A variety of negative transferences may need to be worked through that reflect the patient's anticipation and dread of selfobject failure in relation to the private sense of self. Overall, the negative transference is that the analyst is intrusive, impinging, and disrespectful. Such a negative transference is inevitable since the fundamental rule of analysis is free association, that the patient should say whatever comes to mind without self-censorship. From the perspective of the private sense of self, the patient can only agree to this rule under duress, since the rule seems a fundamental violation of the patient's right of privacy. If agreeing to this rule, which is an implicit abdication of the patient's right of privacy, is a prerequisite for treatment, then the patient will submit to it as a precondition for being in treatment rather than because of a genuine belief in the therapeutic intent or efficacy of the rule. Thus, the treatment contract is established on the basis of a false-self compliance with the fundamental rule of analysis.

Resistance analysis is experienced as the analyst's attempt

to enforce the patient's compliance with the rule. Since the patient agrees to the rule only on a false-self basis, the patient overtly attempts to follow the rule while covertly attempting to maintain the privacy of the self. The analyst is faced with a technical paradox: how to interpret the patient's resistance to free association while respecting the patient's right of privacy. The analyst expects that analysis entails a process of unfolding, of increasing self-revelation and insight. Though it is appreciated that this process is gradual, there is an expected pace and depth of self-revelation, the absence of which is assessed and treated as resistance. Freud believed that without resistance analysis, self-revelation would come to a standstill. Though trust and rapport were thought to be prerequisite to self-revelation, trust and rapport constituted the necessary but not sufficient conditions for self-revelation. Resistance analysis was the additional and essential element that unblocked the flow of free associations. We see that the hidden transference resistance is that the patient complies with the rule of free association under duress and privately feels that the analyst is being overly intrusive and impinging to expect increasing levels of intimate self-disclosure from the patient. As the analyst by virtue of being an analyst expects increasing levels of self-disclosure from the patient and is apt to interpret derivative expressions of concealed attitudes and as the patient views this activity as invasive and violating, patient and analyst are in an adversarial relationship. The patient then asserts the private sense of self in opposition: the more the analyst attempts to expose the private sense of self, the more the patient works to oppose that exposure and thereby maintain and affirm the privacy of the self.

Each character type experiences the analyst as attempting to intrude and impinge on the patient in a particular manner. The obsessive-compulsive fears that the analyst will attempt to control the patient and rob him of his autonomy. The hysteric fears that the analyst will attempt to seduce and betray the patient and thus rob her of her innocence. The depressive-masochist fears that the analyst will enslave the patient and make him feel a fool for being so accommodating. The narcissist fears that the analyst will attempt to competitively defeat the patient and deprive her of her status and prestige. The paranoid fears that the analyst will delegitimatize the patient so that he would be a passive victim without redress. The schizoid fears that the analyst will infantilize the patient and turn her into a needy baby who has regressed to resourceless dependence on the analyst. The antisocial patient fears that the analyst needs to be a "top dog" who will steal from the patient and turn him into a loser who is one of the "have nots" rather than one of the "haves." Thus, each character type fears a particular brand of soul murder through which the sense of identity will be destroyed.

A problem with addressing such negative transferences is that they tend to remain private. To admit to such fears openly in the transference would be tantamount to exposing one's vulnerabilities to the very person with whom it is most dangerous to be openly vulnerable. The patient then must address such transference fears through unconscious or preconscious tests of the analyst, for it would seem to be a strategic error to be openly vulnerable with a person of whom one was unsure was a friend or foe. The obsessive-compulsive may be alternately obsequious and faultfinding in order to reveal the analyst's private attitudes about authority and control. The hysteric may be alternately seductive and innocent in order to reveal the analyst's private attitudes about romantic love. The depressive-masochist may be alternately submissive and complaining in order to uncover the analyst's private attitudes about altruism and self-sacrifice. The narcissist may be alternately exhibitionistic and admiring of the analyst in order to expose the analyst's private attitudes about status and prestige. The paranoid may be alternately accusatory of the analyst and soliciting of the analyst's solidarity with the patient's grievances in order to reveal the analyst's private attitudes about fairness and justice. The schizoid may be alternately coldly aloof and self-consciously timid in order to assess the analyst's private attitudes about closeness, intimacy, and attachment. The antisocial character may alternately brag and gloat over sadistic exploits and attempt to "con" the analyst in order to evaluate the analyst's private attitudes about exploitation and stealing.

The patient may be reticent to reveal these private self-doubts about the analyst's personality, for to do so might seem like an irreverent challenge to the analyst's professional self-presentation. The patient assumes that privately the analyst takes the patient's feedback personally and is insulted by whatever unflattering feedback the patient has to offer about the nature of the analyst's core self as the patient sees it. The patient may feel guilty about making a negative assessment of the analyst's core sense of self. The patient imagines that the analyst feels entitled to receive validation of the professional self-presentation and that the analyst's right of privacy is guaranteed by the fact that the analyst is under no obligation to reveal the analyst's private sense of self to the patient. To imply that the analyst's public and professional self-presentation reflects an incompetent therapist and that the analyst's private sense of self as the patient has been able to discern it reflects someone who is not a good human being at heart is then to engage in the soul murder of the analyst— a guilt-ridden though narcissistically satisfying experience. For the patient to assert the inviolability of the patient's privately maintained sense of identity, the patient may need to expose the analyst's hypocrisy and pretensions in order to destroy the analyst's presumed sense of identity. For the patient to affirm the self, the analyst must be exposed, deflated, and deconstructed. To accomplish such a task, the patient must feel sufficiently courageous to take on the analyst's narcissistic rage at being challenged and guilt if the patient were to rise to the challenge and defeat the analyst.

Winnicott (1971) discussed the importance of the patient's destruction of the analyst in the service of establishing a differentiated sense of identity:

> The subject (patient) says to the object (analyst): " I destroyed you," and the object is there to receive the communication. From now on the subject says: "Hullo object!" "I destroyed you." "I love you." "You have value for me because of your survival of my destruction of you." "While I am loving you I am all the time destroying you in (unconscious) fantasy." [p. 106]

In destroying the analyst's sense of identity and discovering that the analyst survives that destruction, the patient achieves genuine intersubjectivity with the analyst. The analyst is no longer a soul murderer with whom the patient is in an adversarial relationship but a person with whom one may engage in dialogue. Though Winnicott was wary of the deleterious effects of the core of the self establishing communicative contact with the outside world, it would seem that only in surviving an adversarial power struggle with the outside world can a differentiated and distinctive sense of individuality be securely achieved and affirmed. Only in daring to risk the self in exposing it to others and in surviving that exposure can a "real" sense of self be established, a self that is experienced as more than just an illusion. The analyst serves as a role model for this process. If the analyst survives the patient's exposure and critique of the analyst's core sense of self, then perhaps the patient can do the same in identification with the analyst.

The patient must learn to tolerate the destruction of the sense of self-identity to discover that one can survive and recover from the experience of identity loss and that one need not be so quick to defend against apparent threats to the sense of self. Personality change requires tolerating the sense of identity loss in becoming a somewhat different person from whom one had thought oneself to be. Personality change requires role flexibility, a willingness to adopt a new role in life and risk relinquishing the familiar sense of self-identity granted by prior roles. Identity formation is an evolving process in which a dialectic tension must be maintained between becoming different and remaining the same. Overemphasis on self-continuity and stability can lead to stagnation, whereas overemphasis on role flexibility could lead to identity diffusion.

I hope to illustrate in my next case example how the patient's private sense of self is hidden at the beginning of treatment and gradually emerges more overtly over time. In addition, when the patient's private sense of self emerges, the patient feels quite vulnerable in relation to the analyst, easily violated and easily deflated. The analyst must balance maintaining empathy for the identity-affirming function of the patient's private sense of self while also attempting to analyze its defensive function in repudiating self-dystonic aspects of the personality. Concurrently as the patient fears traumatic violation and deflation, the analyst may feel that his or her own private sense of self is under attack as well.

The patient, whom I will call Nelson, was a 30-year-old married man who had taken over his uncle's failing business and was trying to turn the business around. Nelson had been in and out of some sort of psychotherapy since adolescence, tending to suffer from recurrent panic attacks and low self-esteem. Currently, Nelson felt quite overwhelmed by the responsibility of turning his uncle's business around. He felt that he was in over his head and found himself procrastinating to avoid what he expected would be a failed and futile effort. Nelson had never taken work very seriously and worried that perhaps he was not a sufficiently responsible person to have taken on such a large responsibility. Despite his open admission of his insecurities, his overall manner tended to reflect the smug and superior attitude of a narcissistic character.

Nelson grew up in an upper-class, old-money New England family that encouraged "ancestor worship." His mother had grown up rich and raised him as a "spoiled rich kid" with an aristocratic sense of himself. His father came from an upper-middle-class background and had developed a successful career as a lawyer. Nelson experienced his father as a largely absent person who was absorbed in his career and who was a petty dictator on those rare occasions when he was involved with the family. During Nelson's adolescence, the family suffered downward mobility from a life in the upper crust to a life in the upper middle class as a consequence of the father's early retirement due to a heart condition.

Nelson's transfer from private school to public school proved traumatic for him. In private school Nelson had cultivated a cultured, refined persona that did not go over well in the public high school, where the "jock" mentality reigned supreme. Nelson was often teased, as his breeding and social refinement struck other students as effeminate and affected. To be accepted and win friends, Nelson became a "party animal" who drank excessively on the weekends. Whereas Nelson had been a straight A student, his grades began to plummet. During his adolescence, Nelson cultivated an attitude that was cavalier and indifferent, as though he were so above it all that he need not take anything seriously. As a result he was unable to gain admissions to any of the Ivy League schools he wished to attend and went to a small private college attended by affluent but less academically accomplished students.

Nelson did not take college seriously and did not do particularly well. At college he met his wife. She too grew up in a wealthy family that had suffered downward mobility, as her father's business, which had once been extremely lucrative, had been doing poorly. After college, they married and initiated a whirlwind social life. They both obtained jobs and spent money liberally, often finding themselves in debt. They were frustrated that they could not afford to live in the style to which they had become accustomed growing up and to which their friends whose families had not suffered downward mobility from the upper class were still living. Nevertheless, they pretended that they were simply "slumming," living a lesser life for kicks in their youth that they would somehow outgrow as they became more established.

As Nelson's career was not going anywhere, he jumped at the chance his uncle offered him to join the family business and try to turn it around. As the business had made his uncle rich at one time, Nelson hoped that it would make him rich too, solving his financial problems and returning him to a paradise lost to which he felt entitled as a birthright. His wife expected that sooner or later Nelson would provide for her as well as her father had provided for her mother while she was growing up. Yet, as previously stated, Nelson felt overwhelmed by the responsibility of running a business and fell back on his usual cavalier, indifferent, and above-it-all attitude as a defense against his fears of failure. Recognizing that if he did not become a more responsible and hardworking person the business would surely fail, he sought psychotherapy.

Nelson presented himself to me with a generally cavalier attitude. Though he acknowledged that he needed to become more motivated, initiating, and hardworking, he acted as though these would be relatively easy and quick changes to make in his personality once he decided to put his mind to it. He prided himself on being a quick learner with considerable talent, as if to say that his personality problems were rather superficial and passing issues that would not require that much in the way of treatment. Nelson tended to come late for sessions, miss sessions frequently, and accrue a balance. He was always apologetic and nondefensive in regard to his inconsistent participation in the treatment and promised to try to do better.

It seemed to me at the beginning of treatment that his cavalier and indifferent self-presentation reflected his surface-level self-syntonic sense of self and that his sense that he needed to become more responsible and hardworking was a self-dystonic pressure that he wished to deny and repudiate. Nelson seemed to be almost daring me to side with the self-dystonic pressure to be responsible just so he could defy me and prove that he was well above such quotidian expectations. I began to interpret that he felt it was beneath him to have to work for a living, and it offended his dignity to have to lower himself in such a manner. Nelson responded that he wished he had a trust fund so that he could do something that better suited his personality, like being the curator of a museum or a fund-raiser for charity. He educated me that old money, which was inherited, was better than new money, which is self-made. Nelson had always admired his maternal grandfather who had never had to work for a living and had spent his life pursuing artistic interests while living off his trust fund. In contrast, his father, who worked hard for a living, was a sour person who was seen as living a tedious, petty life.

In my recognition of Nelson's aristocratic sense of himself and as he educated me to the ways in which an aristocratic person of his breeding viewed the world, Nelson began to settle into treatment, became less anxious, and began to become more responsible at work. As he became more responsible at work, he reported that marital tensions were easing as his wife began to see him as becoming a more reliable, mature person. In the second year of treatment there was a marked shift in his self-presentation. Nelson let go of the above-it-all aristocratic demeanor and began to conduct himself as a person "on the make." Nelson confessed that he had always had dreams of restoring the family fortune and that perhaps he might become the next Ross Perot.

Nelson began to think of himself as an entrepreneur and empire builder and to express contempt for old-money pretensions. In making his own fortune, he would rise above old-money snobs like most of his friends who did not appreciate the value of money, having always taken it for granted. He would be a self-made person of substance. In contrast, his friends' lives were made by their parents' money and therefore lacked substance. Nelson seemed to see me as the repository of the middle-class work ethic with which he now identified and experienced the treatment as supporting his career efforts. His efforts at work began to pay off as he started bringing in new business and started making more money. His self-esteem and mood were much improved, as were his punctuality and attendance to sessions.

In the third year of treatment, Nelson's wife became pregnant, and Nelson experienced fatherhood as a tremendous responsibility that intimidated him. Nelson seemed extremely identified with the idea that as a father his primary role was to be a good provider and that to be a good provider he needed to raise his children in as affluent if not more affluent a manner than he and his wife were raised. Since Nelson was far from making enough money to raise his child in a way even remotely similar to that in which he was raised, he felt inadequate and became very self-critical. He felt tremendous pressure to make the business considerably more lucrative and quickly so; when he realized that he was unable to accomplish this, he felt quite anxious as well as enraged. To Nelson it was unthinkable that he might not be able to send his child to the best private schools or be able to raise his family in the right neighborhood. His wife should not have to work for a living if she did not want to, and they should be able to afford all the full-time household help they required.

In response to Nelson's self-disparagement, I countered that for an upwardly mobile middle-class professional he did not seem to be doing too badly and that it was only in comparison to an upper-crust lifestyle that he could be seen as falling short. Nelson would argue vigorously with my point of view, attempting to make the case point by point that it was virtually subhuman to raise a child in any other manner than the one to which he aspired. Nelson argued that public school education was inferior, that a child should have a full-time mother who does not work, that a child has to live in the right neighborhood and travel in the right circles in order to be properly connected in society, and so on. Though Nelson never explicitly directed his value judgments at me personally, I began to take his arguments personally, feeling that the adequacy and legitimacy of my own middle-class professional lifestyle was under attack. Whereas previously I seemed to have embodied the virtues of the middle class that seemed morally superior to upper-crust snobbery, now I seemed to be embodying its pathos. I found myself envying the lifestyle to which he aspired and resenting that it was something beyond my reach. Whereas initially in the treatment I felt elevated by my association to the upper crust through my treatment of Nelson, now I felt hopelessly déclassé.

Nelson would make casual remarks that stirred my feelings of inferiority. He noted that his friends all saw psychiatrists who charged significantly more than me, a psychologist, and who had elegant offices on Park or Fifth Avenue on Manhattan's Upper East Side. His friends would never be "caught dead" seeing a "shrink" on Third Avenue where my office was located. When I interpreted that he viewed me as a representative of the professional middle class as well as its advocate and that this was a social class in which he did not wish to become stuck, Nelson responded that it was good for him that I represented that perspective, for even though he always argued with me, that was the position in which he found himself and that he needed to accept even though he aspired to rise above his current station in life. Nelson went on to say that he wanted me to win the debate and convince him that a middle-class life was indeed a life worth living despite his doubts to the contrary. After such a dialogue, Nelson would admit that maybe his life was not so bad after all in having a good marriage, becoming a father, and running his own business at a young age. He worried that he must be sounding awfully bratty and whiney to be complaining about his circumstances, thus trying to demonstrate empathy for what he felt must be my experience of him given my modest lot in life as he saw it.

Nelson's original self-syntonic self-presentation as a cavalier aristocrat who was above taking anything too seriously could be seen in retrospect as a defensive cover for his private wish to become a self-made millionaire who would be superior to bearers of inherited wealth who are incapable of making their own money. Feeling inadequate to actualizing his private dream of making his own money, he would rather act the part of an upper-class snob than be a middle-class "nobody," as he saw it. As the pretense of being an upper-class aristocrat was becoming progressively more difficult to maintain on a middle-class income, Nelson conceded the necessity of having to face the challenge of being an aspiring upwardly mobile professional person. In my recognition of his upper-crust breeding, Nelson felt sufficiently validated to accept responsibility for making a living for himself and his family.

The acceptance of responsibility for making a living led to the revival of the secret dream of becoming a self-made millionaire. Yet no sooner was this aspiration openly acknowledged than Nelson felt traumatically deflated by its apparent unrealizability. In trying to have empathy for Nelson's sense of deflation and disappointment, he began to experience me as the source of his deflation and disappointment, as suggesting that he should settle for being middle class like me, and so he argued with me to prove me wrong. In order to prove me wrong, Nelson began to recount everything that was shamefully inferior about being middle class from an upper-class perspective. In the countertransference, I began to feel that my sense of self-respect as a middle-class professional was under attack. I realized that Nelson was communicating to me how he felt ashamed and humiliated by his downward fall into the middle class and his own difficulty accepting his current social status and its seeming permanence if he were not to become a self-made millionaire.

In many respects Nelson had unconsciously followed in his father's footsteps despite his more surface-level disidentification with his father. His mother's parents had always felt that his mother had married beneath her in marrying his father, and his mother shared that sentiment though she never expressed it openly. Nelson's mother openly adored her own father, who was a sort of free spirit who pursued his artistic interests while free of the pressure to make a living. The father, in contrast, was a grumpy, stuffy person who, although achieving a successful career as a lawyer, could never provide for his wife in the manner in which she grew up. Infusions of money from the mother's family enabled her to maintain upper-crust appearances until Nelson's adolescence, when the father's ill health forced him into an early retirement and the family needed to downsize their standard of living despite the extra money.

Nelson was in many respects his mother's son. She instilled in him a sense of being a child of privilege and a covert contempt for the father who was not seen as a truly successful or high-class sort of person. Nelson identified with his maternal grandfather, whom his mother held out as a male role model, as well as with his mother in her sense of aristocratic entitlement and superiority. In the transference, Nelson was implicitly treating me in the devalued manner in which his mother covertly treated his father but of which she was too well mannered ever to admit openly. Yet privately Nelson also felt that his mother and her values were superficial and pretentious and that his father in contrast had worked hard and had achieved something. Secretly Nelson wished to be a self-made person who would make his mark but felt inadequate as a "spoiled rich kid" to prove himself up to the task. And in Nelson's fantasies, it was not sufficient to become simply a middle- or upper-middle-class professional person like his father. He had to become rich and start a new family fortune like his great-great-grandfather who had established trust funds for his descendants, which had finally run out in reaching Nelson's generation. Nelson would inherit many expensive antiques but would not be able to afford the sort of Park Avenue apartment in which such expensive items seemed to belong.

The trauma for Nelson was in feeling that in the end he was not his mother's "golden boy," in a world in which his mother's upper-crust values reigned supreme, but a déclassé loser like his father despite pretensions to the contrary. This trauma was revived in the transference when it became apparent that even with his best attempts to run his uncle's business, he was not going to become an overnight success story. In my effort to help him assimilate that disappointment, I became the messenger who bears the bad news and who must be killed. In surviving Nelson's implicit attack on my narcissism, I enabled him to accept the blow to his own self-esteem and develop greater pride in what he had accomplished at least from a middle-class perspective. As a result of this process, Nelson began to relinquish many of his own snobbish and pretentious attitudes. Ironically, Nelson mentioned that he believed that the secret scandal in his family's ancient history was that his great-great-grandfather had been Jewish but changed his name, converted, and concealed his Jewish heritage so that perhaps his family was not quite as blue-blooded as they had always pretended to be.

Nelson began to discuss how cold and distant he felt his family had always been. He felt that his mother's side of the family had always treated him and his family with condescension as their poor relations. The lack of concern in his family had become particularly evident to him as he realized that nobody in his family had any interest in the fact that he was soon to become a father. Nelson noted that the only families in which he observed warmth and intimacy while growing up were Jewish families, and he hoped that the family he was initiating would be more like that. Another secret self appeared to be emerging in the treatment, the wish to be a "mensch." Thus in the analysis there was an attempt to maintain empathy with the patient's private sense of himself as an upper-crust aristocrat while noting how that sense of himself served to defend against learning to accept the more middle-class aspect of him that constituted a threat to his sense of identity.

11

Sadomasochism, Perversity, and the Unconscious Sense of Self

The deepest level of character analysis is the analysis of what the patient experiences as the ugliest aspect of his or her personality, the aspect that is most self-dystonic from the conscious self-syntonic sense of self. I would suggest that it is what the patient experiences as perversely sadistic or as perversely masochistic in the self that the patient makes the greatest efforts to repudiate. These aspects of the self tend to be the most destabilizing to the more consciously maintained sense of identity so that analysis is experienced as a grave threat to the patient's narcissistic homeostasis. A dynamic balance must be achieved between maintaining empathy for the patient's need to experience the self as whole and wholesome and the attempt to analyze the patient's resistance to accepting what seems to be the most reprehensible in his or her personality by virtue of its perverse and immoral nature. Empathy for the essential decency of the self must proceed yet be counterbalanced by interpretation of the defensive function of needing to construe the self as entirely decent and wholesome.

Freud (1900) believed that sexuality was the prime element of the personality that needed to be repressed and rendered unconscious. Yet it was not sexuality per se that needed to be repressed but particular aspects of one's sexuality that seemed to be incompatible with socially acceptable notions of mature sexual functioning. Thus one could speak of a manifest sexuality that is socially acceptable and tolerated in conscious awareness and a latent sexuality that is socially unacceptable and repressed. Freud (1905) suggested that it was infantile sexuality in particular that needed to be repressed, for the infant was polymorphously perverse. Repressed sexuality is, then, sexuality that is felt to be perverse rather than wholesome. It is not so much the immature or infantile quality of sexuality that is unacceptable but the perverse quality. Many aspects of infantile sexuality are not considered to be perverse and are therefore quite socially acceptable when engaged in by adults. Infants like to be hugged, petted, and kissed, and it is usually considered a sign of a warm and good person to be physically affectionate in such a manner. Perverse sexuality is sexuality, be it infantile or otherwise, that society deems to be bad, evil, or sinful and should therefore be forbidden.

There is a cultural relativity to what is considered perverse. For example, in Freud's day, masturbation and homosexuality were clearly considered perverse, whereas currently many would construe such sexual behavior as perfectly normal if not wholesome and healthy. Organized psychiatry continues to consider sexual behavior such as voyeurism and fetishism perverse, though it is ironic that those who engage in so-called perverse activity tend to believe that their sexual conduct is a normal, healthy, and perhaps superior form of sexuality in contrast to conventional sexuality, which seems perversely conformist and oppressive in contradistinction.

Perversity is not intrinsic to the sexual behavior itself but rather to the attitude that seems to be conveyed by the sexual behavior. For example, when masturbation seemed to reflect an egocentric turning-away from others, a lack of self-discipline, an addictive pursuit of hedonistic pleasure without redeeming social value, an indulgence in forbidden sexual daydreams, and for the male a sacrilegious spilling of one's seed, one could make a case for its perverse nature. Yet if masturbation is construed as a balm for loneliness, a form of tension relief and self-soothing, a creative exploration of one's sensuality and sexual fantasy life, or a private affair that expresses and affirms one's freedom of choice and personal autonomy, one could make a case that it is a normal, healthy, and growth-promoting activity. It becomes debatable whether any given sexual behavior intrinsically embodies the meaning and significance with which it has been ascribed. Sexual behavior may then function somewhat analogously to a Rorschach, an intrinsically ambiguous yet evocative stimulus that serves as a projective screen for the ascription of personal meanings.

Though it is debatable what kind of sexual behavior should be considered perverse or healthy, it becomes apparent that sexual behavior that is thought to be perverse embodies certain attitudes. Perversity appears to entail the degradation and depersonalization of the object of desire. For example, masturbation, when thought of as a perversion, is considered to be "self-abuse." To the extent that masturbation is seen as a manner of defiling rather than respecting oneself, it seems perverse. To label a sexual behavior as perverse is to hypothesize a particular relationship of the subject of desire to the object of desire, a relationship that is essentially sadomasochistic. The desired other, be it in fantasy or actuality, is treated sadistically, either overtly through abusive, domineering, controlling, and humiliating treatment or covertly through depersonalizing, dehumanizing, and objectifying treatment. It is not only the sadist who is perverse but the masochist as well, for the masochist treats the self sadistically—as a defiled, degraded, and demeaned object to be abused by others.

Sexual behavior that conveys sadistic or masochistic attitudes, be it overtly or covertly, is felt to be perverse. Normal, healthy, and wholesome sexuality would then be defined in contradistinction. Sexual conduct that appears to convey mutuality, reciprocity, equality, respect, dignity, trust, affection, warmth, nurturance, recognition, acceptance, and affirmation is felt to be socially and morally acceptable. Controversy arises when what is presented as wholesome is seen by others as perverse. For example, sexual libertines tend to believe that conventional sexual mores are perverse in that they implicitly reflect a majority domineering, controlling, oppressing, and scapegoating a minority, which is dehumanized by virtue of being made to feel shamefully deviant. Thus, heterosexual intercourse in the missionary position can be construed as perverse if it is seen as the means of enforcing the subordination of women.

People who construe their sexuality as normal, healthy, wholesome, and moral feel offended and indignant when others construe that sexual conduct as perverse. Be it the gay rights movement or the Moral Majority, people organize in order to defend their standards of sexual propriety, as they castigate opposing standards. The assignation of perversity is felt by the recipient of the assignation to be perverse in and of itself, as it is felt to be a slanderous character assassination that betrays a demeaning intent. To be seen as perverse is then an assault on one's sense of normality, health, maturity, wholesomeness, and morality. In terms of the sense of identity, it becomes apparent that an attempt is made to preserve and enhance a sense of oneself as an essentially decent person, especially in regard to one's sexuality, and to repudiate any sense that one might be perverse (i.e., indecent). Though one might play at or pretend to be somewhat indecent or perverse for the thrill and excitement of it, it is nevertheless playacting and not one's "real" self, which remains fundamentally decent and wholesome. Society might label one's sexual conduct perverse, but society is prejudiced and oppressive so that from a more enlightened perspective, one's sexual conduct could be seen as admirably liberated in a manner worthy of emulation. The fly in the ointment, as Freud discovered, is that whatever conscious pretensions we attempt to maintain of possessing a perfectly normal, mature, healthy, and wholesome sexuality, unconsciously we remain perverse, and that perverse sense of self ever threatens to return from repression.

As perversity can be understood as expressing a sadomasochistic relationship and as wholesomeness can be understood as expressing a relationship based on mutuality and

respect, the unconscious sense of self can be seen as organized sadomasochistically, whereas the conscious or preconscious sense of self is organized in terms of mutuality—or
perhaps one should say the illusion of mutuality. Freud
discovered that although one might like to think of oneself as
an essentially decent person who treats others as human
beings, unconsciously one inevitably harbors less humane
tendencies. The unconscious sense of self then stands in
polar opposition to and in conflict with the more conscious
sense of self as a basically decent and wholesome human
being, for if one is basically decent and wholesome, one
would not be a perverse sadomasochist. To the extent the
unconscious sense of self as a perverse sadomasochist returns
from repression, the sense of identity as a moral human being
is undermined. Guilt about wishing to treat others sadistically and shame about being masochistic (i.e., wishing to
treat the self sadistically) constitute the self-evaluatory affects
whose arousal functions as a signal anxiety that triggers
defensive and compensatory activities in the service of maintaining a sense of oneself as a fundamentally humane person
worthy of respect.

The source of unconscious sadomasochism has been debated. There is probably no debate that sadomasochistic family dynamics growing up intensify unconscious
sadomasochistic tendencies in adults through a process of
identification. Yet awareness of the factors that intensify
sadomasochism do not account for its origin. For Freud
(1905), sadomasochism originates in the nature of the instinctual drives themselves (i.e., oral sadism, anal sadism, phallic
intrusiveness, and vagina dentata on the sadistic side and
oral and anal receptivity and genital passivity on the masochistic side). For Kohut (1971), sadomasochism reflects a "breakdown product" as a consequence of selfobject failure. When
there is a failure of recognition, of mirroring of the child's
personhood, the child self fragments and reorganizes itself
on a defensive basis that protects it against the dread of
repeating the traumatic failure of recognition. Sadism reflects
a pathological revivification of the archaic grandiose self in
which the self will be affirmed in dominating, controlling,

and abusing others. Negating the other affirms the self in contradistinction. Masochism reflects a pathological revivification of the idealized parent imago in which the self is secured in submitting to and appeasing an omnipotent but potentially persecutory authority. The self is affirmed vicariously through connection to an omnipotent other. As selfobject failure growing up is inevitable because of the vulnerability of the child's budding sense of self and the realistic limits of parental empathy, a sadomasochistic compensatory response is invariably evoked, more or less intensely, depending on the extent of selfobject failure. As the sense of self is more securely established as development proceeds, the sadomasochistic compensation is split off and repudiated as it proves incompatible with a growing sense of oneself as a related and respected human being. In Kohut's approach, sadomasochism appears to be an innate tendency, as it would seem to be a hardwired adaptation to selfobject failure.

Lichtenstein (1977) construed infantile sexuality as an archaic form of affirming the sense of identity:

> Psychosexual development can be understood as the genetic pattern of changing modes of establishing and supporting the conviction of one's personal existence. If the more advanced, more cognition-based modes of confirming such convictions are poorly developed or break down, the archaic forms are regressively revived, and the conviction of one's existence becomes dependent on orgastic experiences. [p. 267]

Eissler (1958) suggested that the capacity for orgasm served as an ego function as well as a means of drive discharge:

> Descartes' famous "cogito, ergo sum" . . . is after all the genetic product of a long development. The infant, if it had the power to verbalize, would never base incontrovertible truth on such flimsy evidence. Rather, it would say: "I experience pleasure, hence I exist." Since the greatest pleasure available to the human organism is orgasm, I hypothesize that one of the ego functions of orgasm is to ascertain an incontrovertible truth. [p. 238-239]

Sexuality, then, serves as a biologically based mode of affirming the sense of identity, for to experience intense pleasure is to affirm that one exists. When sexuality based on relationships of mutuality and recognition break down, sexuality based on sadomasochistic relationships is evoked as a compensatory means of affirming the self, a mode of compensation that would seem to be an innate adaptation to selfobject failure.

McDougall (1985) discussed how perversions, what she calls "neosexualities," serve to maintain narcissistic homeostasis. She provided the example of a young man who sought homosexual partners every night and who was erotically satisfied only when he had obtained on his penis some trace of his partner's fecal matter.

> As a little boy he had been forced by his mother to go out in the park, where other children were playing, with his soiled underpants tied around his head. The maid, a girl cousin, and the other children would join in the hilarious humiliation of the little boy. In addition, his mother gave him frequent enemas. In his memory these acquired an erotic overtone, in contrast to the drastic punishment of the soiled underclothing. Nevertheless, this intimate contact with his mother through the enema was also experienced by the little boy as a form of phallic-anal castration. One solution was to soil his underpants in advance rather than submit to this maternal castration. The narcissistic mortification engendered by the soiling was felt to be a just, albeit intolerable, punishment for the unconsciously eroticized anal relationship with his mother. In the adult's sexual play, the same painful humiliation [that] was originally an object of horror for his mother became the motivating factor in his sexual arousal, but the height of his triumph came with the fact that it was another person's fecal matter that was now rendered visible. The partner became the one to submit to the fantasized castration and narcissistic mortification he had once experienced. [p. 253-254]

The patient's perversion as a compromise formation serves multiple functions, both self-affirming and defensive. In turning active into passive, the patient achieved a sense of mastery and control over the trauma, a triumph that asserted the patient's phallic narcissism through the achievement of erection and orgasm. Yet on the other hand, the patient's perversion served to defend against an underlying sense of humiliation and emasculation at the hands of his mother. To the extent the sexual experience was felt to be a volitional act of mutual cooperation between consenting adults it was experienced as essentially wholesome and thereby self-syntonic. To the extent the sexual experience was felt to violate the independent volition of either the self (i.e., compulsion) or the other (i.e., coercion), it was felt to be perverse and therefore self-dystonic.

Unconscious sadomasochistic tendencies represent an ever-present, competing mode of affirming the sense of self which coexists with the conscious sense of self that is organized according to a sense of mutuality that validates a sense of oneself as a moral being. Shakespeare's Richard III put it aptly when he declared, "Since I cannot prove a lover, to entertain these fair well-spoken days, I am determined to prove a villain." If affirming the sense of identity as a loving person is ruled out as a possibility, then one will affirm the sense of identity as a hateful person in its stead. Disappointment in love (i.e., failures of mutuality and recognition) awakens a dormant sadomasochistic self-organization that has been deprived self-expression because of its threat to the consciously maintained sense of being a humane and moral being. Benjamin (1988) noted that mutuality in a relationship rests on a precarious balance between self-assertion and recognition and that when this balance breaks down, the result is domination and submission. Mutuality requires asserting one's own desires while granting recognition to the desires of the other. When those desires become conflictual, it becomes problematic as to whose desires will be fulfilled and whose will be frustrated. Hopefully, a dialogue allows for a process of negotiation and compromise. But when negotiations break down, power struggles ensue.

Since everyone possesses an unconscious sadomasochistic self-organization, each character style can be analyzed in terms of its particular style of being sadomasochistic. Obsessive-compulsive characters tend to be unconsciously sadistic in being faultfinding, emotionally controlling, and emotionally withholding. They are unconsciously masochistic in being obsequious and ingratiating. Hysterical characters are unconsciously sadistic in being seductive and abandoning yet unconsciously masochistic in being mindlessly conformist as expressed in their gullibility and suggestibility. Depressive-masochistic characters are unconsciously sadistic in being help-rejecting complainers who induce guilt in others yet are unconsciously masochistic in being submissive, slavishly devoted, and overly accommodating. Narcissistic characters are unconsciously sadistic in attempting to be superior at the expense of the other's inferiority yet unconsciously masochistic in condemning the self to an empty impoverished existence devoid of genuine love and caring. Paranoid characters are unconsciously sadistic in their tendency to intimidate, coerce, and torment others yet unconsciously masochistic in setting themselves up for victimization, abuse, and humiliation. Schizoid characters are unconsciously sadistic in rejecting others by being aloof, detached, cold, and impersonal yet are unconsciously masochistic in provoking others to reject them, dooming themselves to lives of loneliness. Antisocial characters are unconsciously sadistic in their propensity for gratuitous violence and stealing from those whom they envy yet unconsciously masochistic in becoming objects of retribution.

These unconscious sadistic and masochistic tendencies prove incompatible with the privately maintained identity theme of each character type. The obsessive-compulsive does not construe the self as faultfinding but as giving constructive criticism and not as obsequious but as dutiful and conscientious. To recognize that one was faultfinding would undermine one's pride in being morally superior, and to recognize that one was obsequious would undermine pride in being autonomously self-contained. The hysteric does not view the self as seductive but as friendly and not as mindlessly conformist but as maturely accommodating. To recognize that one was seductive would undermine the sense of innocence, and to recognize that one was mindlessly conformist would undermine the sense of being a freely loving and giving person. The depressive-masochist does not view the self as a help-rejecting complainer but as someone who stoically tolerates being unfairly deprived of what one deserves and not as shamefully slavish but as altruistic. To recognize that one was rejecting would undermine the sense of charity that a saintly person should possess, and to recognize that one was shamefully slavish would undermine the sense of the nobility of self-sacrifice for a greater good. The narcissist does not view the self as arrogant and condescending but as admirably exceptional and not as empty and impoverished but as full, indulged, and sated. To admit that one was arrogant would undermine the sense of entitlement to be treated as exceptional, and to admit that one was emotionally impoverished would undermine the sense of having it all. The paranoid character does not view the self as threatening and hostile but as indignantly aggrieved and not as a victim but as a proud survivor. To admit that one was hostile would undermine the sense of self-righteous indignation, and to admit that one was a weak, passive victim would undermine the sense of invincible survivorhood. The schizoid character does not view the self as cold and rejecting but as independent, and not as a lonely and needy outcast but as happily self-sufficient. To admit that one is cold and rejecting undermines the sense of self as a gentle and sensitive human being who has compassion for the ironies of life, and to admit that one is needy and lonely undermines the sense of strength in self-sufficiency. The antisocial character does not see the self as gratuitously violent or a thief but rather as a vehicle for giving people what they deserve for being stupid, foolish, and weak and as taking what is their rightful due that has been unfairly withheld from them. The antisocial character does not see the self as feeling deserving of retribution and punishment but rather sees the self as doing everything humanly possible to avoid being caught. To admit that one is gratuitously violent undermines the sense of being just like everybody else, looking out for number one, as gratuitous violence suggests that one is inhuman in going beyond the universal need for comfortable self-preservation and survival. To admit that one feels deserving of retribution undermines the sense of not caring what others think and of smug superiority to those who are made cowards by their consciences.

The traditional goal of psychoanalysis has been to make the unconscious conscious. It becomes apparent that such a process is resisted because the conscious sense of self reflects the person's sense of identity, his or her cherished and cultivated image of self, and no one wants that self-image to be tarnished. If we are all longing for recognition, if not celebration, of the privately maintained sense of identity, then what motivation could there be for acknowledging the illusory nature of that self-identity and admitting that one harbors many tendencies incompatible with one's sense of identity? I would suggest that just as the privately maintained sense of identity must survive exposure to the outside world to affirm its reality and durability, it must also survive exposure to the unconscious sense of self to ever be experienced as genuine and authentic. To acknowledge opposing desires and aims yet remain committed to one's central identity theme nonetheless constitutes a self-affirmation of who one is as a person. The core identity may be enriched and expanded by inclusion of aspects of unconscious functioning that could be seen as invigorating. As sadism reflects a quest for recognition through mastery and masochism reflects a quest for recognition through becoming part of something greater than oneself, it is possible that even sadomasochism contains affirmative elements that may potentially strengthen the self.

The main reason, though, that the unconscious sense of self becomes accessible to consciousness and that a person may be motivated to address that aspect of self is the phenomenon Freud (1900) called a "return of the repressed." When defenses fail, unconscious content returns into conscious awareness in more or less disguised form, often in the form of distressing self-dystonic symptomatology. At that moment, the analyst may either support re-repression of formerly unconscious material or attempt to enable the patient to acknowledge and assimilate self-dystonic material that has intruded on the patient's conscious awareness.

When it is understood that re-repression of unconscious content is in the service of identity maintenance, it becomes apparent that in the long run it is always futile for the analyst to attempt to oppose the principle of identity maintenance. Thus, confronting a patient with unconscious content will only prove therapeutic when it is consistent with the aims and goals of the principle of identity maintenance. Only a self that has been securely recognized and affirmed by others is a self that is capable of risking itself in the service of confronting self-dystonic elements and affirming itself in opposition to conflicting tendencies.

The most common form of the return of the repressed in the treatment situation is in the transference. The patient projects onto the analyst a disavowed aspect of self. Such an occurrence is most likely when there is a failure of mutuality in the therapeutic relationship as sadomasochistic object relations are revived as a breakdown product. The analyst can attempt to restore mutuality to the therapeutic relationship by discovering the source of the rupture in the therapeutic alliance. The analyst can attempt to analyze the dynamics of the enactment of the sadomasochistic relationship in the hopes of establishing a dialogue about the nature of the patient's relationship with the analyst that includes acknowledgment of self-dystonic elements. To the extent the patient is intolerant of such a dialogue, the analyst may have to contain the self-dystonic elements that the patient has projected without attempting to get the patient to take responsibility for those aspects of the patient's personality. The analyst may be unable to establish or reestablish mutuality in the therapeutic relationship and will have to tolerate the patient's stabilization of the sense of self through sadomasochistic enactments without attempting to suppress such an enactment through interpretation.

The analyst can empathize with the patient's experience of the analyst as sadist or masochist or both alternately and the patient's struggle to maintain a sense of self in working with an analyst who is felt to be responsible for turning the analysis into a sadomasochistic relationship. The patient experiences the analyst as the instigator of sadomasochistic dynamics, whereas the analyst may view the patient as the instigator through the induced countertransference. Though theoretically there is no originator of the relational dynamics, as they are a product of reciprocal influence, experientially the patient perceives the analyst as the instigator and experiences the self as a marionette on a string, the string being pulled by the analyst.

The unconscious has been understood as that aspect of the self for which the patient denies responsibility and self-agency. When there is a return of the repressed in the transference, the patient views the analyst as the agent who is responsible for disavowed aspects of self. The patient then experiences the self as a reactive, passive, and helpless being at the analyst's mercy. An adversarial relationship is set up with the analyst in which the patient establishes a sense of self-agency in opposing what is felt to be the analyst's omnipotent control of the therapeutic relationship. The patient must struggle to experience the self as an agent in relation to the analyst. It is in achieving a sense of agency in relation to the analyst that the patient feels empowered to reclaim repudiated aspects of self.

The patient experiences analysis as a perverse activity to which the patient is subjected. Analysis is felt to objectify, depersonalize, and dehumanize the patient in subjecting the patient to the analyst's interpretive formulas. Though the analyst acts as if the analyst's formulations are implicit in the patient's material, the patient feels that the analyst's formulations are purely a product of the analyst's own imagination and are being foisted on the patient. The analyst is seen as perverse, as a "control freak" who "gets off" in abusing the authority granted by being a therapist and in exploiting the hapless patient. The analyst is construed as analogous to the cinema image of the mad scientist who uses living human beings as guinea pigs for scientific experimentation, experimentation that covertly expresses the scientist's megalomania and cruel indifference to human suffering. The innocent patient must somehow liberate the self from enslavement in a sadomasochistic relationship with a pervert. In extricating the self from enmeshment in the analyst's perversity, the patient affirms the wholesomeness, courageousness, and ethical integrity of the self.

The emphasis in the theory of psychoanalytic technique on the analyst's neutrality and nonjudgmentalness appears designed to put a check on the analyst's unconscious omnipotence, for like the patient, the analyst also possesses an unconscious sadomasochistic organization that could potentially return from repression in the treatment situation. The more the patient proves incapable of mutuality, the more the analyst's own unconscious sadomasochistic tendencies will be stimulated. Unfortunately, the analyst's own sadomasochistic tendencies could return from repression under the guise of analytic neutrality in being excessively silent, abstinent, and nondirective. Any analytic stance or technique could be potentially perverted to covertly express sadistic attitudes.

Though the analyst tends to be experienced as the sadist in the therapeutic relationship because of the hierarchical arrangement granting the analyst authority as a professional, the analyst may be experienced as the masochist in the relationship. After all, the analyst is the patient's employee. The patient pays the analyst for a service and may fire the analyst when the patient feels unsatisfied with the quality of that service. The analyst is then felt to be the patient's servant or slave and as such is less than fully human in the patient's eyes. The analyst is not a person but a function, a service, or a commodity that is purchased and dispensed with once it outlives its usefulness. Analysis, thus, stimulates the patient's narcissism in providing an ever-attentive audience for whom one is a center of attention in a relationship that focuses exclusively on the patient's needs and wishes. Analysis is not mutual, for there is not a mutuality of self-disclosure; it is an inherently hierarchical relationship, though who is seen as the dominant participant in the hierarchy is debatable as well as reversible. Though the analyst's refrainment from self-disclosure is often thought to establish the analyst's dominance in frustrating the patient's curiosity, it might be said that from a narcissistic frame of reference, there is no interest in audience self-disclosure. The role of audience is to listen quietly, and for a member of the audience to speak during a performance is a rude impertinence.

Analysis, through the provision of an empathic, sensitive, and attentive audience, seduces the patient into an entitled narcissistic position with the analyst in the role of masochistic servant to the patient's entitlement. Thus the analyst subtly invites dehumanization, to be treated as a selfobject function, a container, a holding environment, an auxiliary ego, a projective screen for transferences. The more the patient thinks of the analyst as a "real" person with "real" feelings, the more inhibited is the patient in expressing unacceptable aspects of the self in consideration of the analyst's personal feelings. Conversely, the more the analyst is depersonified, the easier it is to express unacceptable aspects of self, as the analyst is not felt to be entitled to personal consideration. Ultimately, the patient must resist the narcissistic seduction of analysis and recognize the analyst's humanity. For the patient to affirm his or her humanity, he or she must grow beyond using the analyst as a "lavatory," as Rosenfeld (1964) put it. The patient asserts the decency of the self in opposing the analyst's masochistic submission to the patient's narcissistic sense of entitlement. The patient must affirm the moral integrity of the self in freeing the analyst from masochistic enmeshment with the patient. Probably it is only in termination that the analyst is truly freed from submission to the patient's narcissistic expectations and the patient can affirm the personal integrity of the self.

In the following case example, I will try to illustrate how the patient's surface-level self-syntonic sense of self reflects a wholesome and morally innocent sense of self. When that sense of self is challenged and narcissistic trauma is revived in the transference, it leads to a return of repressed sadomasochistic object relations in the transference–countertransference dynamic. The patient tends to experience the analyst as a sadist who is objectifying and dehumanizing the patient through character assassination, while the analyst tends to experience the patient as a sadist who is forcing the analyst to see the world only from the patient's point of view, thereby obliterating the analyst's entitlement to a separate perspective and existence. In surviving and working through the revival of sadomasochistic dynamics with role reversals in the transference–countertransference relationship, the patient becomes able to assimilate formerly repudiated aspects of self that heretofore had not seemed compatible with the patient's sense of the self's essential innocence, wholesomeness, and moral integrity. A dynamic balance had to be maintained between empathizing with the patient's sense of essential innocence while analyzing defenses against the recognition of sadomasochistic dynamics. Of course this balance was not always achieved and when achieved had to be reachieved over and over again.

The patient, whom I will call Linda, was a 19-year-old undergraduate when I began working with her. Her presenting problem consisted of a fear of a traumatic abandonment whenever she was alone, especially when she felt deprived of male attention. As a consequence, she behaved seductively toward men, recruiting a stable of adoring admirers. Despite her desperate need for male attention, she avoided committed relationships for fear that men would be possessive, domineering, and controlling in a long-term relationship. She indeed had had that experience in her one long-term relationship with a boyfriend. Nevertheless, if she was rejected by an admirer, especially one with whom she had had sex, she felt devastated, as though she had been madly in love and had been callously jilted. Her character style given these presenting problems appeared to be predominantly hysteric.

Linda largely repudiated her fear of abandonment as well as her conviction that relationships with men boiled down to either seduction and abandonment or seduction and enslavement. Her sense of herself as abandoned or abandoning, seductive or seduced, enslaving or enslaved, and enraged or being raged at were all self-dystonic elements of her personality that she repudiated. Linda was not a rigidly defended person, for her defenses often failed, and these self-dystonic experiences of herself would emerge in her conscious awareness as traumatic states for which she would look to me for reassurance that she was not as insecure, sexually competitive, and angry a person as she sometimes felt herself to be. Instead, she prided herself on being and tried to prove to me that she was indeed a confident, independent person who related to men as equals and friends with whom she sometimes had mutually satisfying casual sexual relations. Linda was an extremely bright, ambitious, and achievement-oriented person who was a top student. As she saw it, as a young woman busy with college and preoccupied with working toward her career ambitions, which constituted her first priority in life, men would be relegated for the time being to the role of an admiring and sexually gratifying audience who would not infringe on her freedom with demands or expectations.

Linda grew up in a family that became quite stormy during her adolescence. Both of Linda's parents were brilliant people who were underachievers because of their emotional problems. Her father suffered from manic-depression that required several hospitalizations. He eventually stabilized at the level of an ambulatory chronic psychiatric patient. As a father, he could be mesmerizingly and brilliantly impressive yet also unpredictably verbally abusive, with an implicit but not acted-on threat of physical violence. Her mother tended to be rather submissive and placating toward the father. Eventually, though, during the patient's adolescence, the mother divorced the father, which restored order to the household. Unfortunately, after the divorce, the mother suffered a serious heart attack from which she was able to recover and return to work. The patient had a sister who was 10 years older with whom she had a good relationship with some degree of sibling rivalry but who was already out of the house by the time of greatest family turmoil.

Linda coped with this family environment through the development of a precocious maturity in terms of both autonomy and sexuality. She responded to her father's abusiveness in a defiant and challenging manner, in reaction to which he backed down. She coped with her mother's passivity and later illness through the adoption of a supportive and sisterly role. In her life outside the family, she became sexually active at age 12 and did extremely well at

BALANCING EMPATHY AND INTERPRETATION

school. She graduated high school at age 17 and went away to college. At age 19 when I began seeing her, she was already a junior at school and at the top of her class.

In terms of conceptualizing Linda's character structure, it became apparent how her character style served both self-affirmative and defensive functions. Her precocious autonomy, self-reliance, and sexuality clearly served as a means of survival in a chaotic, abusive, and abandoning family environment. Her sense of herself as an ambitious, achieving, and sexually active person who will eventually find a soul mate after having attained ambitious career goals reflected her respect for and belief in her own potential for growth and development. At a self-syntonic surface level, she viewed herself as a sort of "girl next door" type of person, essentially innocent and wholesome, who had been forced to relinquish her childhood innocence at an early age but who would refuse to give up her essential optimism about life despite her experiences of traumatic abuse and abandonment. To prove that she would not let herself be defeated by unfortunate family circumstances became a mission for her that she pursued with utmost determination.

Linda's self-syntonic view of herself as a basically independent, high-achieving, and sexually assertive person also served a defensive function. It served to repudiate dependency needs and fears of abandonment in claiming that she was totally independent. It served to repudiate fears of male seductiveness, unreliability, and abusiveness in claiming that she related to men confidently as friends and equals without conflict or compromise. It served to repudiate her own identification with the aggressor and denied her own seductiveness and anger toward men in claiming that she was simply a sexually assertive person who did no more than engage in mutually consenting sexual relations between mature adults.

These multilayered issues played out in Linda's relationship with me. At a surface level, she related to me in a dual manner. On the one hand, she quickly became quite dependent on me for reassurance that she was basically an autonomous, achieving, and appealing person. On the other hand, she seemed to fear that if she became too reliant on me for support and approval, it might stifle her growth and infringe on her freedom, so that she would eventually have to wean herself from me in order to regain her independence. In my facilitation of the unfolding of a mirroring transference in which I was experienced as an admiring but nonpossessive and nonseductive father figure, Linda quickly formed a positive therapeutic relationship with me, with consequent remission of symptoms of anxiety and depression. A substantial portion of each session acquired the form of a progress report to which I was expected to say little more than a few words of recognition and encouragement. Periodically, when events transpired that she experienced as a substantial blow to her self-esteem, I was expected to supply some rather firm and authoritative words of support and encouragement. Occasionally she would call me on the phone between sessions in a state of panic seeking reassurance. Since for the most part she did not experience me as disappointing her in my function as a mirroring selfobject, treatment proceeded relatively smoothly, with Linda feeling that she was making slow, steady progress.

A self-dystonic undercurrent to the surface-level self-syntonic mirroring transference that constituted an ongoing subtext to our work together reflected a less benign if not persecutory view of me. Though Linda always had genuine progress to report in terms of her academic achievement, she presented her relationships with men in a fashion that might be aptly characterized as a pseudo–progress report. She would recount varying interludes with various admiring men as though she were trying to convince me of the maturity and healthfulness of her relationships with men, yet the interludes always struck me as situations in which either Linda had been seduced and abandoned by a potential boyfriend or in which Linda had seduced and abandoned a potential boyfriend.

Linda would always present the beginning of such relationships with much excitement and anticipation. When things did not work out, although she was puzzled and disappointed, she tended to attribute her lack of success to the immaturity of the men with whom she was involved. She did not see herself having much of a role in determining the pattern of prematurely aborted relationships that seemed to be emerging. Linda looked to me for reassurance that her approach to relationships was basically healthy and mature. I knew it would not have been genuine on my part to offer that sort of reassurance. Yet I realized that even tactful introductions of my own point of view—that some sort of self-defeating unconscious repetition of the relationship with the father was being enacted—would be experienced by her as unempathic and questioning her maturity and mental health. When she brought in a new relationship to recount with enthusiasm and excitement and I noted the repetitive pattern at work, Linda felt that I was "raining on her parade." And when the relationship soured, she felt that I was smugly self-satisfied that my prediction of difficulty proved to be an accurate forecast, and she was forced to concede that I had been right all along.

Knowing that I was exposing a narcissistic vulnerability in trying to elucidate her role in her self-defeating pattern of relationships with men, I attempted to frame my interpretations in a manner I hoped would demonstrate empathy for the injury that I knew I would be inflicting. I made interpretations along the lines of "Given the pride you take in your independence, it is difficult to admit to yourself how dependent you are upon male approval" and "Given how hurt you have felt when men have seduced and rejected you, you feel guilty when you realize that you have treated men similarly." Linda usually responded to such interpretations with a huge sigh of relief and verbal agreement couched in a slightly begrudging tone of voice. She would studiously work with such insights, and we would trace them back in terms of her relationship with her father. Yet the tone of such analyses suggested to me that she experienced my apparently correct interpretations of her problems with men as a deflating and sobering reminder of a depressing reality to which she would begrudgingly submit if I forced her. It was as though she were a naughty little girl engaging in forbidden sexual antics that she then exhibited to me with total innocence and to which I, in the role of a stern, moralistic, and sexually

possessive father, would respond with rebuke and prohibi-
tion. Linda would then implicitly promise to be good and
never transgress again, only to repeat the pattern once more.

This brings us to an incident that occurred during the third
year of treatment. I observed that Linda was becoming
progressively and more overtly angry at me as I continued to
"catch" her in her typical pattern of relationship with potential boyfriends despite always presenting these relationships
as though she had finally broken the old pattern and achieved
something more healthful. She also began to complain of
being bored with the treatment and experiencing it as a chore,
so I decided to reflect what I believed to be her surface-level
anger at me for seeing her relationships with men as problematic. Initially, Linda deflected the suggestion that she was
angry with me, saying that she was only angry with herself
for being unable to break her pattern with men after working
on it for several years.

The next session, though, Linda came in and in a tone of
self-righteous indignation announced that now she really was
angry at me for falsely accusing her of being angry at me
when she really was not angry at me at all and had only been
angry with herself. She stated that it was unfair of me to see
her as an angry person when in fact she felt she had been a
hardworking person who always tried to be appreciative of
my helpfulness. Recognizing that my interpretation of her
anger at me had been experienced as a narcissistic injury, I
tried to empathize with her experience of me in the negative
transference, reflecting that it must be difficult to come into
sessions feeling unfairly accused of being an angry person
and unappreciated for her efforts to do the best she could.
Linda then went on to say that she experienced me as an
overly demanding person who would never feel that her
progress was good enough no matter how hard she tried and
that she was tired of trying to keep pleasing a person who
could not be pleased. Linda immediately noted that such
feelings toward me echoed her experiences with her father.
And at the time in my countertransference, I felt like a
moralistic and angrily prohibitive father but guilt-ridden
about feeling that way and trying to be the opposite. Yet I also

felt unappreciated for what I thought was my fairly successful effort to be the opposite—a benign, accepting, and nonpossessive father.

Whenever I relinquished the role of a purely mirroring father figure and attempted interpretation of self-dystonic aspects of Linda's relationships with men, Linda began to experience me as controlling and persecutory, and I began to experience myself in such a manner. Rather than shy away from addressing the self-dystonic and remain in a sort of pseudo-mirroring relationship that denied unpleasant realities, I proceeded to address her self-defeating patterns with men, though remaining ready to empathize with her experience of me as an unreasonably critical and overly demanding person who would never be pleased with her. In response to my exposure that her relationships with men were neither as innocent nor as wholesome as she presented them, I evoked a dreaded narcissistic trauma in the transference, the experience of never being good enough and never pleasing her father no matter how hard she tried to win his approval. He had been quite verbally abusive of her despite her continual efforts to prove herself to him.

Working through this trauma in the transference was a pivotal therapeutic experience for Linda. The next session she came in and announced that she no longer wished to spend most of her sessions giving me a progress report because she realized she utilized this tactic as a way of postponing discussions of what was problematic for her until the end of the session, when I had finally exposed it but it was too late to address the difficulty in depth. She also acknowledged that she had a temper, which I had never seen, but that at school she was known as someone who could be quite cutting if provoked so that people rarely crossed her. Linda admitted that she did not like this side of herself, for it reminded her of her father's verbal abusiveness. Thus she became aware of her unconscious identification with the aggressor and her conflictedness about this identification.

After this session I found myself feeling quite free to make interpretations without trepidation lest I be perceived by Linda as persecutory. A short time later Linda developed her first long-term relationship with a boyfriend in over 3 years, a relationship in which there was considerable open dialogue and that did not seem to reflect the intensity of underlying sadomasochistic dynamics characteristic of her previous relationships with men. I was able to respond in a genuinely mirroring manner to her updates of her progress in this relationship, although more subtle sadomasochistic dynamics began to emerge in her covert contempt for and boredom with her boyfriend when he was seen as being overly nice (i.e., passive, weak, and emasculated by her). Thus, as in her relationship with me, Linda could become unconsciously provocative of phallic aggression to which she would masochistically submit when she became frightened of intimacy with a man willing to gratify her dependency needs.

Linda began to discuss issues related to her identification and disidentification with her mother, whom she perceived as a masochistic person. On the one hand, she did not want to be like her mother, who was seen as passive in relation to her father. Linda hoped to be the opposite of her mother in that regard and be self-assertive and challenging in relation to men. On the other hand, Linda felt that her mother was a good, nurturant, and intelligent person whom she hoped to emulate. Yet Linda found herself in a guilt-ridden position in relation to her mother, on whom she was dependent for financial support. Though overtly her mother seemed to be quite generous and happy to support her daughter, covertly Linda believed her mother resented supporting her and was in fact severely depriving herself to send Linda to college. Linda then felt as though she were exploiting her mother, guilty about that exploitation, and resentful in feeling indebted and indentured to her mother. Thus for Linda, a potentially nurturant man was seen as a masochistic woman like her mother, in relation to whom she would become an abusive and exploitative man like her father. Reparations for this exploitation and abuse would make her indebted and indentured to the nurturant/masochistic man-mother. In order to preserve her autonomy, Linda had to maintain a certain distance from such relationships while covertly requiring such relationships to meet her dependency needs.

12

Role Reversibility and the Bipolarity of Self and Object Experience

Character analysis is complicated by the severity of the patient's psychopathology. There is considerable controversy as to whether the principles of technique that apply to a neurotic character also apply when a patient presents as a chaotically organized person (i.e., borderline personality) or as a very brittle and rigidly defended person who is quite disorganized beneath his or her functional facade (i.e., pseudoneurotic character). Do such persons need to be treated even more sensitively than higher-level patients because their precarious adjustment could be easily destabilized by the analyst's being a "bull in a china shop"? Or do such persons need an even more confrontative approach in order to address their primitive defenses, which will rule the day and preclude growth unless actively and consistently addressed? With more disturbed patients this polarization in psychoanalytic theory has been symbolized by the dynamic tension between the work of Kernberg and that of Kohut (i.e., analysis of primitive defenses versus empathy for archaic selfobject needs). I would suggest that empathy for archaic selfobject needs must precede yet be counterbalanced by the interpretation of the defensive function of archaic selfobject transferences (i.e., transferences that exert some degree of omnipotent control over the object as though the object was experienced as a vital aspect of the patient's self).

In terms of character change, the central dialectic is the tension between identity maintenance and identity formation. Identity maintenance is a conservative force that preserves stability and continuity, whereas identity formation is a progressive force that promotes change, growth, and development. Too much change can lead to identity diffusion, whereas too much stability and continuity can lead to characterological rigidity and constriction. Since the sense of identity is an intersubjective as well as an intrapsychic phenomenon, the dialectic between identity maintenance and identity formation will be influenced by the dialectic between the intrapsychic and the intersubjective. As the sense of self arises on the basis of identification with the other's view of the self, identity remains the same to the extent one is seen in a consistent light by others and identity changes to the extent one is seen in a changing light by others.

When the dialectic tension between identity change and identity maintenance is sustained, a dynamic balance is preserved between change and continuity in psychic life. When the balance breaks down, the result is either identity diffusion or characterological constriction and rigidity or some oscillation between identity diffusion and characterological rigidity. Kernberg (1975) suggested that identity diffusion is characteristic of a borderline level of psychostructural integration. In borderline self-experience, good and bad representations of self and others fail to achieve integration. As a result, there is a constant sense of identity spoilage and loss, as the self is experienced as totally good one moment and totally bad the next, and the objects that mirror the self are experienced as totally good one moment and totally bad the next. As the dialectic between self and other breaks down, healthy role flexibility becomes pathological role fluidity and interchangeability, as role reversals in relationships occur rapidly, sowing the seeds of confusion as to who is assuming what role.

If borderline functioning is considered to be a level of psychostructural integration characterized by rapid and intense fluctuations between antithetical self-experiences and by rapid and intense role reversals in interpersonal relationships, then one might think in terms of borderline styles in order to understand how each character type functions when at a borderline level of psychostructural integration. Obsessive-compulsive characters, when functioning at a borderline level, rapidly oscillate between a sense of moral authority, outrage, and condemnation and a sense of failure, weakness of will, incompetence, and lack of control. In interpersonal relations, confusion exists as to who is entitled to be the critic and who deserves to be critiqued. Hysterical characters, when functioning at a borderline level, rapidly oscillate between a sense of rage and humiliation at being betrayed and a sense of worthlessness, ugliness, and unlovableness. In interpersonal relations, there is confusion as to who has been seductive and who has been seduced. Depressive-masochistic characters, when functioning at a borderline level, rapidly oscillate between a sense of reproachfulness at having been abused and abandoned and a sense of defile-ment and degradation. In interpersonal relations, there is confusion as to who has abandoned whom and who should be feeling guilty for being cold and ungiving. Narcissistic characters, at a borderline level of functioning, rapidly oscil-late between a sense of being enraged at rude, impertinent, insulting, and offensive others and a sense of being pathetic, ridiculous, lowly, and foolish. In interpersonal relations, there is confusion as to who is higher in status and who is lower. Paranoid characters, at a borderline level of function-ing, rapidly oscillate between a sense of being a self-righteous avenger and a sense of being a passive, impotent scapegoat. In interpersonal relations, there is confusion as to who is the abusive party and who is the victim. Schizoid characters, at a borderline level of functioning, rapidly oscillate between a sense of hatred toward impinging and intrusive others and a sense of being inhuman, deviant, and shamefully abnormal. In interpersonal relations, there is confusion as to who is rejecting whom and who is the one who is cruelly indifferent, uncaring, unavailable, and cold. Antisocial characters, at a borderline level of functioning, rapidly oscillate between a sense of murderousness toward exploitative others and terror of being exploited. In interpersonal relations, there is confusion as to who is exploiting whom and who is gaining the upper hand over whom.

Borderline identity diffusion reflects a return of the repressed unconscious, sadomasochistic organization in projected form as an archaic means of compensating for the breakdown of an identity sense based on mutuality and recognition. When the self is construed as acting aggressively, there is a sense of humiliated fury that the other has committed a grievous offense against the self and must be blamed and punished to vindicate the self. The self is not construed as sadistic but rather as a morally justified individual who is meting out well-deserved punishment. It is the other who is construed as sadistic, abusive, overly critical, cruel, mean-spirited, unfair, ungiving, cold, merciless, envious, spoiling, and so on, and as such the other is deserving of criticism and punishment for acting immorally. When the self is construed as the object of the other's aggression, there is no sense of being masochistic but only of being a helpless, passive, impotent, and essentially innocent victim who is being unfairly demeaned and degraded against one's will. When the other is construed as weak, inadequate, helpless, impotent, inferior, needy, and so on, those traits are construed as moral failings that are deserving of contempt, ridicule, and condemnation and undeserving of empathy, consideration, or caring.

In the borderline state, it is the other who is construed as either sadist or masochist. The self is affirmed in contradistinction to the other. If the other is a sadist, then the self is an innocent victim who in a courageous act of self-assertion will punish the sadistic other and thereby vindicate the self. If the other is a masochist who is shamefully needy, inferior, weak, and pitiful, then the self is an admirably superior person who is morally entitled to look down on inferior specimens of the human race. The masochistic other is construed as an immoral malingerer who is making an unreasonable claim for special entitlements and privileges on the basis of being an innocent victim of some affliction or abuse. If the masochist is a moral weakling without self-respect who debases the self in order to abdicate responsibility, then the self can be defined in contradistinction as strong, responsible, and self-respecting. In viewing others as perversely sadistic or as perversely masochistic, the self can be affirmed in contradistinction as moral, strong, whole, and wholesome. An illusion of being a humane, moral, and strong person is maintained but at the expense of the other, who is dehumanized and treated as a scapegoat.

Unfortunately, such a strategy of affirming the self is intrinsically unstable as it requires mirroring selfobjects who will accept the role assignment as either evil sadist or lowly masochist. As others tend to reject such role assignments in the service of maintaining their own self-regard and view the attempt to place them in such a role as an attack on their own self-respect, others may counterattack in self-defense, further destabilizing the person functioning at a borderline level. Even if others were to accept such unflattering role assignments, the self would not be stabilized in the long term, as the other would become an object of omnipotent control and as such could not serve as a genuine source of external validation. To the extent that validation is coerced from the object and is not freely given of the other's volitional choice, that validation is a hollow and inauthentic gesture that at most supports a self-deception. Because a self-identity based on the omnipotent control of others requires sustaining an illusion that denies intersubjectivity, it is an extremely precarious illusion, as others will invariably express their otherhood. In addition, since there is unconscious knowledge that one is exercising omnipotent control over others and in effect negating the true identity of the other, there is an unconscious sense of guilt about the attempted soul murder of the other and, as a consequence, fears of retribution that return from repression in the form of persecutory anxiety, which destabilizes the sense of identity.

Each character type functioning at a borderline level can be understood in terms of the rationalization that is used to justify the projection of sadomasochistic dynamics. The obsessive-compulsive feels justified in being highly critical of the other, as the other seems to deserve being harshly critiqued by virtue of being careless, sloppy, weak-willed, poorly controlled, and holding to low standards. The hysteric feels justified in blaming and abandoning the other as the other has committed the heinous act of seduction and betrayal. The depressive-masochist feels justified in being reproachful and complaining, as the other has proven heartless in being abandoning or abusive. The narcissist feels justified in being devaluatory, ridiculing, dismissive, and derisive, as the other has been rude, impertinent, insulting, and offensive. The paranoid feels justified in being punitive and retaliatory, as the other has been evil, devious, and treacherous. The schizoid feels justified in being coldly rejecting and detached, as the other has been intrusive, impinging, and invasive. The antisocial person feels justified in being exploitative or violent, as the other is equally violent and exploitative, so why let the other get the advantage in acting first?

The treatment approach to borderline dynamics has been controversial. Kernberg's (1975) approach was essentially a defense analysis approach with a knowledge of the operation of borderline defenses such as splitting, denial, projection, introjection, projective identification, idealization, and devaluation. These defenses functioned to ward off recognition of sadistic, hateful, hostile, rageful, envious, and spoiling wishes that evoke persecutory anxiety. These defenses were destabilizing in interfering with and precluding the development of more integrated levels of functioning. For Kernberg, the attempt to maintain a view of the self as innocent victim or normally superior being and a view of the other as immoral sadist or pathetic masochist was essentially a self-deceptive illusion that served as a defense against the anxieties inherent in taking responsibility for one's unconscious sadomasochistic tendencies. Thus, Kernberg tracked all the defensive role reversals that the patient utilized in order to project accountability and blame onto others and thereby divest the self of the sense of self-agency. Kernberg consistently—or, some might say, relentlessly—confronted the patient with his or her evasion of moral self-agency in interpreting the patient's warded-off aggression and fear of retaliation for that aggression. Kernberg appeared to feel that to do otherwise would be to collude with the patient's unconscious omnipotent control, abuse, devaluation, and dehumanization of others. Since patients do feel unconsciously guilty about such conduct, the analyst must demonstrate personal integrity in resisting the patient's omnipotent control and insisting that the patient take responsibility for the disclaimed mistreatment of others.

From the perspective of the principle of identity maintenance, it is clear that Kernberg's approach destabilized the patient's narrowly and precariously established sense of identity as an innocent victim who had to aggressively assert the self against malevolent objects in order to establish self-respect. Since Kernberg viewed such a sense of identity as essentially pathological (i.e., a self-deception that denied personal responsibility while rationalizing the mistreatment of others), he had no problem in confronting and challenging that sense of identity by interpreting its defensive function. Given that a sense of identity based on the revival of sadomasochistic dynamics reflected a compensatory response as a consequence of a failure of mutuality, what was to be expected if that compensatory response was challenged? The result often tended to be a further intensification of sadomasochistic dynamics in the service of compensation, which would only seem to have brought the patient further away from achieving mutuality. The patient was driven either to defy or comply with the analyst's destabilizing defense analysis.

A brief verbatim account of a session from Kernberg and colleagues (1989) illustrates a borderline patient's experience of compliance to the analyst's interpretive approach. The example was used to demonstrate how in the advanced stage of the treatment of a borderline patient the analyst could interpret both sides of a conflict simultaneously that had previously been totally dissociated.

Patient: I just saw *Foreign Affairs* on your desk, which proves you read other things beside psychiatry. You can do all that and I barely manage to go from day to day. I just hate you. I've been resentful of all this, and on top of that you are surrounded by all these secretaries who come rushing in. There is

no privacy here. Why can't I see a therapist who has an office
in town where it's silent, where there's nobody else around,
rather than here with all these mechanical women moving in
and out?

Therapist: I have a sense that your anger with me *really* [italics
added] bridges two contradictory reactions. One, a sense of
intense resentment of me as a powerful male whom you hate
and envy since you feel that men have it made. This feeling is
directly connected to the resentment you have when your
boyfriend tries to approach you sexually and you get dis-
gusted with his erect penis. On the other hand, I think you
have a completely different kind of emotion in which you feel
that you could accept me and tolerate me if you were inti-
mately linked to me in an exclusive woman-to-man relationship, but you feel you don't have a chance with all these
secretaries who *really* own me. I think that these two contradictory reactions to me are bridged by rage at me. That rage
protects you both from feeling resentful, as you get enraged
and try to throw me out of your mind, and from being afraid
of all these women who will not tolerate that I exist for you
alone in a quiet office in town.

Patient: (Listening intently and appearing less angry) Why do
you have to make such long, endless interpretations? I know
most of the stuff anyhow. You don't let me express my
feelings towards you. You immediately have to link it with
other things. You can't tolerate that I should have feelings
towards you. [p. 123]

In the follow-up discussion of this brief verbatim account,
there is no consideration of the patient's response to the
interpretation, as though it could be taken for granted that
this was a well-timed interpretation that was well received by
the patient. After all, the patient listened intently, became
less angry, and agreed with the content in claiming to know
it all already.

Yet given the patient's response, it seems plausible that
although the patient may have agreed intellectually with the
content of the interpretation, the patient appeared to have
experienced the interpretation as a lot of intellectualization
that she was expected to take seriously and that diverted her
from the discussion of what she believed were her more

genuine feelings. A more surface-level and self-affirmative reading of the same material is that the patient complained of being barely able to manage from day to day and envies the therapist, who was obviously an active, successful, and important person. The patient found the ambience of the treatment mechanical and busy and would have liked a therapeutic ambience offering greater privacy and solitude. The request for a change in therapeutic ambience at a manifest level stemmed from her experience of herself as someone with profound difficulty coping from day to day and therefore requiring a more personal and less impinging environment. After the therapist responded to her request with a "deep" interpretation that bypassed the manifest content, the patient complained that the therapist stifled her self-expression. In addition, she entertained the hypothesis that the therapist was unable to allow her to express herself because of the therapist's compulsive need to make connections and inability to tolerate her feelings.

It is not that I would disagree with the accuracy of the therapist's formulation, and certainly the patient did not seem to be threatened by the content in any way. Yet the therapist was not working from surface to depth and seemed oblivious to the most surface-level readings of the material. Perhaps the therapist did not believe it was necessary to work from surface to depth at an advanced stage of the treatment and could bypass discussion of the manifest content at a surface level. The result was a patient pleading with the therapist for greater freedom of self-expression yet sounding somewhat resigned to enduring the therapist's textbook precision and pedantic exposition. The therapist did not even seem to register the obvious manifest content of the patient's communication, as the patient's communication was immediately and expertly translated into its latent content. The therapist then explained to the patient what her anger "really" meant.

The manifest content could just as easily be interpreted in Winnicottian as Kernbergian terms. In Winnicottian terms, the patient appeared to be asking the therapist to provide a holding environment in which the patient's continuity-of-going-on-being would not be disturbed so that the patient may have begun to discover in privacy and solitude her true self rather than continue a stable though false self adjustment based on compliance to external demand. Perhaps the patient's manifest sense of self as a barely managing person who required privacy and solitude in order to express herself may have served a defensive function. Yet prior to interpreting the defensive function of such a self-concept, it must first be recognized. The therapist's interpretation implied that the therapist saw the patient as only resentful, envious, and inappropriately sexually possessive. The therapist did not see or respond to that aspect of the patient that seemed to be reaching out to the therapist to establish a more genuine, open, and mutual dialogue with the therapist despite the therapist's propensity in the patient's eyes for making long, endless interpretations.

Kohut (1971) developed a different approach to working with the revival of sadomasochistic object relations in the treatment situation. He focused on the affirmative function of sadomasochism as opposed to its defensive function. If the patient needed to devalue the analyst, then it was understood to reflect a means of affirming an archaic grandiose sense of self. If the patient needed to submit to the analyst, then it was understood to reflect a means of securing the self by merging with the analyst as an idealized parent imago. If the patient obliterated the analyst's individuality by treating the analyst as identical to the self, then it was understood to reflect a means of normalizing the self and feeling a sense of belonging and commonality in construing the analyst as a twin. Whereas interpreting the defensive function of the patient's sadomasochism appears to stimulate further psychological decompensation with a concurrent intensification of sadomasochistic dynamics, to empathize with the affirmative function of sadomasochistic object relations appears to stabilize the self at least temporarily.

The critique of Kohut's approach has been that it may gain transient symptom relief in bolstering defenses but that it does not lead to long-term structural change. Kohut (1971) developed a theory of structural change based on the concept of transmuting internalizations. Since the analyst's empathy is imperfect, the analyst inevitably fails to affirm the patient's sense of self. If the selfobject failure is not of traumatic proportions, the patient survives this failure and through a transmuting internalization learns to affirm the self in a manner analogous to the way in which the analyst successfully affirmed the patient's self prior to the selfobject failure. The patient internalizes a lost selfobject relationship as a means of preserving it. The problem, though, with Kohut's approach is that at the borderline level of functioning all selfobject failures, no matter how small in the analyst's eyes, are experienced as being of traumatic proportions in the patient's eyes, so that the patient reacts with a pathological compensatory response rather than effecting a transmuting internalization. The patient's omnipotence cannot forgive the analyst for being imperfect or tolerate the loss of omnipotent control without going into a rage or panic. Only restoration of omnipotent control alleviates the rage and panic, a restoration that precludes the establishment of a transmuting internalization. It would seem that Kernberg's approach constitutes an assault on the patient's omnipotent control in relentlessly confronting the patient with the analyst as an external object beyond omnipotent control. Kohut's approach appears to constitute a submission to the patient's omnipotent control in the naive hope that the patient will gradually recognize the analyst's humanity if the analyst serves as a "good enough" selfobject who caters to the patient's sense of entitlement.

A case from Stolorow and colleagues (1987, pp. 108-111) reflects the way in which the self-psychologically oriented analyst may unwittingly confirm the patient's sense of being omnipotently controlled by others in a manner that may in the long run undermine the development of a greater sense of self-agency and mastery. The case was utilized to demonstrate the intersubjective approach to the treatment of "borderline states."

The patient was a 23-year-old college student when he began treatment in a marked state of overstimulation. He had not been able to attend classes or concentrate on his work. At night he would take to the streets, where he had been approached for homosexual purposes. In the sessions he gave the impression of someone desperately wanting to cling to someone or something around which he might begin to reorganize and restructure himself. Yet the patient was frightened that he might be used to fulfill the analyst's needs. When this was interpreted, an early idealizing transference developed, and the patient began to resume a stalled developmental process.

The patient's father had always reacted to any weakness or shortcoming with impatience and contempt. This situation entered the analysis because the patient's father had assumed financial responsibility for the treatment and resented the burden of payment. The son's treatment was a source of shame for the father. As the analysis did not seem to be leading in the direction of making the patient into the son for whom the father wished, there were increased difficulties in the relationship.

After 2.5 years, the analyst notified the patient that he was raising his fees generally though he realized that complications might ensue. The request came at a time when the patient's relationship with his father was particularly strained. The patient's initial response was anger followed by a remark to the effect that of course he knew how the analyst felt because everything was going up in price. The analyst interpreted the patient's tendency to substitute an understanding of someone else's position for an expression of his own and his fear of the analyst's reaction to his own feelings. Gradually over the course of the next few sessions, the patient expressed his hurt, disappointment, and violent anger over the analyst's failure to "ever" consider him first. It revived feelings of always having been a burden, a supplicant who stood in the way of other people's plans or enjoyment. The patient was a twin whose brother had always been exactly the child the parents had wanted.

The patient felt that the analyst had put him in a "bind." The patient had started a new job and had been "forced" to ask his father for money for clothes. It was humiliating to ask for money as he "would have to" face a review of how long he had been in treatment and how long it would take. "How could the analyst, knowing all this, *choose* to put Jeff through it!" (p. 110, italics added) Frequently after expressing himself unabashedly, the patient would huddle up in a corner, wrapping his arms protectively around himself. He was sure the analyst would see him as selfish and be furious. A host of memories emerged of how both father and mother expected considerable conformity to their wishes. The rules to which he was expected to conform were treated as sacrosanct. And some of the expectations were rather extreme, like being expected to urinate before every auto trip and his mother checking on him just to make sure that he did not put one over on them.

The patient's response to these experiences was a feeling of "absolute powerlessness." Once when he threatened to run away from home and his parents made no attempt to stop him, he realized that he was "stuck" because nobody else would want him and he would have to "give in." Thus the patient found it necessary to define himself around what was expected of him and subjugate his self despite his tremendous resentment.

The treatment demonstrated the analyst's capacity to empathize sensitively with the patient's experience of powerlessness and rage in the face of expectations to conform or be treated punitively in a variety of shaming, guilt-inducing, and abandoning ways. In addition, the analyst accepted the patient's wish to be accepted by someone on whom he could depend who would not demand his compliance as the price of dependency. Yet the analyst also seemed to accept at face value if not inadvertently confirm the patient's experience of himself as someone who was "forced" to depend on his father for money, who was "stuck" in a "bind" that the analyst "chose" to put him in, and who in the end had to "give in" to these humiliations. The analyst may have been implicitly mirroring and confirming the patient's sense that he lacked self-agency, whereas the analyst was the only one in the room who possessed freedom of choice. If one had questioned the patient's point of view rather than simply mirror it or empathize with it, one might have noted that the patient could have taken out a loan or borrowed money to pay for the increase in fee, the patient could have tried to get more work income to pay for an increase in fee, the patient could have asked his mother rather than his father to make up the increase in fee, the patient could have attended fewer sessions in order to cover the increased fee, the patient could have asked the analyst to suspend the fee increase in his case because of the circumstances and risk being refused, or the patient could have gone to a low-cost clinic and not have to rely on his father at all for the fee.

The patient could have been plausibly construed as unconsciously making a choice around a variety of options and unconsciously choosing reliance on his father for money despite the humiliation involved. The patient may have felt that he was "forced" to choose between the lesser of a variety of evils if there was perhaps a good reason why each of the aforementioned options did not seem preferable to relying on his father. Nevertheless, the patient made a difficult and anxiety-ridden choice that was denied in having presented himself as a person without a sense of self-agency subject to the omnipotent control of heartless or sadistic others. In fact, the patient set up the relationship with the analyst in a particular manner right from the start. Many college-age students with limited financial resources independent of their parents who wish to establish financial independence from their parents go to a student counseling center or a low-cost clinic when they need treatment. The patient in this case went to a private practitioner for psychoanalysis, placing himself by unconscious choice in a position of humiliating dependency on his father given that it did not seem that in the near or distant future he would be able to pay his own way. The patient apparently was not interested in assuming a burden of debt to pay for his analysis himself.

Perhaps the patient was not so much "forced" into this humiliating arrangement with his father as he unconsciously chose it over other equally viable, more independent, and less humiliating options for obtaining treatment. Was the patient unconsciously invested in maintaining the sadomasochistic tie to his father? Did he feel unconsciously entitled to his father paying for a costly analysis with a private practitioner and enraged about having to assume the responsibility of either paying for it himself through the accumulation of debt or seeking out a treatment at a cost commensurate with his ability to pay for it by himself? Was the father "only" a shaming and contemptuous sadist in relation to his son or "also" in part a guilt-ridden masochist who begrudgingly felt obligated to pay for an expensive treatment in which he did not wholeheartedly believe? After all, might not the son have unconsciously identified with two extremely entitled parents and experimented with turning the tables every now and then in seeing if he could succeed in getting others to submit resentfully to his wishes? Had the patient unconsciously established a sadomasochistic tie to the analyst in which he reproached the analyst as a helpless person without choice who was forced to endure a humiliating arrangement with his father in order to maintain a humiliating dependency on an analyst whom he could not afford on his own?

It is quite possible that in interpreting the patient's denial of unconscious self-agency and choice, the patient would have become enraged at the analyst's lack of empathy for the patient's felt lack of a sense of free choice. The analyst might have been experienced as blaming the victim. The analyst might have been experienced as shaming the patient for his lack of independence and pressuring the patient to assume a level of independence for which he did not feel prepared. Yet such a confrontation may also have enabled the patient to deal more directly with his fears of succeeding independently of his father's assistance. Maybe he had been too frightened to run away from home as a child, but perhaps he was ready to leave home as a young adult out of college. In confronting the patient's denial of self-agency, the analyst was implicitly affirming a sense of the patient as someone who could make difficult choices, establish financial independence from the father, and be strong enough to tolerate a difference of opinion or conflict with his analyst. To avoid such confrontations was perhaps to imply the exact opposite and thus verify the patient's unconscious doubts about his capacity to succeed independently of his father or his idealized analyst.

Perhaps the patient needed not "only" an idealizing selfobject on whom to depend for a sense of security but also a selfobject who would facilitate the development of self-agency in a patient who reproachfully decried the lack of it.

If the problem for the borderline patient is a breakdown of mutuality or a failure to achieve mutuality in the first place, then neither Kernberg's nor Kohut's approach addresses the issue of how mutuality and intersubjectivity is reestablished or established in the first place. Kernberg denied the patient's reality in dismissing it as a defensive organization, and Kohut denied the analyst's separate reality in affirming the patient's reality sense as though the analyst did not exist as a separate person with a separate viewpoint. Benjamin (1988) suggested that mutuality and intersubjectivity are achieved when a balance is struck between assertion and recognition. Kernberg's approach was too much assertion and Kohut's, too much recognition. An intermediate stance is to affirm the patient's reality while asserting the analyst's separate reality and then address the issue of how it is that two individuals who seem to see the world and each other in such discrepant ways can find some common ground. Of course, the patient will resist the analyst's efforts to initiate a mutual relationship despite the patient's sadomasochistic provocations.

Kernberg and colleagues (1989) did advocate an approach that began to approximate this intermediate stance. They suggested that unconscious material could not be interpreted until a common view of reality was established between the patient and the analyst. When the patient and analyst see things differently, there must be an attempt to clarify the nature of their incompatible realities until the difference is clearly delineated. With a paranoid psychotic patient, it may mean noting that the difference in perception of reality implies that one of us is sane and the other is crazy. With a psychopathic patient, it may mean noting that the difference in reality means that one of us is lying and the other is telling the truth. The analyst can then go on to explore what it means for the patient to be working with a therapist who is experienced as a paranoid psychotic or psychopath.

Though it is commendable to go so forthrightly right to the heart of the patient's most primitive persecutory anxieties in the transference, for Kernberg it was a forgone conclusion as to whose version of reality would be accepted in the end. "There can be no interpretation of unconscious material unless the patient *agrees* with the therapist on the "reality" of what is being observed. The only *distortions* of reality that can be interpreted are those that are ego-dystonic" (p. 62, italics added). Does the analyst never act out the countertransference unconsciously even in subtle ways which lend at least a kernel of truth to the patient's perception of the analyst? Does the analyst not possess some of the pathological personality traits that the patient ascribes to him or her at least as unconscious tendencies? Could the analyst's perceptions of reality be occasionally inaccurate in comparison to the patient's? And are the analyst's perceptions of reality only one construction of reality among many that are based on the analyst's particular theoretical preconceptions? Though Kernberg was astute in clarifying the nature of the difference between his reality and that of his patients and of having some empathy for the patient's experience of that difference, he seemed overly confident in the ultimate validity of his sense of reality.

I would suggest that a common view of reality has been established when patient and analyst establish a consensus that they both view the world differently and that they can still continue to work meaningfully with each other despite this difference of opinion. I am not so sure that the patient has to agree with the analyst's perception of reality before work can proceed, as Kernberg seemed to imply, or that the analyst has to be experienced as completely in tune with the patient's perception of reality, as Kohut implied. Perhaps the relationship can tolerate and contain living with a difference of opinion when it does not seem that both parties can be "right" simultaneously. Maybe that is what is curative, living with difference and discovering that neither party has to submit to or be defined by the perceptions of the other party. The analyst must have empathy for the patient's experience of difference but should not necessarily feel that difference is a problem that must be resolved by the establishment of sameness.

Winnicott (1971) differentiated between subjective objects, objective objects, and transitional objects. Subjective objects are objects over which one possesses omnipotent control, such as the objects of one's fantasies or daydreams. Objective objects are objects over which one cannot exert omnipotent control and are therefore considered to exist outside of the self in external reality. Transitional objects are objects of which it is ambiguous whether or not they are subject to omnipotent control and therefore appear to exist in a space intermediate between the subjective and the objective. It would seem that Kohut's idea of a selfobject reflects an object that like Winnicott's transitional object is neither fully self nor fully other, neither fully subjective nor fully objective. It is a part of the self in that it performs a vital self-regulatory function on which the self is dependent, yet it is outside of the self in that it is beyond omnipotent control in contrast to a fantasized object. Selfobject success sustains the illusion of omnipotent control of the object, and selfobject failure shatters the illusion of omnipotent control of the object. As healthy selfobject relationships reflect some balance between optimal responsiveness (i.e., good-enough attunement) and optimal frustration (i.e., nontraumatic misattunement), the selfobject is never unambiguously established as either self or other. Mutuality can be seen as a selfobject relationship in that the other is part self (i.e., exists to recognize the self) and part other (i.e., exists as a separate entity which asserts itself in its own right and demands recognition of its individuality). Mutuality breaks down when the other is either only a subjective object or only an objective object.

At the borderline level of functioning, the fear of becoming an extension of the other, subject to the other's omnipotent control and thus deprived of a sense of recognition, leads to the attempt to make the other an extension of the self by subjecting the other to omnipotent control and depriving the other of its identity. In the treatment situation, the analyst attempts to counter the patient's omnipotent control and inculcate mutuality in reflecting the patient's self verbally but reflecting the analyst's own separate attitudes nonverbally. For example, if the patient is in a panic, the analyst may verbally reflect an appreciation of the patient's sense of imminent danger; but to the extent the analyst remains calm and relaxed, a nonverbal message is conveyed to the effect that the analyst "really" thinks that the patient is overreacting and that the patient is not "really" in a desperate or urgent situation. If the analyst were to express that nonverbally conveyed attitude verbally, the patient might be offended that the analyst does not believe the patient and is dismissing the realistic basis of the patient's distress. The analyst verbally mirrors the patient's panic-stricken self-state while nonverbally challenging that self-state in reflecting a calm that is expected to soothe the patient. The analyst's metacommunication is "I know you're frightened, but trust me, it's nothing to worry about." The patient attunes to the analyst's mood rather than vice versa. If the analyst were to go into a panic in response to the patient's panic, the analyst would fail as a soothing selfobject, as the analyst has lost an independent sense of self in becoming submerged in the patient's panic-stricken sense of reality.

In creating a nonverbal ambience of safety and calm and maintaining that ambience in the face of the patient's anxiety and aggression, the analyst is implicitly challenging the patient's sadomasochistic sense of reality whether or not the analyst verbally mirrors or challenges that sense of reality. Yet because the analyst does not possess omnipotent control of his or her own sense of reality and relates in part to the patient as selfobject, the analyst cannot help but respond in the countertransference to the patient's sadomasochistic provocations in kind, thus confirming the patient's illusion of omnipotent control. The analyst tends to become continually enmeshed in the patient's personality organization and then must struggle to extricate the self to reestablish a separate perspective.

In order to attempt to maintain mutuality despite the fact that the analyst is responding in a sadomasochistic manner in the countertransference, it may be necessary for the analyst verbally to acknowledge construing the situation differently than the patient, though not necessarily implying that the analyst's perspective is the objective one. The metacommunication is "Even though I am acting out in a sadomasochistic manner with you, I am aware of the enactment and take responsibility for it; yet I would still like to have a different kind of relationship with you." What is important is not whether the analyst's perspective is objective or biased but whether it is different from the patient's. There is no answer to the question of the analyst's relative objectivity or subjectivity, but there is no doubt that the analyst's perspective is different from the patient's regardless of the question of its accuracy. In the framework of borderline functioning, the question of who is right and who is wrong is vital, as the answer to that question decides who is blameworthy. From the perspective of mutuality, the question is one of how two people who view the world in such discrepant manners can find some common ground. How is a connection formed between someone who is looking to establish hierarchy through the assignation of blame and innocence and someone who is looking to establish mutuality through the bridging of difference? The analyst is in the position of someone who is attempting to negotiate a peace with an enemy who does not want peace but victory and for that reason would prefer to go on fighting despite the costs.

The analyst may encourage the establishment of mutuality in functioning as a selfobject who facilitates perspective taking. The analyst does not challenge the validity of the patient's view of reality as though the question were one of correct or incorrect perceptions. Instead, the analyst demonstrates that alternative and multiple perspectives exist. Kernberg's approach encouraged perspective taking to the extent it enabled the patient to look at his or her rapidly oscillating self-experiences and rapid role reversals in broad perspective. It discouraged perspective taking to the extent it established a hierarchy of normal, objective perceptions that were nondefensive in nature and pathological, distorted perceptions that were defensive in nature. Kernberg's clear-cut differentiation between normal and abnormal object relations reflected a sort of splitting that denied the relativity of the self. After all, who can say with absolute certainty that the world is not a confusing, chaotic place full of danger in which the sense of identity is ever precarious and in flux, as borderline individuals would have it?

Kohut's approach encouraged perspective taking through identification. To the extent that the patient identified with the analyst's empathic immersion and affirmation of the patient's subjective experience, the patient may have been predisposed to do the same for others. Kohut's approach discouraged perspective taking to the degree that the analyst masochistically submitted to the patient's narcissistic entitlement and thus discouraged the patient from discovering the analyst as a separate or "real" person, a person outside of the patient's omnipotent control. Kohutian selfobjects have sometimes been presented as objects that seem devoid of self-agency as well as separate desires, intentions, and perspectives. Yet it would seem that for a selfobject to facilitate the development of a sense of self-agency, initiative, autonomy, self-delineation, individuality, and self-reflection, it would need to possess those qualities itself.

Though it may be true that others may not understand how the borderline-level patient views the world, neither does the borderline-level patient understand how others view the world or even acknowledge that others possess a different perspective than the patient. The idea is not so much to condemn the patient's egocentrism and encourage greater empathy for others, as though the patient were only a selfish and self-centered person who needs to be reformed and reconstituted as a more sensitive and considerate person. The reason that the patient requires a sense of perspective is that only when the other's independent subjectivity is granted is the other's validation of genuine worth. The coerced validation of an omnipotently controlled object is of no real value. Thus, genuine mirroring and affirmation is only possible when the object is recognized as possessing feelings, thoughts, desires, intentions, and perspectives of its own. To the extent the other is depersonalized, be it through devaluation or idealization, its power to affirm the self realistically is diminished. Affirmation coerced from an omnipotently controlled object, be it idealized or devalued, cannot be experienced as real, authentic, or genuine. The patient will possess private doubts about affirmation that is coerced rather than freely given of the analyst's own independent volition. Paradoxically, the patient at a borderline level desperately wants to be loved and respected and therefore attempts to coerce love and respect from others. Yet it is the attempt to coerce love and respect from others that guarantees that the patient will not receive it except on a compliant false-self basis.

In the next case example I will illustrate how the borderline state reflects a crisis mentality. To engage the patient in the crisis state, the clinician must achieve a dynamic balance between accommodating the patient's omnipotent control and challenging the patient's omnipotent control. In addition, the analyst must tolerate and attempt to understand confusional states generated by role reversals in the transference–countertransference relationship. Despite the apparent breakdown of psychological structure, the analyst must discern the method in the madness, the hidden coherence in apparent chaos. To this end it is useful to understand that the patient in the borderline state possesses and is attempting to affirm a surface-level self-syntonic sense of self that has been severely challenged while attempting to re-repress self-dystonic elements that have returned from repression in projected form, resulting in the experience of traumatic states of abandonment and persecution. The analyst must begin to grasp the fine structure of the fragmentation state in order to enable the patient to achieve a metaperspective into which the traumatic state can be assimilated. In trying to analyze the coherent structures of the traumatic state, it is quite likely that the patient will experience the analyst as traumatogenic.

The patient, whom I will call Harriet, was 56 years old when I began to work with her in what was to be a more than 9-year treatment at once and twice weekly sessions. Harriet was a married woman who worked full-time as a secretary. Her husband had been on disability for several years because of cancer in his brain, which was in remission. Her son was a drug addict in his mid-twenties who lived at home and did not work. Although Harriet had been in and out of therapy all her life, at this point she was seeking treatment to help her cope with her son. He had recently overdosed on drugs at home, and Harriet had discovered him and rushed him to the hospital, and his life was saved. Her husband was rather passive and removed in regard to his son's addiction, and Harriet felt on her own and overwhelmed in dealing with him. She was concurrently attending Al-Anon meetings but did not feel she was being helped there. Harriet could be characterized as functioning on a moderately to severely borderline level of psychostructural organization with histrionic and depressive-masochistic features.

Harriet had for her entire life been prone to panic attacks and temper outbursts. Since late adolescence she was prone to hypochondriacal fears of dying from cancer. Every time she had a headache, she worried it was brain cancer; every time she had a stomachache, she worried it was intestinal cancer. Harriet was constantly visiting her doctors for one reason or another. She did have a moderately severe case of rheumatoid arthritis in her knees and hands that made getting to work and doing her typing torturous for her. Feeling continually at her breaking point, Harriet often lost her temper at what might seem to others to be minor irritations or annoyances, such as not getting a seat on the subway or feeling ignored by friends at a social gathering.

Harriet had always been unhappy with her marriage of over 30 years. She and her husband regularly had bitter arguments in which she would be screaming at him as he withdrew in cold detachment. She had had extramarital affairs throughout her marriage about which she felt quite guilty but that she was unwilling to give up since it seemed her only source of validation as an attractive person to whom others might cater. Yet she also felt used by her lovers and humiliated and for that reason experienced her affairs as somewhat of an addiction that she wished she could break.

Harriet was also frustrated by her extremely limited financial situation. Between her husband's disability income and her modest salary as a secretary, they could barely make ends meet. They had already expended a considerable amount of their savings on expensive residential treatment programs for their son, which had proven ineffective. Harriet frequently compared their own situation to those of their friends who were much more comfortable and had secure arrangements for their retirement. She was also quite envious of the success of her friends' children, all of whom seemed to have become successful married professionals with children. These comparisons were a source of searing shame, and Harriet often found herself lying about her son's situation to her friends to make it seem better than it really was. She worried about looking a fool and one day being caught in a lie.

Harriet also reported what seemed to be transient quasi-psychotic episodes. Sometimes at night, especially if she was alone, she began to imagine that there were burglars in her backyard who were going to break into the house and rape her. She would be full of terror and dread until she could make contact with others for reassurance. It emerged that a number of years before such an incident had actually occurred, so Harriet was suffering from posttraumatic stress disorder in addition to all her other emotional difficulties.

Harriet carried around a piece of her deceased mother's wedding dress as a magical charm. When feeling endangered, she would rub this piece of fabric and pray to her mother in heaven to watch out over her. When her son was out late at night, she would go into a panic that he had been murdered by drug pushers and would scream at her son when he came home for causing her to worry. On the whole, night was a scary time for Harriet when she would feel herself overcome by all sorts of fears and anxieties.

Others tended to treat Harriet as a hysterical woman who was deemed inconsolable and not to be taken too seriously. Both husband and son treated her contemptuously as someone who made mountains out of molehills, and she treated them as failures who could not make something out of themselves of which she could be proud. Harriet had always felt her husband was a poor provider and had fantasized that her son would vindicate her by becoming a great success in life of whom she could boast. She could never see her son's addiction as a disease and felt that he was a "lowlife" who was a disgrace to the family. Her mission in life was not only to save her son from his addiction but to go on to turn him into a great success. Her son always rejected his mother's agenda, defiantly proclaiming that he could live his life any way he wished regardless of what his mother thought of it.

Growing up, Harriet had always felt ashamed of her family. Her father was a gambler and a womanizer who did not provide reliably for the family. Her mother was a rather depressed and insecure person who dared not leave her husband. Her mother did not have the support of her own family, who treated Harriet and her family as their poor relations. Harriet had an older sister who suffered from epilepsy, low intelligence, and poor impulse control, with whom the mother was often frustrated and overburdened. Harriet was often sick for one reason or another growing up. She had been hospitalized a number of times and experienced herself as a sickly person who could die at any moment. She experienced her mother as a protective person without whom she would be lost and maintained a rather dependent and clinging relationship to her mother until her mother's death from breast cancer when Harriet was in her forties and her mother was in her sixties. Her father was still alive at the time I began working with Harriet. He was in his nineties, rather senile, and still as frustratingly self-centered as ever.

Harriet was a fairly bright person who was "college material," but she never followed through on her potential. She did begin nursing school but found herself so frightened that she might develop the illnesses she was learning about that she dropped out. Harriet as a young adult was a very attractive woman and was often pursued by men. She picked her husband because he seemed to be a stable, reliable, and trustworthy person, though she never felt romantically inclined toward him. At some level she sensed that her husband was someone who would never demand or expect much from her, for he was a rather detached person, and who would put up with just about anything to which she might subject him. Nevertheless, she experienced his emotional detachment as a humiliating sexual rejection for which she could never forgive him and his lack of career ambition as a chronic humiliation because she would never have the material comfort that her friends possessed. Her one claim to fame would have to be her son. Because of fertility problems, she never had more than one child, though she wanted more children. Largely viewing herself as a housewife and mother, she never pursued her own career. When her husband became ill and went on disability and the family became reliant on her income, she bitterly resented having to work for a living with her arthritis. Harriet was just counting the days until she could retire, though she knew she would be retiring on extremely limited means.

Harriet's sessions with me quickly assumed a typical form. She would walk into the session and as soon as she sat down would burst into tears, wailing and sobbing uncontrollably. Sometimes she did not know why she was crying, and at other times she recounted the most recent crisis with her son. After 5 to 10 minutes of crying, Harriet would work herself into an enraged state in which she started screaming, recounting the latest indignation to which she had been subjected in life. Therapists in adjoining offices would often tell me that their sessions with patients were interrupted by my patient's screaming and that sometimes it was so loud that they would just sit and wait until it passed. Usually by the end of the session, Harriet would begin to calm down but often left the session letting me know that things were no better for having ventilated her feelings. I would try to say things to empathize with her feelings, but most of the time it seemed she did not even hear me, and I could have just as well remained silent and have had the same effect. As I got to know Harriet better, I often would remain silent until the affect storm subsided on its own, and Harriet would be more attentive to what I had to say.

From the beginning, Harriet was oriented toward getting me to give her advice about how to handle her son. It was as though her son was the "real" patient, I was the supervisor, and Harriet as my supervisee was also her son's therapist. Harriet as the novice therapist would allow me to treat her son indirectly through her if I only gave her the right instructions. She spent considerable session time hypothesizing what her son's dynamics were and how she might intervene. At this point her son was quite resistant to seeking treatment for himself, as his mother had over the years dragged him recalcitrantly to various therapists and programs. Harriet often expressed the wish that I would see her son, to which I responded that I was her therapist and not his.

I responded to her affect storms and her desire for me to help her son with what I hoped would be experienced as empathy. I made interpretations along the lines of reflecting how overwhelmed and overburdened she felt, how confusing the situation was, how alone she felt, how frightened she felt, how important her son was to her, how desperate she felt to save her son, how despairing she felt about being able to succeed, how enraged she was at the unfairness of it all, and her disappointment that I did not provide her with immediate solutions. On the one hand, Harriet appreciated my attempts at empathy, for I seemed to be the one person in her life who was not treating her dismissively and impatiently as a hysterical female who should just contain herself and become a more rational person. On the other hand, though being understood did soothe her and calm her down, it did not solve anything, and she was looking for concrete solutions to solve an immediate and desperate situation in which her son's life was on the line. Harriet felt that if her son died, her life would become meaningless, and she would just as well commit suicide.

In addition to being reflective, I also tried to encourage some degree of introspection by asking her questions that focused on exploring her own dynamics. Though it seemed that Harriet's use of the sessions for catharsis and ventilation was helpful, I felt that catharsis and ventilation alone would be insufficient to help her if she did not develop some insight into herself and her situation. It seemed to me that she was stuck in a variety of repetitive and self-defeating patterns of relationship to both her husband and her son that contributed to a chaotic situation. I soon realized that any attempt to encourage self-examination and understanding of her role in the situation was experienced as blaming and put her on the defensive in relation to me. Harriet already felt that she ruined both her husband's and her son's lives at the same time she blamed them for ruining her life. Harriet protested that it did no good to recount all the mistakes she had made in the past when she wanted to embark on a new beginning to fix things and put things right if I would only point her in the right direction.

I found myself resisting the pull to take charge of her life and give her advice and direction. In part I resisted this interactional pressure because I was confused and felt her situation was hopeless. In addition, I felt that giving in to her pressure would be tantamount to acting out the induced countertransference. I did not want to be held responsible for her decision making and then be held accountable for bad advice that did not work out. It seemed that Harriet wanted me to rescue her and that it would have been an effort at omnipotence on my part to make the attempt. Curiously, despite my attempt to refrain from giving advice and to stick with empathy and analysis, Harriet often experienced my interpretations as containing implicit advice and would often check with me to test whether I was really making the recommendations that she thought were implicit in my comments. When I interpreted Harriet's desire for me to advise her and her frustration that I did not advise her in a clear-cut way, Harriet would reassure me that she did not expect me to have all the answers and that it was of value just to have someone to talk to, but that if I did have any ideas about what to do, it would be appreciated.

As the first year of treatment wore on, it did not seem that the treatment was making much progress. I felt as if we were just waiting for disaster to strike—when her son would overdose once more and finally kill himself. I also found that my resistance to giving Harriet advice was being worn down. As I found myself almost begrudgingly making a few suggestions, I was surprised to discover that Harriet perked up with enthusiasm and hopefulness. Though I felt I was doing something unanalytic that perhaps I would later regret,

Harriet's positive reinforcement was encouraging me progressively to become the sort of authoritative, directive kind
of clinician she wished me to be. As I gave more advice,
Harriet informed me that the treatment was becoming more
helpful and that she wished to begin attending sessions more
frequently. In the past when I had suggested increased
sessions, she claimed that it would be "too much." We
embarked on the second year of treatment with Harriet
feeling that she had finally found a therapist who would
really help her and with me feeling somewhat relieved that I
had finally established a therapeutic alliance with Harriet but
worried at what price. Even though I encouraged Harriet to
come more frequently for sessions, at some level I also
wished she would just drop out of treatment because she
seemed so difficult to treat.

At the time I began working with her, I did not think in
terms of working from surface to depth in the same manner
as I do currently, and I was not as interactively flexible as I
currently aspire to be. In retrospect from my current theoretical perspective, it is clear that I was unwittingly invalidating
her surface-level self-syntonic sense of self. Harriet construed
herself as a normal mother doing what any normally dedicated and loving mother would do for her son. It was
irresponsibility in her eyes to just let her son self-destruct
without her active intervention in his life. It was therefore
reasonable and commendable that in a crisis situation she
would seek a therapist who as an expert could tell her what
to do in this confusing situation. Harriet could not live with
herself if she abdicated this responsibility. My interactive
style/interpretive stance said to her in effect, "You made this
mess, so you take responsibility for fixing it all by yourself."
Viewing her as pathologically enmeshed with her son, avoidant of taking responsibility for herself, and overly blaming
of others, I was unwittingly invalidating her self-syntonic
view of herself as a normal mother. In my countertransference, I experienced Harriet as the opposite of a normal
mother, just the sort of monstrous castrating witch-mother
from whom any normal male would recoil in horror. Once I
began to act as though her wish for advice was a legitimate

request that I might attempt to satisfy, I was implicitly affirming her self-syntonic sense of herself as a normally devoted, caring, and responsible mother who would not abandon her son in a crisis. To the extent I began to share responsibility for crisis management, Harriet felt that she was no longer alone in her moment of desperation and that I was on her side and working on her behalf rather than simply remaining a sympathetic bystander who did not really want to get involved.

As the second year of treatment proceeded and I made a conscious decision to experiment with being an authoritative and advice-giving therapist, I decided to recommend that Harriet kick her son out of the house. It seemed to me that her son exploited Harriet for free room and board so that he had disposable income for drugs and that he might do better if he had to assume responsibility for fending for himself. It also seemed that Harriet was incapable of setting limits without being alternately overly strict and overly lax. Her son readily manipulated Harriet by making her feel guilty or frightening her with his self-destructiveness. She would eventually retaliate by screaming at him and belittling him. As it seemed that Harriet would never be able to alter this pattern no matter how much insight she possessed into it, it seemed the only way to remedy the situation was to separate the two.

Harriet responded to my recommendation with a sense that this was probably the right thing to do since her Al-Anon group had been advising her to do this for years, but, on the other hand, she worried that the very day she kicked her son out of the house he would simply commit suicide by overdosing and then it would be as if she had killed him with her own hands. For me to suggest that she kick him out of the house was like telling her to abandon her son; it seemed a heartless thing to do. Harriet insisted that there must be some other way she could help her son short of that alternative. I challenged Harriet to come up with another method of helping her son besides the ones she had tried already, which had not worked. Harriet was stumped as to what she could do differently but felt too frightened to implement my recommendation.

Though Harriet was frightened by my recommendation in feeling that I was leading her to do something risky and dangerous and felt that I was somewhat heartless in encouraging her to do something that might eventuate in her son's death, my recommendation focused the treatment and gave it coherence. Exploring Harriet's fears of implementing my suggestion became the focus of treatment. As Harriet's defenses against her fears of causing her son's death by separating from him began to emerge, it became possible to begin to articulate the self-dystonic elements of her character structure—that is, all the ways in which she did not seem to be a normally caring and responsible mother. And, of course, assimilating these self-dystonic elements was very painful for Harriet, for she possessed tremendous shame and guilt in relation to all the ways she felt she was not a good mother.

If kicking her son out of the house was what a "good" mother would do, then Harriet had to come to grips with the possibility that holding on to her son so that she could save him might be what a "bad" mother would do. As her son had become suicidal and overdosed a number of times under her care, Harriet was not so sure of her efficacy as a good mother. Yet on the other hand, if she kicked him out and he killed himself, there would be no doubt at all that she was a bad mother. And there was no question that her entire sense of self was invested in being a good mother and that she had no sense of her life having any meaning or value beyond her function as a good mother. To not be a good mother was unthinkable and unspeakable, the annihilation of all purpose and meaning in life.

The transference to me remained essentially positive even though I gave her advice that she worried was misguided: at least I was willing to share her burden in having to make what seemed like a life-or-death decision for her son. I worried that perhaps it was misguided to give her advice at all and that perhaps the advice I was giving would result in a successful suicide attempt by the son for which I would be blamed and held accountable, maybe even in a malpractice suit, as I imagined it. Yet I found that interpretations of Harriet's fears of kicking her son out and of her resistance to implementing my advice were interpretations that Harriet took seriously and with which she was willing to work. It seemed that making recommendations, and especially making a recommendation that seemed to require Harriet to do something that evoked her greatest unconscious fears, allowed me to establish an alliance with her desire to be a good mother and to begin to analyze her fears and defenses against not being a good mother. What had begun as crisis management was gradually evolving into a character analysis of Harriet's style of being a parent, which was also generalizable to the ways in which she related to people overall.

Though at one level Harriet seemed to have a need to control, dominate, infantilize, and emasculate her son, at another level she was quite dependent on her son for meeting her needs for intimate attachment, and she felt lost and abandoned whenever she felt she might lose him. As her entire sense of belonging and self-esteem was dependent on her relationship to her son, she felt quite endangered by any threats to that tie and became enraged at him for anything he did that put that vital tie at risk. Harriet then became frightened that her own hostility toward her son might destroy him and that she would be cruelly punished by the traumatic loss of the emotional tie that was her sole reason for living. Harriet had to exert omnipotent control over her son to avert the most horrendous tragedy imaginable: the infanticide of her son. I was making a recommendation that might make that potential tragedy a reality; on the other hand, I seemed to be predicting that if she did not follow my recommendation, her worst nightmare might become true anyway, and then she would despair for not having followed my advice. Harriet was in anguish about what seemed to be the most important decision of her life, a decision that she felt I had forced upon her and that she felt inadequate to make despite my having taken sides on the issue.

The next several years of treatment centered on working through this conflict in a variety of ways. Harriet would threaten to kick her son out if he did not conform to her demands. Of course, her son would promise to meet her demands and then would not, and Harriet could not find the heart to follow through on her threat. Harriet would then berate herself for being inconsistent and caving in. Finally, Harriet did succeed in kicking her son out temporarily but would let him back several weeks or months later on the presumption that he was only returning to live at home briefly, only to discover that her son was settling back into living at home permanently. It did give her confidence that he could survive for at least brief periods of time independent of her without killing himself or being murdered. In the fourth year of treatment, Harriet kicked her son out. He took this as an opportunity to move out of state, as home had become a very unpleasant place for him.

Harriet confronted her son so relentlessly that once he was provoked to start choking her to shut her up. Her son as well as Harriet was quite unnerved by her son's aggression. The son apparently left to avoid the possibility of matricide, and Harriet began to become fearful that he might kill her when he was high. This incident also highlighted to Harriet that perhaps she was being masochistic in her relationship to her son to let him exploit and abuse her. I interpreted that being a good mother could involve expecting her son to act like an adult and to treat her with respect for her wishes and that in being a good role model for her son, perhaps she should stand up for herself. Perhaps a good mother has to push her child out of the nest so that the child can become independent.

Once her son was out of the house, Harriet demonstrated significant symptomatic improvement, as her son clearly had a regressive effect on her psychological functioning. When she did not receive a phone call from him for an extended period of time, she would begin to panic and imagine the worst. Nevertheless, it seemed like an impasse had been transcended, though she dreaded the next time he might show up on her doorstep in a crisis demanding to be allowed to come home to live once more. In terms of the transference-countertransference dynamic, I had accommodated to her need to control me omnipotently in giving her advice. That acquiescence to her omnipotent control allowed her to feel that I was emotionally connected and involved with her. Yet

I challenged her omnipotent control in recommending she do something that evoked her worst fears of loss of control. In making the recommendation, I began to feel in relation to her the way in which she felt in relation to her son. I felt I was making a life-or-death decision for which I felt ill prepared but for which I would be held accountable nevertheless. Harriet acted like her son in behaving as though I was forcing her to do something beyond her ability, from which she should be excused if I were only a genuinely understanding person. In reversing roles in the transference, I discovered what it was like to be in her shoes—to feel totally responsible for another's life without any sense of control in the situation.

In the fifth year of treatment while her son was living out of state, Harriet's husband unexpectedly died. Harriet felt devastated, for now she seemed to be all alone in the world with no husband, no son, no money, no friends, no family, no longer young, and no longer healthy. The future seemed bleak as she said explicitly that she only had me for support, and that was not enough. At this time her son came back into town, feeling that he needed to move back in to take care of his mother now that she was a widow. Shortly before a session, I found a message from Harriet on my answering machine, saying that she was bringing her son in to see me because she could no longer deal with the situation and that I had to do something about it. I knew that she had often told her son that she kicked him out on my recommendation, so I had the fantasy that her son blamed me for kicking him out of the house and that perhaps he might attack me for having ruined his life. I decided that to avoid a volatile scene in the waiting room, I would see him.

I decided to see her son by himself in order to assess his mental status. Her son stated that he was worried about his mother all alone in the house and thought that perhaps he should move back in to help her. I suggested that his mother could take care of herself but that indeed he was right to be concerned because his mother had serious emotional problems that would only be exacerbated if he moved back in. I suggested that now that she was bereaved, she could not handle the stress of having him live there. Though I expected that her son would be angry with me, to my surprise he nodded in agreement with everything I said. He told me that he always knew his mother was "crazy" but that she had always made him feel like he was the only one who had any problems. It was good to hear from his mother's therapist that what he suspected all along was valid. He claimed that in the past he had only lived at home because he believed his mother needed him there, adding he was quite capable of living independently from her and was relieved in being out of the house and not having to be constantly scolded by her.

I then brought Harriet into the room and recounted our dialogue. Harriet started screaming at me at the top of her lungs that I should have focused on his problems rather than hers and why does everything have to be her fault. I countered that I was her therapist and not his and that he could worry about his own problems. I noticed that as Harriet was screaming at me, her son was sitting there with an amused smirk on his face as if to say, "I told you she was crazy—look what I have had to put up with all these years." After this incident, the son moved back out of state, found a girlfriend, had a child with this girlfriend, became either drug-free or relatively drug-free, maintained an independent living situation, and assumed responsibility for raising a family. Four years later the son's situation seemed to be relatively stable, though for the most part he did not share much of what was going on in his life with his mother so it was difficult to know for sure.

The sixth through the ninth years of treatment involved Harriet's adjustment to widowhood and her feelings about growing old. Harriet was able to retire early on disability because of the severity of her arthritis. In some ways, Harriet's husband's untimely death had a similar effect on her as she had had on her son by throwing him out of the house. They both were forced to either sink or swim in learning to take care of themselves. Harriet, to her surprise, rose to the occasion and found it a relief not to have to care for her disabled husband, not to have to argue with him, and not to have to be disappointed with him. She felt lonely and guilty that her emotional mistreatment of her husband might have somehow contributed to his untimely death. Harriet began to make friends with other women in the neighborhood who were also widows in order to have a supportive social network. She found this very difficult because she was ashamed of her life and did not want anybody to get to know her too well.

The transference shifted significantly as I was no longer needed for advice, for now that her son was out of the house, she had no life-shaking decisions to make. When she was not worrying about how her son was doing and feeling frustrated being largely shut out of his life, Harriet became progressively more absorbed in worrying about her physical health and who would take care of her if she became disabled. She had taken care of her father until he had died, about a year before her husband's death. She had also taken care of her mother when her mother was stricken with terminal cancer. Harriet was resentful that she had been there for her husband, father, and mother in illness and dying but that she would die alone, with nobody to take care of her now that her son had abandoned her.

I experienced her complaints as covertly reproachful of me for having forced her to relinquish her relationship to her son. I felt as though I was expected to be the son she never had and take care of her in her old age, as I began to wish that maybe the son would come back to take care of his mother now that he seemed to be better adjusted. I seemed to be in the position of advocating that she had to take care of herself as best she could, which seemed a heartless thing to advocate now that she was a widow with health problems, limited finances, and no family support. Our sessions assumed a pattern in which she would complain inconsolably about her depressing life situation for most of the session but would end the session with an anecdote or two suggesting that her life was improving in some respects. The sense of life-or-death urgency that had characterized our first years working together was greatly diminished.

In many ways I assumed the role of a supportive mother who firmly and definitively encouraged autonomy and responsibility. In this respect, I was unlike Harriet's mother who had instilled in her the sense Harriet need not learn to take care of herself because her mother would always be there to protect her, even from heaven after she died. To Harriet, her mother was a good mother, and she would be a good mother like her mother to her son, a fiercely protective mother who is a lifesaver. In contrast, a mother who facilitated autonomy and separateness was a bad mother, an infanticidal mother, a mother who would abandon her child to die from neglect left alone in the cold cruel world. In the countertransference, I often felt like an infanticidal mother who would be persecuted and punished for being a horrible person. In the transference I was simultaneously her mother and herself, and she was both her mother and herself. In addition, I was the "good" son who had to save his "crazy" mother, and I was the "bad" son who had to escape the clutches of his "crazy" mother in order to save himself.

Progress in terms of character analysis meant that Harriet had to tolerate a reversal of what was self-syntonic with what was self-dystonic. Perhaps a mother who aimed to be a lifesaver was an overprotective mother who was infantilizing so that her child did not develop the skills necessary to survive on one's own, and was therefore a "bad" mother. And perhaps a mother who firmly encouraged autonomy and separateness was a mother who enabled her child to learn to assume adult responsibility and was therefore a "good" mother. Treatment continually revived the narcissistic trauma that the mother on whom she depended for her existence may have been a "bad" mother who undermined her autonomy and that she too may have been a "bad" mother who undermined her son's autonomy, thus threatening his independent existence. And if she were a bad mother who ruined her son's life, then she should be punished by his death, for which she had only herself to blame—the most unspeakable horror imaginable. Yet to the extent that treatment enabled her to become a good mother who would facilitate autonomy and allow her son to separate from her, she could save his life and in so doing save her own.

Once Harriet had saved her son in kicking him out of the house, she had to confront her own sense of aloneness and abandonment in life, from which no one could save her but herself. I had to bear her covert reproachfulness for not becoming the caretaker-son who would spare her the fate of what might be an old age in which there would be no one to take care of her or watch out for her. Yet in gradually assuming such a responsibility for herself, Harriet began to develop a supportive network of women in the same boat as her. She felt proud of finally beginning to feel like a mature and responsible adult at the ripe age of 65, and at least she had become a grandmother so that her son had given her something of which to boast to others after all. I felt that Harriet had taught me a lot about how to work with her and people like her and was grateful that the treatment had not ended tragically, which had been the anxiety I had had to endure for much of the treatment. Perhaps I had not been such a bad son after all.

In contrast to the chaotic situations that arise in working with borderline patients, an opposite situation arises in working with pseudoneurotic patients in which treatment becomes boringly routine and predictable. Characterological rigidity can be seen as a defense against as well as a compensation for a breakdown of mutuality, with its attendant revival of sadomasochistic object relations. To defend against the dread of identity diffusion, the person becomes wedded to a stereotypic role that defines the self in a clearly delineated though simplistic, unidimensional, unipolar, and inflexible manner. Role rigidity and inflexibility gives the personality a stable though constricted form. Persons who define the self in terms of stereotypic roles could be seen as *pseudoneurotic*. They seem neurotic to the extent that they may be asymptomatic and functional individuals. They are pseudoneurotic to the extent that their relationships with others are superficial and impoverished, being choreographed according to stereotypic role relationships. Such an adjustment tends to be brittle and readily destabilized in emotionally charged, complex, and ambiguous situations for which a stereotypic response proves insufficient. Substance abuse, perverse sexuality, hypochondria, and eating disorders may be resorted to as a means of bolstering a precarious pseudoneurotic adjustment. Failure of the pseudoneurotic adaptation may lead to a regression to a borderline level of functioning.

Patients at a pseudoneurotic level of psychostructural integration present certain therapeutic challenges. Such patients tend to be remarkably concrete. They are not insight oriented, psychologically minded, introspective, or self-reflective. They tend to be unaware of their fantasy life, dream life, or feelings. Their childhoods tend to be recalled as uneventful, as are their daily lives. As a consequence, they often do not know what to talk about in the treatment situation. They are unable to free-associate. They tend instead to report updates of their daily lives, focusing on daily problems in living for which the analyst might give a few words of advice. If there is no daily problem to be solved, there is nothing to discuss. Emotional distress is felt to be externally and situationally determined by stressful life events. The self is experienced as essentially a reactive being coping as best one can to events beyond one's volitional control.

Such patients tend to take things at face value. There is no sense of symbolic, latent, covert, or unconscious meanings to psychic events. For pseudoneurotic patients, a cigar is always a cigar and never a symbolic representation of a breast, penis, or feces. Pseudoneurotic patients are implicit behaviorists. Life is a problem of behavioral management for which one needs to discover practical and pragmatic strategies. The behavioral focus arises from their overidentification with their public sense of self, their social role that has been stereotypically defined. There is no sense of possessing an unconscious sense of self, for all that seems to exist to them is what is surface, concrete, tangible, visible, and can be taken at face value. Appearance is what counts because appearance is obvious, apparent, objective, and therefore real. There is little sense of a private sense of self, for what is private is an idiosyncratic perception to be dismissed. Only perceptions that are consensually validated by the popular majority are considered valid. A conformist mentality assimilates to the popular majority in order to feel normal, and the achievement of a sense of normality confers a sense of security and self-esteem.

In the transference, the pseudoneurotic patient looks to the analyst as a representative of the views of the popular majority. The patient is eager to be in treatment with an authoritative analyst whose advice and guidance, whether communicated explicitly or implicitly, is sought. The patient wants to be in treatment with an expert behavioral manager who will teach the patient the arts of impression management. To the extent the patient acknowledges an inner life that is problematic, there is a desire to improve one's habits of mind through the power of positive thinking. The patient wants the analyst to tell the patient how one should think, and the patient will then practice that form of mental self-management. The patient wants to possess a normal mind and needs the analyst's instruction as to how a normal person should think and feel.

As analysts tend to resist gratifying the patient's wishes for an authoritative, advice-giving, and directive treatment provider, the patient is destabilized as the analyst fails as a normalizing selfobject. Some patients who need the analyst to function as a normalizing selfobject will simply hear the analyst's interpretations as implicit instructions conveying normative standards of social conduct to which the patient will subscribe. For such patients, analysis is a sort of magical initiation ritual from which one will emerge a normal and healthy individual. Most pseudoneurotic patients, though, prove incapable of being a compliant analysand even though they would like to. The compliant analysand who is capable of going through the motions of analysis must be at least somewhat imaginative and insightful. The typical pseudoneurotic patient, as a result of not remembering dreams, fantasies, and emotion-laden childhood experiences and of being unable to analyze and interpret implicit motives and intentions in interpersonal relations, cannot even pretend to be a good analysand despite the desire to do what the doctor orders. The result, then, is that the patient tends to become repetitive or silent. Treatment becomes routine, boring, superficial, trivial, and stalemated. The patient feels frustrated with treatment, either feeling a failure as a patient or feeling that he or she needs to be in treatment with a more directive and opinionated therapist who will make things happen. Defense and resistance analysis tend to evoke feelings in the patient that he or she is either a very stubborn and opposi-tional person without knowing it or a rather dull and empty person who is dreadfully understimulating to the analyst. The patient may accept the analyst's formulations as plausible interpretations, the truth of which cannot be denied. Yet the patient does not possess a sense of conviction and is only taking the analyst's word on the matter on the basis of respect for the analyst's authority.

Just as one might think in terms of borderline styles, one could think in terms of pseudoneurotic styles. A pseudoneu-rotic style would reflect the particular stereotypic role to which the person is wedded. At a pseudoneurotic level of functioning, there is no sense of intrapsychic conflict. The person either feels a taken-for-granted goodness of fit with the social surround when things are going well or a sense of conflict with the social surround when things are not going well. The patient would prefer to change the social surround rather than the self to solve the problem. In contrast, at a genuinely neurotic level of functioning, there is a sense of intrapsychic conflict, of being identified with multiple and contradictory roles and not knowing which one to act on or how to achieve some integrative compromise. The neurotic is aware of thesis and antithesis but cannot arrive at a creative synthesis. The pseudoneurotic is only aware of the thesis but not of the antithesis so does not even appreciate the need for synthesis. When in conflict with the social surround, the pseudoneurotic experiences the social surround as embod-ying the antithesis to the patient's thesis. For this reason the social surround needs to be neutralized in order to preserve the integrity of the patient's thesis.

The obsessive-compulsive at the pseudoneurotic level is completely rule-bound. There is a sense that there is a right/proper way and a wrong/improper way, and the obses-sive-compulsive knows the right/proper way. All events in analysis are judged in terms of correct and incorrect, precise and imprecise. The hysteric at a pseudoneurotic level is completely absorbed in the apparent drama of trivial and superficial social relations, which seem to comprise the warp and woof of existence. In analysis the patient's discourse may strike the analyst as social chit-chat or gossip. The depressive-masochist at a pseudoneurotic level is absorbed in complaining and soliciting sympathy. The depressive-masochist strikes the analyst as a grievance collector who never ceases to whine. The narcissist at a pseudoneurotic level is completely absorbed in comparing the self to others in terms of status and prestige. The paranoid at a pseudoneurotic level is completely absorbed in injustice collecting by ferreting out hidden hypocrisy and deceit. The schizoid is completely absorbed by the ironic absurdities of mundane daily existence, which may be recounted in every quotidian detail. The antisocial person at a pseudoneurotic level is completely absorbed in keeping score as to who has the upper hand in a situation.

At first blush, these attitudes may seem to represent the standard resistances of these character types to analytic treatment, so that each patient seems to be a standard neurotic character for whom a little resistance analysis would help the analysis unfold to a deeper level. What makes such attitudes pseudoneurotic rather than simply neurotic is not only the extreme tenaciousness of the characterological resistance but the absence of any other personality characteristics. There are no conflicting or competing personality traits to the stereotypic attitudes that the patient presents, nothing self-dystonic. The personality seems to lack depth and breadth. There are no higher-level traits such as irony, a sense of humor, empathy, playfulness, creativity, or insightfulness, nor are there apparent lower-level traits as found at a borderline level such as panic, rage, desperation, dread of abandonment, fear of persecution, and confusion. The meat and potatoes of analytic work tends to be to bring the higher-level traits to bear on the lower-level traits. Yet all the pseudoneurotic patient displays are the midlevel personality traits associated with social adaptation.

In terms of technique, given how rigid and constricted the

pseudoneurotic patient is, it is tempting to attempt to encourage greater role flexibility, in both a progressive direction
in terms of stimulating a more self-reflective attitude and a
regressive direction in terms of stimulating the patient's
awareness of the archaic affect for which the pseudoneurotic
adjustment serves as a defense. Often, though, such attempts
result in a sort of "pulling teeth" stalemate. The analyst seems
to take all the initiative and do all the work to make
something happen and runs into what Rosenfeld (1964) called
a "narcissistic stone wall." There is a sense of "chipping
away" at some impenetrable "character armor" in which one
never seems to make a dent. Such resistance analysis does
not so much result in an adversarial relationship, as the
patient does not overtly fight back—a phenomenon that the
resistance-minded analyst might construe as passive-
aggressive. Instead, the result seems to be stalemate, as the
patient does not seem to move or budge from the stereotypic
attitudinal position with which the patient began treatment.

The patient who is aware that the analyst sees the patient
as impenetrable, boring, superficial, repetitive, dense, insuf-
ferable, understimulating, unimaginative, stuck, passive-
aggressive, frustrating, and annoying begins to suffer low
self-esteem as a result of being seen in that light by a mental
health professional whose authority to evaluate and judge the
patient is unquestioned. The analysis becomes one more
situational stressor that makes the patient unhappy. The
patient may terminate treatment at that point or stay on in the
hopes that the treatment will normalize the patient over time,
so that he or she should just patiently endure the discomfort
of the treatment situation until the cure takes effect. Such
patients are readily seduced by the allure of more directive
treatment approaches with more authoritative therapists.

An alternative to employing aggressive defense analysis to
which the patient is impervious or to attempting to outwait
the patient with one's infinite patience for the timelessness of
unconscious processes until the patient takes a spontaneous
initiative toward self-exploration is to actively enter, explore,
and empathize with what I have called the "world of the
concrete" (Josephs 1989). Rather than attempt to increase the

patient's role flexibility to encompass the role of an introspective, analytic patient, the analyst can accept the patient's role rigidity as an experiential parameter within which the analyst must learn how to work. The analyst must learn how to see the world in the same narrow-minded, literal, unidimensional, and stereotypic manner in which the patient construes the world. The analyst must learn to appreciate the inner coherence, fine points, and subtle nuances that exist within a stereotypic worldview. The analyst must learn to perceive depth in superficiality.

For example, to enter the world of the pseudoneurotic obsessive-compulsive, the analyst must appreciate the world of rules, propriety, precision, and duty. The analyst must understand that rules are complex, that propriety expresses dignity, that imprecision is not to be taken lightly, and that duty is a sacred dimension of human existence. To enter the world of the pseudoneurotic hysteric, the analyst must appreciate the world of friendly social relations. Within such a world, the analyst must grasp the intricacies of shifting alliances and divided loyalties. The analyst must comprehend the implicit rules of social etiquette and manners through which shifting alliances are covertly expressed. To enter the world of the pseudoneurotic depressive-masochist, the analyst must appreciate the world of the would-be altruist and its inevitable disappointments. The analyst must understand the innumerable rebuffs that an altruist suffers in a world of selfish and self-centered people for whom the depressive-masochist attempts to care. To enter the world of the pseudoneurotic narcissist, the analyst must appreciate the importance of status hierarchies and the subtle ways in which status is established and expressed in social relations. To enter the world of the pseudoneurotic paranoid, the analyst must be attuned to the world of social injustice and the hypocrisy of those in authority who are the source of oppression. To enter the world of the pseudoneurotic schizoid, the analyst must appreciate how the world looks to an ironic spectator who disidentifies with the social surround and tries to approach the world as an existentialist might. To enter the world of the pseudoneurotic antisocial, the analyst must grasp the fine points of strategies of getting one up on rivals with whom there exist no rules of fair play.

Every role relationship, no matter how stereotypic or narrow-minded, can nevertheless be appreciated as an entire world unto itself with depth and breadth, complexity and nuance. The analyst's entry into this world has the effect of stabilizing and affirming it. It may seem contraindicated to affirm a point of view or an attitude that is stereotypic and therefore inevitably harbors many biases and prejudices. Nevertheless, it is in the affirmation of the pseudoneurotic patient's constricted adjustment that the patient develops the resilience as well as the inclination to stretch the boundaries of the self beyond its familiar borders. Of course, depending on the resilience of the patient, the analyst may enter the world of the concrete as well as challenge that world with the usual sorts of defense–resistance analysis in order to enable the patient to become decentered from his or her egocentric frame of reference.

Sometimes the concern has been expressed that to empathize with a point of view or to enter a worldview is tantamount to the analyst implying that he or she views the world in a similar manner, so that the way in which the patient sees the world is then the "only" way in which the world "could" or "should" be seen. Given that any worldview can serve a defensive function denying other worldviews, it may seem that to empathize with and affirm a worldview is akin to colluding with a defensive attitude. I would suggest, though, that the patient is always aware that the analyst possesses a separate perspective even when the patient acts disinterested in that perspective. Even in psychotic states, patients are aware that others hold a different point of view. For example, when a mental status examination is given to a psychotic patient and the patient is asked whether the patient hears voices that others do not, it is understood that even the hallucinating patient knows that others do not hear the same voices. That understanding is distressing to the patient, because then somebody must be crazy, if everybody lives in the same perceptual reality. Likewise, the pseudoneurotic patient knows that the analyst sees the world differently but is unprepared to handle the intersubjective disjunction that occurs when two opposing worldviews collide.

The analyst must be like a stranger in a strange land who is trying to understand the customs and has no desire to convert the natives to his or her own culture. The patient from the beginning has no doubts that analysis is a cross-cultural exchange, despite the fact that initially the patient has little interest in learning about the analyst's culture but only wants the analyst to learn about the patient's own. The analyst is always experienced as an outsider looking in, more or less successfully. Even with the pseudoneurotic patient, the patient is likely sooner or later to express curiosity about what the analyst thinks and at some point in the analysis pose the question, "What do you think? I'm glad you know what I think, but now I want to know what you think."

13

Ambience and
Interpretation

Much debate in psychoanalytic theory has centered on what
is the essential curative element—interpretation leading to
insight or relationship leading to new experience? To some
extent, this is a false dichotomy because interpretation implicitly expresses the analyst's emotional relationship to the
patient, and the nonverbal emotional ambience of the treatment is experienced by the patient as an implicit interpretation. As the emotional ambience constitutes an implicit
interpretation, it behooves us to examine the nonverbal
atmosphere in which the treatment is conducted as an aspect
of the analyst's technique. The emotional ambience that the
analyst creates implies an implicit characterization of the
patient that the patient may find affirming or threatening,
just as the analyst's verbal interpretations reflect characterizations of the patient that the patient may find affirming or
threatening. Not only must the analyst's verbal interpretations reflect a dynamic balance between empathy and analysis, so must the nonverbal ambience of treatment convey an
implicit dynamic balance between empathy and analysis. The
nonverbal ambience of treatment must initially be experienced as empathically holding, containing, and mirroring the
patient prior to being counterbalanced by an experience of the
nonverbal ambience of treatment as abandoning, persecutory, or challenging.

To focus on the technique of character analysis is to focus
on what might be called the strategy or tactics of interpreta-

tion. Questions of timing, depth, phrasing, and focus are highlighted—questions on which the success or failure of the treatment seem to hinge. Treatment then seems to become a technical enterprise that one must conduct correctly rather than a human relationship developing and evolving with a high degree of unpredictability and surprise. Technique focuses on the cognitive and planned element in the conduct of treatment but seems to downplay the emotional, intuitive, spontaneous, and personal. The split between the analyst's cognitive and emotional functioning in the treatment situation echoes the old debate over whether insight or a corrective emotional experience is the essential curative element in the treatment situation. As with most other false dichotomies, the answer need not be either/or. Freud (Breuer and Freud 1895) made it clear from the beginning that cure was in the integration of affect and ideation and that either insight alone (i.e., intellectualization) or affect alone (i.e., isolation of affect) was a defensive bifurcation of what in health should be an integrated unit. In discussions of the analyst's therapeutic function, it remains useful to highlight one or another function (i.e., verbal versus nonverbal communication), though the analyst always operates as an integrated unit who simultaneously executes multiple functions (i.e., communicates verbally and nonverbally simultaneously).

Ferenczi's (1925) active technique and Alexander and French's (1946) corrective emotional experience reflected the earliest attempts to develop noninterpretive approaches to treatment that complemented rather than replaced Freud's technique of interpretation. Ferenczi attempted to give patients the love they never had, whereas Alexander and French tried to act in ways that would challenge the patient's distorted perception of them in the transference. The basic premise of noninterpretive treatment approaches is that it is the relationship which the analyst establishes with the patient that is curative and that the analyst must therefore develop and implement a therapeutic strategy of relating to the patient. The main critique of such approaches is that they harken back to Freud's pressure techniques, such as hypnosis and the laying of the hands on the forehead. A pressure technique is one in which the analyst intentionally exerts an interactional pressure on the patient to respond in a certain manner. A transference relationship is enacted rather than analyzed, raising the specter of the analyst and the patient succumbing to acting out a pathological repetition-compulsion in the treatment situation. To guard against this possibility, Freud (1915) advised that the analyst should remain both abstinent and neutral, confining his or her participation to interpretation. The principles of abstinence and neutrality seem to suggest that it would be taboo for the analyst to exert any interactional pressure on the patient.

Despite the principles of abstinence and neutrality, even the classical analyst exerts interactional pressure on the patient. Abstinence and neutrality constitute a nonverbal interactional pressure that induces regression through frustrating the patient. In the regressed state, the patient will project his or her infantile conflicts onto the analyst so that unconscious conflict is enacted in the transference. Freud (1912a) realized that the patient would not tolerate the privations of an analysis without some degree of unobjectionable positive transference to the analyst. Some degree of rapport and attachment needed to develop before meaningful interpretive work could be conducted. Freud implicitly proposed a nonverbal ambience that the analyst had to create in order for the interpretive work to be effective. The analyst had to establish an attached, trusting relationship so that the patient would tolerate frustration in the therapeutic relationship without breaking off the treatment. The purpose of frustration was to induce a regression that would expose the patient's infantile conflicts, which could then be addressed and resolved through verbal interpretation. The relationship was not what was curative in and of itself. Rather, the relationship via the transference was the vehicle for bringing unconscious conflicts to light; it was the emotional insight into unconscious conflicts that was effected through interpretation that was curative.

For Freud, the analyst had to maintain a balance between frustrating and gratifying the patient. Too much gratification reduced the patient's motivation to change, and too much frustration may have provoked an unanalyzable negative transference-resistance. An optimal balance between frustration and gratification had to be maintained as a precondition for interpretive work. Not only was a certain quality of relatedness with the analyst a precondition for interpretive work, but the relationship was also the main subject matter of the interpretive work. The patient repeated infantile conflicts in the transference rather than remember them (Freud 1914), so that the transference was a royal road to the unconscious. The transference relationship then became the main subject matter or content of interpretive work. The analyst had to succeed in inducing the patient to regress through frustration so that a transference neurosis would develop. Otherwise, the analyst would not have had any meaningful content to interpret, which would have brought a sense of emotional conviction. Freud (1914) believed that only insight gained in the here-and-now immediacy of the transference relationship to the analyst would bring a sense of emotional conviction, insight that integrated affect and ideation.

For Freud, the relational components of analytic technique were fairly straightforward. To develop rapport, one only needed to listen attentively and sympathetically. To be neutral, one only needed to listen without being judgmental. To be abstinent, one only needed to refrain from gratifying the patient. The only arduous aspect of the relationship was to refrain from acting out the countertransference, as the patient's transference was likely to be experienced as an unconscious provocation. As the relational components of analytic technique were mainly passive, of exercising restraint, the active component of technique, verbal interpretation, was what required considerable attention and thought. Freud's technique papers, Reich's and Fenichel's character analysis, Anna Freud's ego–defense analysis, Sterba's establishment of an observing ego, and so on, reflected strategies of verbal interpretation in which the analyst's noninterpretive participation in the treatment could be taken for granted if the analyst was following the prescribed principles of abstinence and neutrality.

In the work of Stone (1961), Winnicott (1965), and Balint (1968), in particular, the nonverbal ambience of treatment began to be seen as a therapeutic element in and of itself rather than as merely constituting a necessary precondition for verbal interpretation. These theoreticians implied that the classical analyst all along had provided this facilitating and therapeutic ambience or atmosphere without ever being quite fully aware of the therapeutic role of the psychoanalytic situation (Stone 1961) or holding environment (Winnicott 1965), in and of itself independent of interpretation. Yet in the work of Winnicott and Balint, an interesting reversal of priorities appeared to take place as they began to warn of the deleterious effects of certain forms of interpretation on the therapeutic ambience of analysis. Premature interpretations, too-frequent interpretation, too-intrusive interpretation, too much focus on resistance, too much focus on transference, too much focus on unconscious infantile drive-wishes to the exclusion of object relational needs, and so on, might disrupt and spoil the atmosphere of analysis. If it was the ambience or atmosphere that was curative, then it was the ambience that had to be cultivated, facilitated, maintained, and protected. Classical strategies of interpretation began to emerge as a potential danger to the unfolding of the facilitating environment.

This shift in sensibility of the role of interpretation and ambience was well illustrated in Guntrip's (1975) comparison of his analyses with Fairbairn and Winnicott. Guntrip noted the irony that although in terms of theory Fairbairn had made a radical break with Freud, which Winnicott had not, in terms of technique it was exactly the opposite. Fairbairn's consulting room and manner were described as formal and austere, and his interpretations were described as precise, logical constructions. During sessions, Guntrip experienced Fairbairn as like his rejecting schizoid mother, but after sessions when they would discuss theory face to face more informally, he experienced Fairbairn as like a good father. Guntrip made the point that it was the intellectual precision of Fairbairn's interpretive style that fostered the negative transference. Nevertheless, Guntrip did feel that he gained much understanding of himself through his analysis with Fairbairn, which was helpful although he did not feel he reached the deepest levels of his own schizoid pathology because of the limitations of Fairbairn's personal style.

In contrast, Guntrip described Winnicott's consulting room and manner as simple, restful, friendly, and cheery. Winnicott's interpretations were characterized as intuitive, imaginative, and going right to the heart of the matter. Winnicott was experienced as the good mother he never had, which allowed him to reexperience and work through the trauma of his mother's unrelatedness and his brother's death when Guntrip was 3 years old. Though the examples of Winnicott's interpretations were certainly complex, employed theoretical terms, and had elements of obscurity, the interpretations tended to have an affirmative tone and highlight the personal nature of their relationship. At one point, Winnicott noted that analyzing Guntrip made him feel good about himself, whereas the "chap" before Guntrip made Winnicott feel that he was not any good at all.

What is interesting in this comparison is the apparent correlation between the content of the interpretation and the tone or style of its delivery. Fairbairn in content emphasized Guntrip's attachment to his mother as a bad object as well as his hostility toward his mother as a bad object. His mother had been physically abusive as well as emotionally rejecting. His withdrawal was seen as a defense against the revival of this bad object relationship. To confront a patient with his investment in keeping a sadomasochistic relationship alive would seem to call for a fairly cool and matter-of-fact style of delivery as it is the sort of bad news for which the messenger is usually killed. In contrast, the content of Winnicott's interpretations centered on Guntrip's heroic effort to maintain the vitality of his true self in the face of traumatic emotional abandonment. Such interpretations call for a tone of solace and consolation in their delivery, as the implication of such interpretations is that the analyst will be reliably available to support the patient's shattered self. Thus different contents require different styles of delivery so that it is difficult to separate the therapeutic effect of the content of the interpretation from the tone or style of its delivery.

When the ambience of treatment is seen as the essential curative agent, interpretation comes to serve a new function other than the acquisition of insight. Interpretation comes to serve the function of cultivating, maintaining, and protecting the ambience. This function of interpretation can be seen most clearly in the work of Kohut (1971). For Kohut, the analyst's functioning as a selfobject is the curative factor in the analytic relationship, yet the patient's dread of selfobject failure in conjunction with failures of the analyst's empathy may prevent the analyst from being experienced as an effectively functioning selfobject. Interpretation then serves to repair ruptures in the therapeutic relationship. Insight is useful to the extent it allows a curative ambience to be reestablished. Kohut (1984) noted that the experience of being understood allows for a relationship that is curative. Empathy is both a cognitive/emotional understanding of another's subjective experience as well as a form of intersubjective relatedness to that person. Accurate empathy is necessary to achieve empathic relatedness, and it is in achieving and reachieving that quality of relatedness that analysis is curative. Whereas for Freud relationship is in the service of insight, for Kohut insight is in the service of relationship.

Gill (1982) adopted the Sullivanian notion that the analyst is always a participant-observer, or should we say participant-interpreter. According to Gill, the analyst is always interacting with the patient in some manner, intentionally or unintentionally. That participation is always having some impact on the patient, perhaps facilitating of the analysis and perhaps not. It behooves the analyst to attempt to explore and interpret the impact of the analyst's participation on the patient. Since the analyst is always participating or interacting with the patient in some manner and since highly restrained, silent, and intentionally frustrating conduct is indeed a very powerful form of participation, Gill suggested that the analyst may as well act more spontaneously, naturalistically, and freely, and focus interpretation on analyzing the impact on the patient of that style of participation. Gill noted that verbal interpretation is also a form of interaction whose impact must be assessed. Interpretation is not simply a neutral delivery of information but is indeed an interpersonal event that a patient could experience as accepting or rejecting, empathic or critical, supportive or attacking, and so on.

Sandler (1976) noted the analyst's role responsiveness to the patient's transference. The analyst inevitably responds to the patient's transference with a countertransference, a countertransference that is invariably expressed in some manner in the analyst's attitude toward the patient. In other words, the analyst cannot refrain from acting out the countertransference in implicit attitude, though the analyst may succeed in refraining from acting out the countertransference in a more overt and explicit manner. According to Racker (1968), patient and analyst enact a transference–countertransference neurosis reflecting a repetition-compulsion. It is in the analysis of this enactment that both parties may be freed from it to relate to each other in a new manner. Thus, there are always two elements to the interactional ambience of the treatment situation: One aspect reflects a certain type of empathic relatedness that is curative in and of itself in supporting the developmental unfolding of the sense of self. Another aspect, in reflecting a pathological repetition compulsion, is undermining of the unfolding of the sense of self.

A problem in technique arises as it may not be so easy to differentiate healthy empathic relatedness from a pathological repetition-compulsion. If what is in fact a healthy empathic relatedness is misunderstood and misinterpreted as a repetition-compulsion, then that sense of empathic relatedness may be undermined, thus thwarting the developmental unfolding of the sense of self. On the other hand, if a pathological repetition compulsion is misunderstand and misinterpreted as a healthy empathic relatedness, then the analyst would be inadvertently colluding with a pathological enactment from which the patient may never break free. Given that any interaction is comprised of some admixture of these two components, in what light should the interaction be managed and interpreted?

In returning to Guntrip's analyses with Fairbairn and Winnicott, it is surprising how many unanalyzed irregularities in terms of the frame of a classical analysis were present in both of his analyses. For both analyses, Guntrip took extensive notes of all of his sessions. With Fairbairn he had regular face-to-face theoretical discussions after each session, and with Winnicott he only had a few sessions a month and only 150 sessions over a 6-year period. Guntrip reported that he did not resolve the infantile amnesia for his brother's death until after his analysis with Winnicott was over and Winnicott had died. One could suggest that these irregularities may have become the vehicle for unanalyzed transference resistances and the unconscious repetitions of pathological object relations in the transference. Perhaps Guntrip treated Fairbairn and Winnicott in the emotionally withholding and exacting manner in which his mother had treated him, a dynamic that Guntrip did not cite having been analyzed in either of his analyses. Yet at least from Guntrip's perspective, it was exactly the flexibility around frame issues that both Fairbairn and Winnicott exhibited that provided for the relational atmosphere he believed was ultimately curative.

As usual in terms of the sequence of interpretation, the affirmative function of an enactment should be interpreted prior to its defensive function with which it is counterbalanced. In terms of interactional management, an interaction should be managed initially as though it were an apparently wholesome affair to which the analyst readily accommodates prior to its being managed as a pathological transaction to which the analyst attempts to refrain from accommodating so as to avoid collusion. For example, the first time a patient arrives late for a session, the analyst might take the patient's excuse and apology at face value. In managing the lateness, the analyst implicitly affirms that the patient is entitled to the common social courtesy of having one's excuse and apology for a minor discourtesy accepted at face value. After several late arrivals, the analyst might express some skepticism in regard to the patient's excuse, question its validity, and begin to suggest possible defensive functions of arriving late. The analyst implies that chronic lateness is unacceptable, though such an implication could be construed as affirming the patient's potential to be a more reliable and considerate person in the therapeutic relationship.

All interactions are to some degree consciously and intentionally managed by the analyst. Some components of the therapeutic interaction are unintentional in the sense of being unconsciously determined—some combination of the analyst's induced countertransference and of the analyst's own unconscious personality dynamics. Yet independent of the analyst's unconscious contribution to the therapeutic interaction, the analyst's participation is also always a conscious phenomenon that reflects theoretical beliefs, rational planning, anticipation, strategic thinking, and volitional intent. The analyst always possesses a strategy of interactional engagement and management that complements and operates in tandem with the analyst's strategy of verbal interpretation. The classical strategy is one of restraint and frustration. Gill's strategy was one of spontaneity and naturalness, as was that advocated by Fenichel (1941). Winnicott, Balint, and Kohut appeared to have advocated a strategy of management in which the analyst molded to the patient in such a manner as to allow the patient the experience of an undisturbed illusion that served a purpose in enabling the developmental unfolding of the sense of self. Alexander and French implied a strategy of engagement in which the analyst acted in a manner opposite to the patient's transference image of the analyst in order to dispel it. A contemporary application of Alexander and French would be that once the analyst discerned the induced countertransference and role responsiveness, the analyst would adopt a role counter to the role responsiveness. To some degree all analysts attempt to do this. When patients are in a panic, the analyst attempts to respond calmly, though the countertransference is one of anxiety. When the patient is blaming and accusatory, the analyst attempts to respond nondefensively in openly exploring the patient's criticisms, though the countertransference is to counterattack.

Just as interpretations are experienced as interactions that communicate the state of the analyst's relationship with the patient, interactions are experienced as implicit interpretations that contain informational value as to the analyst's assessment of the patient's dynamics. When the analyst responds with calm to the patient's panic, it can be experienced as the equivalent to the verbal interpretation "Your panic is not a realistic response to the current objective reality, but rather it is a product of your own intrapsychic conflicts which you are projecting." When the analyst responds to the patient's accusations nondefensively, it can be experienced as the equivalent to the verbal interpretation "Your accusations against me are ungrounded in reality so I have no need to defend myself, so that your accusations are in actuality projections of your own intrapsychic conflicts that you are avoiding by being provocative." Every communication, be it verbal or nonverbal, contains a metacommunication that is implicit. Implicit in every verbal interpretation is a statement about the state of the relationship between analyst and patient, and implicit in every nonverbal communication is a statement about the analyst's interpretation of the patient's intrapsychic dynamics. Interactions are implicit interpretations, and interpretations are implicit interactions.

I would suggest that the main way in which an ambience is established in the treatment situation is through the use of language. Though it is true that facial expression, tone of voice, and body posture constitute a powerful means of nonverbal and often unconscious communication through which basic affective attitudes are expressed, analysis is foremost a "talking cure." The patient is bathed and immersed in a sea of words, words evoking affect and imagery. Nonverbal communication largely serves as a cue that tells the listener how to interpret verbally conveyed meanings. If nonverbal communication is consistent with verbal communication, the speaker is interpreted to "really" mean what is said. If the nonverbal communication is inconsistent with verbal communication, the speaker is interpreted to not "really" mean what is said or at least as being ambivalent about whether the speaker "really" means what she is saying. Thus, the analyst creates an atmosphere through a style of interpretation that is either amplified or undermined by the analyst's nonverbal communication.

In the following case example, I will illustrate how interpretations are experienced as implicit interactions and how interactions are experienced as implicit interpretations. Though my interpretations were empathic to the patient's state of panic, my relatively calm nonverbal behavior challenged her anxiety-ridden state of mind by implying that her fears might be unfounded, at least from my point of view. The overall metacommunication was to the effect that I was not as worried about her situation as she was but that I would not try to persuade her of my own point of view but try to articulate hers instead. Thus a dynamic balance was maintained between empathy and analysis by being verbally empathic yet nonverbally challenging.

The patient, whom I will call Kathy, was 31 years old when I began working with her in a more than 5-year treatment. Kathy worked as a secretary, was single, and lived at home with her parents. Her presenting problem was that she was having severe panic attacks, felt on the verge of a nervous breakdown, and believed that perhaps she needed to be hospitalized. Kathy believed that the source of her anxiety derived from an incident in which she was walking by a baseball field in a local park and just narrowly missed being hit in the head by a line drive. For her this was a near-death experience or at least one in which she might have become brain damaged for life. Kathy was full of dread that her life hung in the balance. Every time she drove her car she feared she might die in a car accident.

Kathy had completed a 10-year classical psychoanalysis several years before that she felt had been quite helpful. Her only complaint was that her psychiatrist did not believe in medication. Currently she did not feel she needed to be reanalyzed and just wanted some counseling and referral to a psychiatrist for medication. I referred her for a psychiatric consultation, and she was placed on a minor tranquilizer. Her acute panic attacks subsided in the next several months, but Kathy remained unnerved by how close she felt she had come to a nervous breakdown. She worried that she had the potential to become a chronic mental patient who would either be permanently institutionalized or homeless. In fact, Kathy had the demeanor of a chronic mental patient, and other patients of mine who saw her in the waiting room would tell that me that they were relieved that they were not as disturbed as her. The consulting psychiatrist did not think she was psychotic but worried about some sort of subtle neuropsychological problem that accounted for her stiff and affectless demeanor. Kathy could be aptly characterized according to DSM criteria as a schizotypal personality disorder.

During the first year of treatment, Kathy recounted innumerable fears of personal disaster. What if because of her panic attacks she was fired from her job? What if her parents died and she could not take care of herself? What if she had a nervous breakdown? What if she were in a car accident? What if she could not hold down a job? What if she could only be a secretary and that was not enough money to live independently of her parents? What if her parents died and did not leave her any inheritance? Kathy had a profound sense of being unable to take care of herself and a dread that she would be abandoned to fend for herself in a world indifferent to her welfare.

Kathy felt she did the best she could with her limited resources. From an early age she felt she was a social outcast who was different from others. She had always been teased at school and had few friends. Kathy withdrew into a fantasy world in which she could live a different kind of life. In her fantasy life her family members were animals. Her mother was a coyote, her father was a monkey, she was a monkey, and her two older brothers were wolves. They all lived a happy and carefree life in the jungle. Kathy felt that her analysis had taught her how to separate fantasy from reality and learn to live in the real world—as depressing, frightening, and angering as she found the real world to be. She felt her analysis had taught her to take responsibility for herself. She had initiated her analysis in late adolescence when she fought constantly with her parents and did poorly at school. In her twenties she began attending community college and assuming responsibility for a full-time job.

It became apparent that for Kathy, fantasy was a realm of pure wish fulfillment and that reality was a realm in which her most terrifying nightmares would come true. For Kathy, real life was a place of fear and trembling, and fantasy life was a pleasant though unrealistic escape from a terrifying reality. It was clear that Kathy would have been intolerant of any suggestion that reality might not be as immediately life threatening as she imagined it to be. Any attempt at reality testing, in the hopes of reassuring her that either she possessed more coping skills than she gave herself credit for or that she had more social support and more of a safety net than she believed she had, was experienced as a major lack of empathy for her sense of acute endangerment.

It seemed to me that Kathy probably did suffer from an underlying psychotic process but had achieved a stable social adjustment through the help of her previous analysis and family support. It was also clear that her family felt Kathy was a burden that they resented. I hypothesized that the underlying trigger to Kathy's sense of decompensation was that her parents had begun to speak of retiring, moving to Florida, and leaving Kathy behind to fend for herself. Her parents did not like to think of Kathy as a seriously emotionally disturbed individual but rather as an immature adolescent who needed to be pushed out of the nest in order to grow up. Kathy resented this characterization, seeing herself instead as a damaged and defective person who was trying to do the best she could with her limited emotional resources. She protested that she would love to be college educated, have a good job, live independently of her parents, and be married with children, but that did not seem to be within her capacity.

I was worried that Kathy might require psychiatric hospitalization, especially if her parents ever left her to fend for herself. After a few months it became apparent that although her medication was helpful, it only took the edge off her worst fears, which still plagued her and left her feeling at the precipice of a sense of psychological collapse. I was uncertain how to support her as I soon discovered that she experienced efforts to reassure her, focus on the positive, or encourage better coping as pollyannaish and unempathic attempts to avoid facing the horrible reality in which she was required to live her life. Kathy experienced reassurance as dismissal of her experiential reality.

I discovered that the only type of intervention to which Kathy was receptive was when I reflected and stood witness to the horror of her life situation. I interpreted that she felt like Humpty Dumpty who would fall off the wall, shatter into a thousand pieces, and never be put back together again. I reflected that in an individualistic society in which everybody is expected to support herself, there is little sympathy or support for those who cannot support themselves and who are then forced to live marginal lives as social outcasts. I reflected that the world is a dangerous place in which accidents and tragedies occur unpredictably. I reflected that the world is an outrageously unfair place in which injustice goes unpunished. When I made interpretations along these lines, Kathy would close her eyes, raise her head, open her mouth, and silently nod in agreement as though being given communion. It was as though I were feeding a hungry and agitated infant with my interpretations, which left her feeling soothed and pacified.

I was not telling Kathy anything she did not already know, so my interpretations were not a source of novel insight. I was simply articulating a sense of reality that was as familiar to her as the air she breathed but that she felt nobody else understood. Kathy felt that others were privileged to be spared her unhappy fate and that in their privilege they were selfish and self-centered. Even though I existed in the world of privilege, at least I was willing to acknowledge her reality and in a sense offer consolation and solace in witnessing and validating her tragic sense of reality. My interpretations, therefore, were experienced as an interaction, a concrete provision of solace and consolation that did not solve her problems or save her but were a source of comfort and emotional support nevertheless.

Concurrently as my interpretations suggested acceptance

of her sense of impending doom, my interactive style communicated another message. Though I was worried that Kathy might decompensate, I knew that I did not have absolute control of the ultimate outcome of our work together and tried to remain calm and composed in the work. I felt that she did have social support and a safety net if she were to fall apart, so that from my perspective, I did not think it likely she would become a homeless person without resources. Her parents were upper middle class, and Kathy had already saved over a hundred thousand dollars in preparation for that time in the future when she would be on her own. My interactional demeanor suggested implicitly the interpretation "Although I know you feel like you are doomed, I have some confidence that you are not and that perhaps your worst fears do not reflect an invariant external reality beyond your control but reflect in part the externalization of inner fears and fantasies that we may be able to ameliorate through psychological understanding." I knew I could not make such an interpretation explicitly without being experienced as dismissive, and I did not feel we had a sufficient alliance to work through experiences of me as invalidating her.

During the first year of treatment, Kathy attributed any improvement in her condition to her medication, as though psychological understanding could not ameliorate her problems. Nevertheless, the fact that Kathy continued to participate in insight-oriented psychotherapy and was a great believer in psychoanalysis suggested that she possessed latent hopefulness that her troubles could be addressed psychologically. During the second year of treatment, Kathy's worries about the return of her panic attacks began to subside, and fears of imminent personal doom became less pressing. Sessions began to assume the form of weekly updates in which she would check in with me to inform me of the good news that the week had proceeded uneventfully. Kathy would use the sessions to recount the various events of the week about which she had various feelings, but none of which portended crisis or calamity. For the most part Kathy reported these events in a rather affectless manner. As I was not expected to say much, I sometimes had difficulty staying alert during the sessions, but Kathy did not seem to notice or mind.

During the third year of treatment, Kathy began to share with me more of her private fantasy life and also began to discuss her sex life. She told me about what she called the "doody world," which was full of doody brown objects such as doody brown chocolates, doody brown clothing, doody brown people, and so on. One of her friends was a photographer who liked to take photographs of toilets with feces in them, and she found him quite amusing to listen to because of his like-minded obsession with feces. In her fantasy world in which she and her father were monkeys, she fed her father bananas and then changed his diapers like a baby when he made a doody.

In recounting these fantasies in our sessions, I noticed for the first time in our work together that Kathy's frozen, affectless, and masklike facial expression began to crumble, revealing a person who was quite amused and somewhat embarrassed by what she was telling me. When I saw that Kathy was trying to resist her temptation to break into laughter and remain serious in talking about the "doody world," I decided to enter the doody world by indulging in some coprophagic humor, making a joke about how surprised chocolate lovers would be to realize that they were enjoying nothing other than doody brown chocolate. Kathy burst into laughter, saying that she loved chocolate, and I found myself laughing as well as we indulged in "black" humor. Though it felt somewhat perverse to encourage and indulge her in her scatological fantasies, it seemed like a breakthrough in the treatment for Kathy to be emotionally expressive, related, happy, and enthusiastic in my presence. Here was a powerful demonstration that life need not be all doom and gloom as well as fear and trembling. I had a sense that we had connected in a more person-to-person and genuine manner.

Kathy also told me that she had had a long-standing affair with an older married man, but not too long after the previously discussed incident she developed a relationship with a boyfriend. The boyfriend was an unemployed and emotionally disturbed psychologist who was friendly with her photographer friend who was obsessed with feces and toilets. I could now see that Kathy was not an entirely unrelated and affectless person but that her affect and relatedness were reserved for her secret private life in which she found others with whom she could be involved in unconventional ways that might seem perverse by conventional standards. It was only in my interacting with her in a manner that suggested that I was not above indulging in or a stranger to the sort of anal humor and fantasies that she found so enjoyable that I was also able to make a life-affirming connection to her. In mirroring, matching, and amplifying her anal excitement, I was making an implicit interpretation that her anality need not be hidden out of fear of social censure.

As Kathy described the doody world in more detail, I tried to explicitly interpret its psychological function. The doody world reflected a kind of "gallows humor." Though basically Kathy experienced the world as a horrible place in which she would come to a tragic end, she did not have to take her fate lying down and passively. Kathy could laugh in the face of death and be proudly defiant by reducing life to an absurd fecal joke. Her anal universe also expressed her disdain for and defiance of conventional social reality. Kathy felt that conventional reality and especially conventional reality as reflected by her parents was superficial and denied life's essentially tragic nature. In making a mockery of conventional values through anal humor, Kathy felt she could expose the hypocrisy of those who tried to impose a clean, sanitized, and expurgated view of the human situation to which she was expected to respond with a compliant false self. For Kathy, her anally defiant self was her true self, a brutally honest self that had personal integrity, passion, and vitality. Interpretations along these lines were met with agreement and further associations illustrating their validity.

Treatment had begun at the level of Kathy's surface-level self-syntonic sense of self. Kathy saw herself as a fragile and vulnerable person in a world that would let her perish if she had to fend for herself. There was no basis of any therapeutic relationship with her whatsoever if I did not recognize and validate this sense of herself. Even with such affirmation, the beginning of treatment reflected the revival of a narcissistic trauma in the transference, the trauma of psychological collapse in the presence of a sympathetic but essentially powerless witness who will stand by helplessly and watch as Kathy's life ends tragically. As Kathy's ability to endure and contain a tragic sense of life was stabilized, Kathy began to share her private, secret self that lived in a doody world. Her hidden anal self was the carefully protected repository of her sense of aliveness and pleasure in living. Her anal self was a survivor self who laughed in the face of hopelessness and adversity.

In the third year of treatment, her eldest brother, who was married with children and was somewhat of a benign surrogate father whom she expected would look after her after her parents died, developed cancer. In the fourth year of treatment, he died. Kathy was full of rage and a horrendous sense of loss during his illness and after his death. Though I feared she might decompensate, Kathy instead seemed to become more solid and stable. Though her fear of being all alone in the world after her parents died seemed to be more of a sure thing than ever before, she now seemed to be able to face that eventuality with some degree of equanimity. She felt that her parents, lost in their grief over their deceased son, had forgotten that they had a daughter. Her surviving brother, who was a rather irresponsible and immature person, was indifferent to her. The brother she lost was the only person in her family who she felt had ever treated her like a human being.

What emerged more sharply after her brother's death was that in a variety of ways her parents treated her as though she did not have a right to exist as a person in her own right. Whenever Kathy expressed her feelings or her own viewpoint, such as feelings of grief or anger in regard to her brother's death, she felt treated as selfish, inappropriate, audacious, and immature. It was as though her parents felt that her brother's death was a tragedy that had happened only to them and not to their daughter. For Kathy to be anything other than a wallflower was treated as though she

were imposing an unwanted burden that her parents resented. To be treated as though she did not and should not
exist made Kathy feel as though there must be something
horribly wrong with her if she did not deserve to exist as a
person in her own right.

The self-dystonic element that began to emerge was the
sense that a person as selfish, angry, and burdensome as her
did not deserve a life of her own and that she probably should
be punished for being such a worthless person. As Kathy
came to realize that her sense of badness reflected a way she
had been seen and not necessarily the way she was, she
began to express the fantasy of moving out of the house in
several years because she did not like her parents' attitude
toward her and did not want to have to put up with their
invalidating attitude indefinitely. Kathy began to understand
herself as the family scapegoat, the family's emotional "toilet." If she was going to be used as a "toilet" and treated like
feces, then she would find a way to "turn shit into gold," take
something life denying and transform it into something life
affirmative no matter how socially unacceptable that was to
others. Yet to be treated as an emotional scapegoat also left
her feeling emotionally shattered and left for dead.

In terms of technique, there was no clear boundary between interpretation and interaction. Verbal interpretations
were experienced as provisions of consolation, solace, and
comfort to someone who experienced her life as inescapably
tragic. Interactions were experienced as interpretations that
suggested that despite her sense of the tragic, she might
possess hidden strengths, hidden capacities to survive and
persevere, and hidden potentials for vital and passionate
living. When I interacted with her in ways that evoked and
elicited these hidden aspects of herself, these aspects became
amenable to verbal interpretation once they were out in the
open. As the years went by without the return of panic
attacks despite the hardship of her brother's death, Kathy
began to feel that perhaps psychological understanding and
insight did have an ameliorative effect after all. Thus it is
important to recognize that even the analyst who at the level
of verbal interpretation completely refrains from confronting

the patient may at a nonverbal level be responding in a way that represents a significant challenge to the patient's sense of reality. Conversely, even an analyst who is relentlessly confrontative at the level of verbal interpretation may convey an opposite message nonverbally, to the effect that one is in the safe hands of a firm, authoritative, and protective person so that there is no need to feel unsettled by the analyst's provocative verbal interpretations.

CONCLUSION

In my case histories, it is probably apparent that certain preferred story lines emerge in my clinical work. I believe that these typical narratives emerge as a result of the interpretive framework/interactive style which I employ. This style generates a typical sort of therapeutic process that, although differing for different patients, nevertheless embodies some common features. The beginning phase of treatment is characterized by my attempt to ally myself with and affirm the patient's surface-level self-syntonic sense of self. To the extent the patient resists this clinical overture, treatment tends to be slow going or perhaps prematurely terminated. To the extent the patient is receptive to this clinical overture, a positive therapeutic relationship is established concurrent with significant symptom remission. Thus in the beginning phase of treatment, success or failure hinges on the analyst's capacity to work through the patient's resistance to the establishment of an affirmative connection to the patient's surface-level self-syntonic sense of self.

The middle phase of treatment transpires when this initial positive connection to the patient becomes a resistance to deeper work. Thus I try to work dialectically with the patient's positive alliance with the analyst, both as a necessary ingredient of a therapeutic relationship to be empathically affirmed yet as a resistance to deeper work that must be analyzed, for it may embody a repetitive enactment of one sort or another. The patient, on the one hand, resists the analyst's attempts to interpret anything that is self-dystonic and therefore disturbing of the surface-level alliance. The patient experiences interpretation of the self-dystonic as a lack of empathy and a rupture of the therapeutic relationship. On the other hand, to the extent the analyst avoids interpreting the self-dystonic and continues to mirror the self-syntonic, the patient begins to feel that the treatment is becoming boring, repetitive, and superficial. The patient may begin to feel that the analyst expects the patient to be no more than his or her surface-level self-syntonic sense of self. Working through this apparent and recurrent therapeutic stalemate is the essential process of the middle phase of treatment. And working through such ruptures requires constantly reachieving a dynamic balance between empathy and analysis in the clinical work.

The therapeutic stalemate can be more readily worked through if it is understood as a regressive revival of a childhood narcissistic trauma in the transference. The analyst has to fail the patient so that the patient can relive and reexperience core traumatic experiences. If the patient dreads repeating childhood trauma in the transference and keeps the treatment at a surface level, the patient may terminate prematurely, preserving the symptomatic improvement of the beginning phase without the benefit of a deeper repair of the patient's underlying narcissistic vulnerability. To the extent the patient feels sufficiently resilient and has sufficient trust in the analyst, the patient can tolerate the regressive revival of narcissistic trauma in the transference and productively work it through.

The middle phase reflects a return of repressed self-dystonic aspects of self that are projected onto the analyst. As a consequence, in this phase it is useful for the analyst to interpret self-dystonic aspects of self as these are expressed in the negative transference as the patient's experience of the analyst as a moralistic character assassin. I believe that during this phase the patient requires at times an adversarial selfobject who will challenge the patient's point of view with alternative perspectives. Failure to do this is to deprive the patient of a needed form of facilitation. Thus the analyst must balance empathy for what is self-syntonic with analysis of defenses against what is self-dystonic.

The patient's experience of the analyst as a moralistic character assassin may express itself in a variety of persecutory experiences of the analyst that may be expressed both implicitly and explicitly. The patient may feel that the analyst (i.e., head shrinker) is stereotyping or typecasting the patient on the basis of preconceived notions and thereby annihilating the patient's individuality. The analyst is felt to be an egocentric person who can only see the patient through the light of the analyst's all-purpose psychoanalytic theories that reduce the patient to a theoretical formula. The patient may feel that the analyst uses the cleverness of a detective and the prosecutory zeal of a litigator in order to catch and convict the patient for being a fundamentally weak, flawed, and unsavory character. The analyst is seen as a "soul murderer" who takes perverse pleasure in the sadistic omnipotent control of the patient.

The analyst may have difficulty tolerating being seen as a moralistic character assassin, for most analysts imagine themselves to be the exact opposite in their conduct of an analysis: respectful of the patient's individuality, sensitive to the patient's point of view, and nonjudgmental in attitude toward the patient's character. Thus it is tempting for the analyst to assiduously avoid evoking such negative transferences. And when such negative transferences are evoked, it is tempting to interpret them primarily in terms of their defensive functions to the neglect of their self-affirmative functions. To avoid character analysis is to avoid having to deal with such negative transferences, whereas to attempt character analysis is to evoke such negative transferences and have to discover some balance between empathy and analysis in working them through.

As narcissistic trauma is worked through, the patient begins to expand the boundaries of the surface-level self-syntonic sense of self by incorporating formerly repudiated self-dystonic aspects of the personality into it. The analyst repairs the ruptured therapeutic relationship by having empathy for the patient's experience of the analyst as a moralistic character assassin and by forming an affirmative alliance with the "new and improved" version of the surface-level self-syntonic sense of self, which has incorporated formerly repudiated aspects. The analyst must balance empathy with the patient's experience of the negative transference with analysis of its multiple functions (i.e., defensive and repetitive functions). The middle phase, therefore, consists of working through repeated ruptures to the therapeutic relationship in which childhood narcissistic trauma is relived, repudiated self-dystonic elements of self return from repression, and the analyst is experienced as some sort of moralistic character assassin. As the rupture is repaired, the patient establishes a more complex and multidimensional sense of self that incorporates multiple perspectives, and the patient begins to discover that the analyst's existence as a separate subjectivity provides an enriching source of novel perspectives.

Inevitably the dynamic balance between empathy and analysis will be lost, leading either to ruptures in the therapeutic relationship (i.e., too much analysis) or analytic stalemate (i.e., too much empathy). In regaining the dynamic balance between empathy and analysis, the therapeutic process is facilitated, and the twin dangers are avoided of either a treatment that remains stuck at a superficial level or a treatment that the patient experiences as undermining and hurtful. Of course, despite the best balancing act that the analyst can maintain, many moments of the treatment will be stuck at a superficial level, and many moments will arise in which the patient feels the treatment is more hurtful than helpful. Despite the analyst's best effort to apply a balanced approach, it is quite likely that analysis will oscillate between those two extremes as the analytic dyad struggles to find a balance between affirmation and change.

As a general principle of technique, I have argued that empathy for the self-affirmative function of whatever is being subjected to analysis precede yet be counterbalanced by analysis of the defensive function of whatever is being analyzed. Linear/hierarchical modes of clinical reasoning (i.e., working from surface to depth) must take precedence over yet be counterbalanced by dialectical modes of clinical reasoning (i.e., articulating repetitive cycles of reciprocal influence and of rupture and repair as the dyadic system struggles to achieve an evolving homeostatic balance). One must balance working in a manner that reflects a systematic and orderly sequencing of interpretive activity with working in a manner that reflects a spontaneous response to the largely unconscious give-and-take of the therapeutic relationship. Paradoxically, one must respond in a systematic and orderly manner (i.e., secondary process) to a fluid dyadic system, of which one is a participant, that is to a large extent unconsciously organized according to the nonlinear analogical logic of the primary process.

There is no clear-cut termination phase. As the patient's sense of self becomes progressively more complexly defined and as a consequence more resilient, the analysis begins to become superfluous, and the patient is able to terminate. Though one could spend a lifetime in analysis incorporating self-dystonic elements, for there is a bottomless reservoir of self-dystonic elements in the unconscious, at the point of diminishing returns the patient begins to seal over and in so doing stabilizes a surface-level self-syntonic sense of self that is considerably more multidimensional and well integrated than at the beginning of treatment and that seems sufficiently adaptable to living a reasonably satisfying life.

The genre of clinical narration I have been developing tends to focus attention on and highlight certain dimensions of the analytic situation and therefore cannot help but draw attention away from and deemphasize other dimensions of the analytic situation. A focus on here-and-now characterological functioning tends to deemphasize complex genetic or developmental formulations of the origins of here-and-now characterological functioning. There is no reason, though, that my approach could not be complemented by and enriched through the formulation of more comprehensive reconstructions of the origins of the patient's character structure. In addition, my approach has a place for both resuming aborted and arrested development in the transference as well as for reenacting and reliving pathological object relations and narcissistic trauma in the transference. A focus on character analysis, though, tends to highlight the latter rather than the former due to its exposure of the patient's narcissistic vulnerability.

My formulations of character structure tend to highlight self-syntonic surface structure, a focus that tends to reflect secondary process social realism and therefore tends to deemphasize that aspect of self-dystonic deep structure that reflects archaic primary process fantasy life. Again, there is no reason why my approach could not be complemented by and enriched through a more comprehensive elucidation of unconscious conflict in its most infantile and fantastic forms. Any approach that highlights and elucidates a neglected area is vulnerable to the potentiality of overemphasizing the importance of that area of neglect.

From a more interactive point of view, I have placed central emphasis in my clinical narratives on the interactive effects of my preconceived theoretical framework as it manifested itself in my approach to interpretation and my interactive style. As a result, there is a relative deemphasis of the interactive effects of countertransference and my own personality dynamics, which I could have delineated in greater detail if that was to be my central focus. Certainly, choice of theoretical orientation can be seen as derivative of one's own idiosyncratic personality organization. Regardless of the source or sources of one's theoretical orientation, I believe that we all possess preconscious theories of therapeutic technique that exert an organizing influence over the progression of the analysis and that this organizing influence is often obscured to the extent that analysts believe that they are only discovering rather than also creating their findings. Theoretical orientation can be appreciated as a major organizer of how one understands one's own idiosyncratic personality and countertransference.

To some degree, receptivity to the genre of clinical narration I am developing will depend on its aesthetic appeal. Since most genre of clinical narration can be subsumed under the genre of "success stories," it is sometimes difficult to argue with success. Yet analysts, including myself, are well known for arguing with success, so that one analyst's success is another analyst's superficial false-self compliance that avoids grappling with deeper issues that were never adequately addressed. Clinical validity can only be assessed according to particular criteria of validity, and in psychoanalysis there is considerable difference of opinion as to what constitutes valid criteria for evaluating clinical validity. To some extent, each approach provides its own criteria of validity. From the vantage point of my approach, I have been able to critique the clinical adequacy of other approaches to the extent they either succeed or fail to effectively recognize and address the issue of the patient's surface-level self-syntonic sense of self. I have also been able to assess other approaches in terms of how they manage the implicit dynamic tension between empathy and analysis.

I would like to address what I anticipate the criticisms of my approach would be from the various theoretical perspectives. I suspect that classical analysts would view my approach as advocating excessive interactive freedom for the analyst. Classical analysts have warned of multiple dangers arising from interactive excess. Interactive excess may be akin to manipulating the transference rather than analyzing it. Interactive excess may reflect undue avoidance or undue provocation of the negative transference. It can reflect a seduction into some sort of dependent, erotic, or narcissistically gratifying transference. In addition, excess interaction concurrent with face-to-face treatment at once or twice weekly sessions may curtail sufficient regression to allow for the emergence of primitive mental states in the transference.

I do not think that I am advocating significantly more interactive freedom than those ego psychologists who recommend establishing a therapeutic or working alliance or who recommend that unconscious character resistances need to be actively addressed. I see myself as refining those recommendations in suggesting that the alliance is with the patient's surface-level self-syntonic sense of self and that character analysis proceeds after the patient's surface-level self-syntonic sense of self is sufficiently resilient to tolerate being challenged by self-dystonic elements. To the extent I recognize that the alliance with the patient's self-syntonic sense of self will over time become an important transference resistance to be analyzed, I think it diminishes the danger that treatment will be reduced to an unanalyzed transference manipulation. Transference analysis in my approach very much revolves around analyzing resistance to the formation of the alliance, resistance to allowing the therapeutic relationship to go beyond the sense of alliance, repairing ruptures to the alliance, and establishing new forms of alliance as the therapeutic relationship evolves. Likewise, the patient's experience of the analyst as an active analyzer of character is also addressed, recognizing that character analysis is often experienced as some sort of narcissistically wounding character assassination.

The possibility that my approach would curtail regression can be countered in noting that regression to the reliving of narcissistic trauma in the transference is very painful for the patient. Narcissistic trauma generates profound feelings of shame, helplessness, confusion, and impotent rage. In the transference there is intense persecutory anxiety, hatred of the analyst for being traumatogenic, and guilt over hating the analyst with whom one had formerly been in a relatively nonambivalent alliance. This is clearly a volatile situation in which the patient may be retraumatized and damaged by the analysis. I believe that my approach manages the regressive revival of narcissistic trauma in the transference in a judicious manner that is neither unduly provocative nor unduly avoidant of such regression. In recognizing that astute character analysis goes right to the heart of the patient's narcissistic vulnerability and regressively revives narcissistic trauma, the analyst is able to have greater empathy for the patient's experience of character analysis.

The limitation of the classical approach, from my point of view, is the insufficient interactive freedom that the analyst is allowed. The classical approach, despite claims of neutrality, does reflect an interactive style that exerts an interactive pressure. Sustained silence, abstinence, frequent sessions, and use of the couch constitute a powerful pull toward a hostile, dependent relationship with the analyst. The patient is implicitly encouraged to participate in and tolerate a relationship that is simultaneously intense and frustrating. The intensity induces regression to dependence, and the frustration induces hostility. A hostile, dependent relationship emerges unless the analyst interacts with the patient in other ways that decrease the intensity of the relationship and are more gratifying, thus attenuating the emergence of hostile dependence. Different patients will defend against regression to hostile dependence in different ways, yet those differences in the ways different patients respond to the classical stance do not negate the fact that the classical stance exerts a particular interactive pressure. To the extent the classical stance induces a hostile, dependent relationship, it may be experienced as undermining of the patient's surface-level self-syntonic sense of self. Such a stance is not neutral but is taking sides in a conflict. It is implicitly taking the side of what is self-dystonic against the side of what is self-syntonic.

To undermine the surface-level self-syntonic sense of self prior to having recognized and affirmed it can be a prescription for therapeutic stalemate. This is a frequent problem I have found among classically oriented analysts in training whom I have supervised. Elements of the classical approach such as extended silence, abstinence, high session frequency, and use of the couch may make many patients with "garden variety" neuroses less rather than more analyzable due to excessive destabilization of the self-syntonic sense of self. Though many classical analysts claim from so-called empirical experience and personal authority that more is better, I could also claim from empirical experience and personal authority that many patients who had years of classical analysis with limited benefit went on to do better in a less frequent, face-to-face, more freely interactive psychoanalytic treatment. I am sure that classical analysts could supply just as many anecdotes reporting the exact opposite. All this says to me is that we are constructionists who organize the data of analysis in keeping with our own theoretical preconceptions.

What I would hope that classical analysts might appreciate in my approach and even attempt to utilize is my refinement of the technique of working from surface to depth. My approach to character analysis extends a Freudian tradition that has been refined by Reich, Fenichel, Brenner, and Schafer, to name a few classical notables whom I have quoted and incorporated in my own fashion. To think of the mind in terms of a surface structure that is self-syntonic and a deep structure that is self-dystonic enables one to see more precisely what is on the surface of the mind, to see the world from the tip of the iceberg facing a particular direction. This sort of pinpoint accuracy is very useful if one's aim is to work systematically from surface to depth. I believe that my explicit conceptualization of surface structure is clinically useful and that surface structure has tended to be vaguely delineated in psychoanalytic theory in general, which has tended to be overly fascinated by and overvalue work with deep structure. For this reason, it has tended for the most part, with a few notable exceptions, to bypass, minimize, and devalue as defensively avoidant or superficial more extensive work with surface structure.

Perhaps classical clinicians might feel that I am overemphasizing the issue of the patient's narcissistic vulnerability in making the self-syntonic self-dystonic and not giving sufficient attention to the interpretation of other dynamic issues like the interpretation of derivatives of infantile sexual and aggressive fantasies. I hope that I have demonstrated that although I give a major emphasis to this issue, I do not give it an exclusive emphasis. I believe that it is a greater error in technique to underemphasize than to overemphasize this issue. Insensitivity to the patient's narcissistic vulnerability is more difficult to remediate than is oversensitivity to the patient's narcissistic vulnerability. This is not to say that insensitivity to the patient's narcissistic vulnerability is a horrific mistake, as the analyst can always attempt to remediate the effects of the analyst's insensitivity in empathizing with the patient's experience of the analyst's insensitivity. If the analyst is insensitive to the patient's experience of the analyst's insensitivity, a situation has been created that is ripe for a negative therapeutic reaction. On the other hand, if the analyst is consistently overly sensitive to the patient's narcissistic vulnerability, the treatment may remain somewhat superficial in certain respects, yet that deficiency can be easily remedied if the analyst begins to interpret more deeply.

I anticipate that the major criticism of my approach from self psychology is that any approach that challenges or questions the patient's point of view or any approach that utilizes objectifying characterizations of the patient is incompatible with an empathic stance as many self psychologists seem to define empathy. I believe that the analyst must extend empathy to multiple and conflicting points of view that the patient possesses and that one often repudiated point of view is that of the patient as an object and a character in the eyes of others, including the analyst. I believe that self psychologists tend to lack empathy for certain frames of reference in tending to focus their empathic efforts primarily on what I would label the patient's surface-level self-syntonic sense of self.

This heightened empathic focus on a particular dimension of the patient's self-experiencing is a virtue as well as a weakness of self psychology. The virtue of the self-psychological approach is in its effectiveness in stabilizing and affirming the patient's surface-level self-syntonic sense of self. The weakness is that there is relatively less empathy for self-dystonic and conflicting dimensions of self-experience, which tend to be repudiated, especially unconscious identifications with hated aspects of the parents and, in particular, identification with hated aspects of the parent of the opposite sex. These identifications are often enacted as role reversals in the transference, which self psychologists are less inclined to recognize, tending to view the analyst as a parental selfobject.

The patient's perennial curiosity toward and fear of the analyst's separate subjectivity and preconceptions tend to be minimized by self psychology or are seen as arising only as a developmental achievement late in the analysis, as though more disturbed patients lack curiosity about the analyst's independent perspective. To the extent I see my approach as expanding the range of the analyst's empathy and increasing the range of the analyst's interactive freedom to facilitate self-development, I believe my approach is in many respects an extension of Kohut's self-psychological sensibility, though I realize that many mainstream self psychologists might see my character-analytic approach as retrograde or deviant, perhaps intrinsically incompatible with the tenets of self psychology.

It seems to me that when empathy is defined as consistently understanding the world from the patient's subjective point of view, there is a presumption that the analyst is capable of eventually making a clear-cut demarcation between the analyst's viewpoint and the patient's viewpoint.

Stolorow and Atwood (1992) have suggested in their intersubjective approach that the analyst's and the patient's viewpoints interpenetrate in the analytic situation. The idea that
the patient has a separate perspective independent of the
particular intersubjective context in which the patient's perspective is embedded can be seen as reflecting what Stolorow
and Atwood called the "myth of the isolated mind." The
dichotomy of labeling one viewpoint as subjective and another as objective, one as self and one as other, one as inner
and another as outer, as well as one as the patient's and one
as the analyst's is to some extent arbitrary. All viewpoints can
be understood as condensations of subjective and objective
perspectives, self and other vantage points, and inner and
outer realities. The experience of boundaries between these
dichotomous aspects of self-experience is a psychological
phenomenon that has a developmental history and is intersubjectively constructed.

If the boundaries between self and other, inner and outer,
and subjective and objective are not fixed in any absolute or
ultimate manner but are fluid and malleable, then notions of
what is empathic are relative to fluid and shifting perspectives. If there is no such thing as a purely subjective frame of
reference that is not thoroughly infiltrated and interpenetrated by otherness and externality, then we might speak of
the "illusion of empathy." People do indeed have experiences
of being understood, but people also have experiences in
which in retrospect from a new vantage point and as a result
of new experience, they reinterpret the past experience of
being understood as an illusion of having been understood
that reflected their prior suggestibility, naiveté, gullibility, or
lack of experience. What is empathic from one perspective
can be felt as unempathic from another perspective. As
patients possess multiple and conflicting perspectives that
evolve over time, there is no guarantee that what was
experienced as empathic at one particular point in time
through the filtering lens of one particular perspective will be
at a later date construed as empathic in the light of an
alternative perspective. Similarly, an interpretation that at the
moment was experienced as unempathic may at a later date

be reinterpreted as having been quite empathic in the light of a different perspective, perhaps understanding that one had been too defensive at the time to have been open to an alternative point of view.

Kleinian concepts such as projection, introjection, projective identification, and introjective identification seem to capture the essential fluidity and reversibility of self and other as well as inner and outer points of view. Perceptions of external reality can reflect projections of inner states, while perceptions of internal reality can reflect incorporations of the perspectives, values, attitudes, and beliefs of others with whom one is identified. There is no perception of a pure objective reality that is not filtered through the lens of a personal subjective viewpoint, and there is no experience of a pure subjective reality that is not contaminated by identifications with the external viewpoints of others. I would suggest that we are inevitably identified with the perspective of others and that we learn to see ourselves (i.e., we become a subject) through identification with how we are seen in the eyes of others. The self is a "looking glass self," as a sociologist like Mead (1934) would put it.

Empathic constructions say as much about the analyst's point of view as about the patient's point of view so that the analyst is creating as well as discovering the patient's subjectivity. Analytic cure in part reflects the patient's identification with the analyst's creative formulations of the patient's subjectivity and in so doing making those modes of understanding the patient's own. Self psychology's understanding of empathy seems to minimize the analyst's creativity in the analytic situation. Are selfobject transferences created as well as discovered, and what does it mean if the analyst is creating a selfobject transference rather than some other kind of transference?

Perhaps the belief that the patient's perspective can be clearly differentiated from and understood apart from the analyst's perspective serves in part as a defense against "interpenetration anxiety." There is inevitably a fear that the integrity and wholesomeness of the surface-level self-syntonic sense of self will be violated, defiled, and usurped by unsolicited and unwanted invasion by alien mentalities. I believe that despite dread of an annihilating encounter with the alien unknown, there is also curiosity about the nature of the alien unknown. And it is only in satisfying that curiosity that the boundaries of the self can be enlarged and become more inclusive of what had previously been experienced as alien and anathema to what was presumed to be the intrinsic nature of the self.

My impression of the self-psychological approach to treatment is that it embodies considerable ambivalence in regard to the issue of the analyst's interactive freedom. In comparison to classical analysts, self psychologists seem to advocate greater interactive freedom in the service of affirming the patient's sense of self. Not wanting to be perceived as too stodgy, formal, detached, or poker-faced by patients, self psychology suggests a greater willingness to inject emotional responsivity, enthusiasm, humor, and the exchange of social amenities into the analytic encounter. Yet there is also a fear of interactive freedom, that the overly active analyst could infringe on and derail the natural developmental unfolding of the patient's sense of self. The overly interactive analyst may not allow selfobject transferences silently to unfold undisturbed; instead, the patient will develop a compliant false self that will submit to the interactive style of an overbearing analyst. I would say that the patient who is so disposed could develop a compliant false self to any interactive style be it passive or active, supportive or confrontative, and similarly the patient who is so disposed could oppose any interactive style.

To some extent, self psychology contains an implicit characterology that objectifies the patient in terms many patients may find both flattering and unflattering. Self psychology tends to judge and evaluate patients in terms of whether their selves are strong or weak, whole or fragmented, developmentally evolved or developmentally arrested, vital or depleted, grandiose or deflated, resilient or vulnerable, actively initiating or passively traumatized, and so on. I imagine some patients might experience it as a form of character assassination to be seen as weak, fragmented, developmentally arrested, depleted, deflated, vulnerable, and traumatized. And other patients might experience it as a form of character affirmation to be seen as strong, whole, developmentally evolved, vital, resilient, and actively initiating.

In terms of object relations theory, I would wonder whether there would be a sense that my emphasis on the surface structure of the mind is somehow avoidant of the deep structure of the mind and its manifestations in the unconscious transference–countertransference dynamics of the analytic dyad. My impression of object relations theory in practice is that the focus is on elucidating the unconscious repetition of pathological object relations in the transference–countertransference relationship. Clinical events such as projective identification, induced countertransference, role responsiveness, and role reversal seem central in the object-relational understanding of the analytic process. I have no problem with this model as a means of understanding the deep structure of the patient's mind and how it expresses itself unconsciously in the transference. Perhaps from the vantage point of object relations theory, my approach seems fearfully wedded to surface-level social realism at the expense of a deeper-level appreciation of atavistic and fantastic relational terrors.

My problem with object relations theory is that I see little awareness of surface structure and therefore minimal interpretive work at that level of mental functioning. In not working from surface to depth, the object relations clinician runs the risk of premature interpretation. The result of the premature interpretation of self-dystonic repetitions in the transference of pathological object relations is that the surface-level self-syntonic sense of self is destabilized rather than affirmed. To the extent the surface-level self-syntonic sense of self serves as a resistance to the experiencing of unconscious self-dystonic elements, to bypass its interpretations is to interpret content before resistance and thus ignore a split-off surface-level resistance that continues to be opera tive despite apparent access to deeper material. My approach can provide object relations theorists with a relational model of working from surface to depth.

Object relations approaches tend to overemphasize dialectic reasoning (i.e., articulating repetitive transference–countertransference configurations as they spontaneously arise in the clinical encounter) to the exclusion of linear/hierarchical clinical reasoning that highlights orderly interpretive sequences (i.e., working from surface to depth or interpreting defense before drive-wish). Paradoxically, the object relations approach may reflect a breakdown of dialectical balance in failing to counterbalance dialectical reasoning, which it overutilizes with linear/hierarchical modes of organizing the clinical material, which it underutilizes. This is probably why there is not nearly as much written on principles of technique from the object relations perspective as there is from the Freudian perspective. Recommending a principle of technique only makes sense if one can envision an analysis as unfolding in an orderly, predictable sequence of events. It can be a skewed approach to *always* and *only* think dialectically, just as it may be a skewed approach to *always* and *only* think in linear/hierarchical modes.

When narcissistic traumas of childhood are regressively revived in the transference, one also sees the emergence of the sort of primitive mental states that object relations theorists have often described. In the traumatic state, there tends to be blurring of self and other boundaries, rapid role reversals, confusion, persecutory anxiety, split and polarized experience of self in relation to others, affect flooding, and intense countertransference evocation. Such traumatic states are not infrequently elicited by the attempt to analyze character. Thus I believe that I get to the same place that object relations theorists attempt to get to, but perhaps it takes me longer to get there because I spend more time and emphasis exploring and interpreting surface structure. I believe that sustained immersion in surface structure makes in the end for a more meaningful experience of deep structure. It provides a broader context in which the experience of deep structure can be embedded and as such constitutes part of the containing and holding functions of the analysis.

In terms of interpersonal theory, I am sure that I have a greater proclivity for reifying structural metaphors than interpersonalists in the tradition of Sullivan who prefer to speak of process rather than structure. My concreteness in this respect, I believe, is adaptive because I think it is difficult to capture intrapsychic complexity without the use of structural metaphors. Descriptions of interpersonal complexity alone do not require structural metaphors, as an interaction between two people can be readily described as a process of mutual influence in which social roles are fluid, interchangeable, and ever evolving. To the extent the person is seen as a reflection of an ever-changing social scene, there is little need to conceptualize the person or the person's inner experience in terms of invariant properties. To the extent the person is seen as an independent center of initiative that shapes as well as is shaped by the social surround, there is a need to formulate the relatively stable organizing principles through which the person aims to influence and shape the environment so that the environment accommodates to the person.

As noted previously, I tend to focus more on the interpersonal impact of the analyst's preconceptions than on countertransference or the analyst's personality. I believe that preconceptions shape countertransference and that preconceptions shape the way in which the analyst formulates his or her own personality. I believe that sometimes interpersonal analysts become naive realists in their approach to examining the impact of the analyst's personality and the impact of the analyst's countertransference on the analytic process. They do not always see how their depictions of interactional (i.e., transference–countertransference configurations) dynamics are shaped by their own theoretical preconceptions.

Though the narrative that arises through psychoanalytic dialogue is co-authored and thus a collaborative enterprise, I suspect that every analytic narrative reflects in part the analyst's personal signature. I think that the fear that an overbearing analyst can impose a viewpoint on a hapless patient who accommodates to the analyst's procrustean bed tends to obscure the fact that analysis is always interpenetrated by the analyst's viewpoint, to which the patient's subjective universe is assimilated. This is not to say that analysts do not also have to accommodate their theoretical preconceptions to the individual patient, as psychological understanding is always a process of assimilation and accommodation.

Each orientation can be thought of as a self-syntonic system of thought to its practitioners, in relation to which competing orientations seem self-dystonic. To the extent I make unflattering as well as flattering characterizations of a particular orientation that is self-syntonic to the reader, I am in a sense conducting a character analysis of the orientation that could be experienced by its advocates as a sort of slanderous character assassination that tendentiously misrepresents and caricatures the orientation. Oftentimes comparative psychoanalytic dialogue seems to proceed by comparing an elegant and subtle version of the favored theory with a crude and simplistic version of the rival theory, thereby setting up a straw man that is then unfairly knocked down. Though I aspire to present a reasonable characterization of the views with which I disagree, it seems characteristic of theoretical debates in psychoanalysis that the subject of the critique feels grievously misunderstood. It is as though most psychoanalytic criticism is experienced by the subject of that criticism as a form of crude and unempathic character analysis.

To the extent, though, that my argument has persuaded the reader of the usefulness of an alternative point of view, the scope and multidimensionality of the self-syntonic theoretical orientation of the reader will be enlarged. To the extent my argument fails to persuade, confuses, or offends, the process is stalled at the point of empathic failure, and it may be difficult to move on to a consideration of the next point of disagreement. I hope that in empathically appreciating the strengths of each theoretical orientation, I have been able to create a climate in which the limitations as well as the strengths of each point of view can be openly and fairly analyzed. In the final analysis, the process of theoretical integration in psychoanalytic scholarship is not so different from the process of characterological integration in the treatment situation, posing similar challenges yet offering similar rewards.

REFERENCES

Alexander, F., and French, T. M. (1946). *Psychoanalytic Therapy*. New York: Ronald.

Apfelbaum, B., and Gill, M. M. (1989). Ego analysis and the relativity of defense: technical implications of the structural theory. *Journal of the American Psychoanalytic Association* 37:1071–1096.

Anzieu, D. (1989). *The Skin Ego: A Psychoanalytic Approach to the Self*. New Haven, CT: Yale University Press.

Arlow, J. A., and Brenner, C. (1964). *Psychoanalytic Concepts and the Structural Theory*. New York: International Universities Press.

Atwood, G. E., and Stolorow, R. D. (1979). *Faces in a Cloud: Subjectivity in Personality Theory*. New York: Jason Aronson.

—————— (1984). *Structures of Subjectivity: Explorations in Psychoanalytic Phenomenology*. Hillsdale, NJ: Analytic Press.

Balint, M. (1968). *The Basic Fault: Therapeutic Aspects of Regression*. New York: Brunner/Mazel.

Beck, A. T., Freeman, A., and Associates. (1990). *Cognitive Therapy of Personality Disorders*. New York: Guilford.

Beebe, B., and Lachmann, F. (1992). A dyadic systems view of communication. In *Relational Perspectives in Psychoanalysis*, ed. N. Skolnick and S. Warshaw. Hillsdale, NJ: Analytic Press.

Benjamin, J. (1988). *The Bonds of Love: Psychoanalysis, Feminism, and the Problem of Domination*. New York: Pantheon.

Bion, W. R. (1967). *Second Thoughts: Selected Papers on Psycho-Analysis*. New York: Jason Aronson.

Blechner, M. (1993). Homophobia in psychoanalytic writing and practice. *Psychoanalytic Dialogues: A Journal of Relational Perspectives* 3:627–638.

Bollas, C. (1987). *The Shadow of the Object: Psychoanalysis of the Unthought Known*. New York: Columbia University Press.

—————— (1989). *Forces of Destiny: Psychoanalysis and Human Idiom*. London: Free Association Books.

Brenner, C. (1979). Working alliance, therapeutic alliance, and transference. *Journal of the American Psychoanalytic Association* 27:137–158.

—————— (1982). *The Mind in Conflict*. New York: International Universities Press.

Breuer, J., and Freud S. (1895). Studies on hysteria. *Standard Edition* 2.

Ehrenberg, D. B. (1992). *The Intimate Edge: Extending the Reach of Psychoanalytic Interaction*. New York: Norton.

Eissler, K. R. (1958). Notes on problems of technique in the psychoanalytic treatment of adolescents: with some remarks on perversions. *Psychoanalytic Study of the Child* 13:223–254.

Ellis, A. (1985). *Overcoming Resistance: Rational-Emotive Therapy with Difficult Clients*. New York: Springer.

Erikson, E. (1959). *Identity and the Life Cycle: Selected Papers*. New York: International Universities Press.

Fast, I. (1984). *Gender Identity: A Differentiation Model*. Hillsdale, NJ: Analytic Press.

Fenichel, O. (1941). *Problems of Psychoanalytic Technique*. New York: Psychoanalytic Quarterly.

—— (1953). *The Collected Papers of Otto Fenichel: First Series*. New York: Norton.

—— (1954). *The Collected Papers of Otto Fenichel: Second Series*. New York: Norton.

Ferenczi, S. (1925). Contra-indications to the "active" psycho-analytical technique. In *Further Contributions to the Theory and Technique of Psycho-Analysis*, pp. 217–230. London: Hogarth, 1950.

Freud, A. (1936). *The Ego and the Mechanisms of Defense*. New York: International Universities Press.

Freud, S. (1953–1974). *Standard Edition of the Complete Psychoanalytic Works*, ed. and trans. James Strachey. London: Hogarth. (Hereafter cited as *Standard Edition*.)

—— (1900). The interpretation of dreams. *Standard Edition*, vols. 4 and 5.

—— (1905). Three essays on the theory of sexuality. *Standard Edition* 7:125–245.

—— (1909). Notes upon a case of obsessional neurosis. *Standard Edition* 10:155–249.

—— (1910). "Wild" psycho-analysis. *Standard Edition* 11:219–227.

—— (1911). The handling of dream-interpretation in psycho-analysis. *Standard Edition* 12:89–96.

—— (1912a). The dynamics of transference. *Standard Edition* 12:97–108.

—— (1912b). Recommendations to physicians practicing psycho-analysis. *Standard Edition* 12:109–120.

—— (1913). On beginning the treatment (further recommendations on the technique of psychoanalysis I). *Standard Edition* 12:121–144.

—— (1914a). On narcissism: an introduction. *Standard Edition* 14:73–102.

—— (1914b). Remembering, repeating, and working-through (further recommendations on the technique of psychoanalysis II). *Standard Edition* 12:145–156.

—— (1915). Observations on transference-love (further recommendations on the technique of psychoanalysis III). *Standard Edition* 12:157–171.

—— (1916). Some character-types met with in psycho-analytic work. *Standard Edition* 14:159–171.

—— (1917). Mourning and melancholia. *Standard Edition* 14:237–258.

—— (1923). The ego and the id. *Standard Edition* 19:1–66.

—— (1926). Inhibitions, symptoms and anxiety. *Standard Edition* 20:75–175.

—— (1937a). Analysis terminable and interminable. *Standard Edition* 23:209–253.

—— (1937b). Constructions in analysis. *Standard Edition* 23:257–269.

Friedman, L. (1969). The therapeutic alliance. *International Journal of Psycho-*

Analysis 50:139–153.

Gill, M. (1982). *Analysis of Transference*, vol. I. New York: International Universities Press.

Glover, E. (1955). *The Technique of Psycho-Analysis*. New York: International Universities Press.

Goffman, E. (1959). *The Presentation of Self in Everyday Life*. New York: Anchor.

Goldner, V. (1991). Toward a critical relational theory of gender. *Psychoanalytic Dialogues* 1:249–272.

Gray, P. (1994). *The Ego and the Analysis of Defense*. Northvale, NJ: Jason Aronson.

Greenson, R. (1967). *The Technique and Practice of Psychoanalysis*, vol. I. New York: International Universities Press.

———— (1974). Transference: Freud or Klein. *International Journal of Psychoanalysis* 55:37–48.

Grossman, W. (1982). The self as fantasy: fantasy as theory. *Journal of the American Psychoanalytic Association* 30:919–938.

Guntrip, H. (1969). *Schizoid Phenomena, Object Relations and the Self*. New York: International Universities Press.

———— (1975). My experience of analysis with Fairbairn and Winnicott. *International Review of Psychoanalysis* 2:145–156.

Hartmann, H. (1939). *Ego Psychology and the Problem of Adaptation*. New York: International Universities Press.

———— (1951). Technical implications of ego psychology. In *Essays on Ego Psychology*, pp. 142–154. New York: International Universities Press, 1964.

Horney, K. (1950). *Neurosis and Human Growth*. New York: Norton.

Josephs, L. (1989). The world of the concrete: a comparative approach. *Contemporary Psychoanalysis* 25:479–500.

———— (1992). *Character Structure and the Organization of the Self*. New York: Columbia University Press.

Kanzer, M. (1981). Freud's "analytic pact": the standard therapeutic alliance. *Journal of the American Psychoanalytic Association* 29:69–87.

Kernberg, O. (1975). *Borderline Conditions and Pathological Narcissism*. New York: Jason Aronson.

———— (1984). *Severe Personality Disorders: Psychotherapeutic Strategies*. New Haven, CT: Yale University Press.

Kernberg, O., Selzer, A., Koenigsberg, H., et al. (1989). *Psychodynamic Psychotherapy of Borderline Patients*. New York: Basic Books.

Kohut, H. (1959). Introspection, empathy, and psychoanalysis. *Journal of the American Psychoanalytic Association* 7:459–483.

———— (1971). *The Analysis of the Self*. New York: International Universities Press.

———— (1977). *The Restoration of the Self*. New York: International Universities Press.

———— (1979). The two analyses of Mr. Z. *International Journal of Psycho-Analysis* 60: 3–27.

———— (1984). *How Does Analysis Cure?* ed. A. Goldberg. Chicago: University of Chicago Press.

Kris, E. (1951). Ego psychology and interpretation in psychoanalytic therapy. *Psychoanalytic Quarterly* 20:15–30.

Lesser, R. (1993). A reconsideration of homosexual themes. *Psychoanalytic Dialogues: A Journal of Relational Perspectives* 3:639–642.

Levy, S. T., and Inderbitzin, L. B. (1990). The analytic surface and the theory of technique. *Journal of the American Psychoanalytic Association* 38:371–391.

Lewis, H. B. (1971). *Shame and Guilt in Neurosis*. New York: International Universities Press.

Lichtenberg, J. D., Lachmann, F. M., and Fosshage, J. L. (1992). *Self and Motivational Systems: Toward a Theory of Psychoanalytic Technique*. Hillsdale, NJ: Analytic Press.

Lichtenstein, H. (1977). *The Dilemma of Human Identity*. New York: Jason Aronson.

Loewald, H. (1960). On the therapeutic action of psychoanalysis. *International Journal of Psycho-Analysis* 41:16–33.

_____ (1962). The superego and the ego-ideal. II. Superego and time. *International Journal of Psycho-Analysis* 43:264–268.

Loewald, H. (1980). *Papers on Psychoanalysis*. New Haven: Yale University Press.

Loewenstein, R. M. (1951). The problem of interpretation. *Psychoanalytic Quarterly* 20:1–14.

_____ (1954). Some remarks on defences, autonomous ego and psychoanalytic technique. *International Journal of Psycho-Analysis* 35: 188–193.

_____ (1956). Some remarks on the role of speech in psycho- analytic technique. *International Journal of Psycho-Analysis* 37:460–468.

McDougall, J. (1985). *Theaters of the Mind: Illusion and Truth on the Psychoanalytic Stage*. New York: Basic Books.

Mead, G. H. (1934). *Mind, Self, and Society from the Standpoint of a Social Behaviorist*, ed. C. W. Morris. Chicago: University of Chicago Press.

Mitchell, S. A. (1988). *Relational Concepts in Psychoanalysis*. Cambridge: Harvard University Press.

_____ (1991). Contemporary perspectives on self: toward an integration. *Psychoanalytic Dialogues: A Journal of Relational Perspectives* 1:121–148.

_____ (1992). Commentary on Trop and Stolorow's "Defense Analysis in Self Psychology." *Psychoanalytic Dialogues: A Journal of Relational Perspectives* 2:443–453.

_____ (1993). *Hope and Dread in Psychoanalysis*. New York. Basic Books.

Ogden, T. (1982). *Projective Identification and Psychotherapeutic Technique*. New York: Jason Aronson.

Ornstein, A. (1974). The dread to repeat and the new beginning. *Annual of Psychoanalysis* 2:231–248. New York: International Universities Press.

Piaget, J. (1954). *The Construction of Reality in the Child*. New York: Basic Books.

Racker, H. (1968). *Transference and Countertransference*. London: Maresfield Reprints.

Reich, W. (1928). On character analysis. In *The Psychoanalytic Reader*, ed. R.

Fliess, vol. 1, pp. 129–147. New York: International Universities Press.
_____ (1933). *Character Analysis*. New York: Pocket Books.
Rosenfeld, H. (1964). On the psychopathology of narcissism: a clinical approach. *International Journal of Psycho-Analysis* 45:332–337.
Sandler, J. (1976). Countertransference and role-responsiveness. *International Review of Psycho-Analysis* 3:43–47.
Schafer, R. (1983). *The Analytic Attitude*. New York: Basic Books.
Schwartz, D. (1993). Heterophilia—the love that dare not speak its aim. *Psychoanalytic Dialogues: A Journal of Relational Perspectives* 3:643–642.
Shapiro, D. (1989). *Psychotherapy of Neurotic Character*. New York: Basic Books.
Shengold, L. (1989). *Soul Murder: The Effects of Childhood Deprivation and Abuse*. New Haven, CT: Yale University Press.
Spence, D. P. (1987). *The Freudian Metaphor: Toward Paradigm Change in Psychoanalysis*. New York: Norton.
Sterba, R. (1934). The fate of the ego in analytic therapy. *International Journal of Psycho-Analysis* 15:117–126.
_____ (1953). Clinical and therapeutic aspects of character resistance. *Psychoanalytic Quarterly* 22:1–20.
Stern, D. (1985). *The Interpersonal World of the Infant*. New York: Basic Books.
Stolorow, R. D., and Atwood, G. E. (1991). The mind and the body. *Psychoanalytic Dialogues: A Journal of Relational Perspectives* 1:181–196.
_____ (1992). *Contexts of Being: The Intersubjective Foundations of Psychological Life*. Hillsdale, NJ: Analytic Press.
Stolorow, R. D., Brandchaft, B., and Atwood, G. E. (1987). *Psychoanalytic Treatment: An Intersubjective Approach*. Hillsdale, NJ: Analytic Press.
Stolorow, R., and Trop, J. (1992). Reply to Richards and Mitchell. *Psychoanalytic Dialogues: A Journal of Relational Perspectives* 2:467–473.
_____ (1993). Reply to Blechner, Lesser, and Schwartz. *Psychoanalytic Dialogues: A Journal of Relational Perspectives* 3:653–656.
Stone, L. (1961). *The Psychoanalytic Situation*. New York: International Universities Press.
Strachey, J. (1934). The nature of the therapeutic action of psycho-analysis. *International Journal of Psycho-Analysis* 15:127–159.
Sullivan, H. S. (1950). The illusion of personal individuality. *Psychiatry* 13:317–332.
_____ (1953). *The Interpersonal Theory of Psychiatry*. New York: Norton.
Trop, J., and Stolorow, R. (1992). Defense analysis in self psychology: a developmental view. *Psychoanalytic Dialogues: A Journal of Relational Perspectives* 2:427–442.
Wachtel, P. L. (1993). *Therapeutic Communication: Principles and Effective Practice*. New York: Guilford.
Waelder, R. (1930). The principle of multiple function: observations on overdetermination. In *Psychoanalysis: Observation, Theory, Application*, ed. S. A. Guttman, pp. 68–83. New York: International Universities Press, 1976.
Weiss, J., and Sampson, H. (1986). *The Psychoanalytic Process: Theory, Clinical*

Observation and Empirical Research. New York: Guilford.

Winnicott, D.W. (1960). Ego distortion in terms of true and false self. In *The Maturational Processes and the Facilitating Environment*, pp. 140–152. New York: International Universities Press, 1965.

———— (1963). Communicating and not communicating leading to a study of certain opposites. In *The Maturational Processes and the Facilitating Environment*, pp. 83–92. New York: International Universities Press, 1965.

———— (1965). *The Maturational Processes and the Facilitating Environment*. New York: International Universities Press.

———— (1971). *Playing and Reality*. London: Tavistock.

Wolf, E. S. (1988). *Treating the Self: Elements of Clinical Self Psychology*. New York: Guilford.

Zetzel, E. R. (1956). Current concepts of transference. *International Journal of Psycho-Analysis* 37:369–378.

INDEX

Abreaction, defense analysis,
236–237
Abstinence, nonverbal interaction,
377, 378
Alexander, F., 182, 376, 384
Alliance. See Therapeutic alliance;
Working alliance
Ambience. See also Interpretation
establishment of, 385–386
interpretation and, 379–381
Antisocial character. See also
Character type and style
borderline-level functioning,
331–332
defense analysis, 247
impression management, 216
pseudoneurotics, role
reversibility, 370
Anxiety, interpretation, sequence
of, 108–109
Anzieu, D., 100
Apfelbaum, B., 94, 95, 96, 97
Arlow, J. A., 78, 81, 84, 106
Atwood, G. E., xiii, 108, 128, 143,
144, 277, 408
Authority
positive transference and, 19
transference and, 17
Autonomy, ego, therapeutic
alliance and, 49

Balint, M., 108, 379, 384
Beck, A. T., 249
Beebe, B., xxii
Benjamin, J., 312, 344
Biology
human nature and, 276–277
identity maintenance and, 284
sadomasochism, 310
sexuality and, 311
Bion, W. R., 86, 127, 219
Blechner, M., 135

Bollas, C., 202, 203–205, 276
Borderline character
defense analysis and, 235
defenses and, 93–94
holding environment, 337–338
identity diffusion, 330–331
interpretation, case report,
335–337
self psychology, 338–339
treatment, 334–335
Borderline-level functioning
crisis mentality, case report,
350–366
interpersonal relations, 346–347
role reversibility and, 331–334
world view, 349–350
Brenner, C., 52, 53, 54, 78, 79, 81,
84, 86, 87, 88, 89, 90, 91, 92,
106, 107, 235, 405
Breuer, J., 376

Case reports
borderline patient, interpretation,
335–337
Brenner, 86–93
confrontation, 148–154
countertransference analysis,
183–190
defense analysis, 129–135,
242–245, 263–273
identity maintenance, 281–283,
295–304
as illustration, 20
impression management, 220–231
interpretation, 386–395
Joe case
countertransference analysis,
191–194
introduced, 20–23
Reichian character analysis
perspective on, 36–41
self-syntonicity and, 137–142

Case reports (*Continued*)
  structural model and, 102–104
  therapeutic alliance perspective
    on, 71–75
  transference analysis, 164–168
  lavatory transference, 157–162
  Mr. Z case (Kohut), 115–120
  normality concept,
    normopathic/normotic
    illness, 203–205
  perversity, 319–327
  role reversibility
    borderline-level functioning,
      crisis mentality, 350–366
    self psychology, 339–344
  Schafer, 124–127
  stages and, 397–398
  summarization and, 3–4
  theory and, xv
Change, role reversibility and, 330.
  See also Role reversibility
Character
  narrative and, xxi
  self and, xvii
Character analysis
  benefits of, xxiii
  dangers of, xxiii–xxiv
  decline in interest in, xxvii–xxviii
  defense analysis and, 233
  defined, xxii–xxiii
  empathic character analysis
    compared, xi
  empathy and, 400–401
  here-and-now, xxix–xxx
  interactive excess, 403
  interpretation and, xviii, 375–376
  narcissistic injury and, 399–400
  negative transference and, 43–44
  perception and, xx
  Reichian, 25–41. *See also* Reichian
    character analysis
  relational context, xx–xxi
  relevance of, xxvi, xxvii
  self presentation and, 207
  severity of psychopathology and,
    329
  stages and, 397–398

therapist as character assassin,
  398–399
Character armor, 276
  defense analysis, 233–234,
    235–236
  Fenichel on, 43
  normality concept and, 217
  Reichian character analysis, 26–27
Character resistances, Reichian
  character analysis, 26–27. *See
  also* Resistance
Character type and style. *See also
  entries under specific character
  type*
  borderline-level functioning and,
    331–334
  defense analysis, 238–240
  identity maintenance and,
    285–287, 292–293
  perversity and, 312–314
  pseudoneurotics, role
    reversibility, 369–370
Childhood sexuality, Rat Man case,
  14–15
Compliance. *See* Patient compliance
Compromise, normal/pathologic,
  89–90
Conflict
  interpretation and, 79
  multiple selves, 110–111
  neutrality and, 89
  personality and, 80
  structural model and, 80–81
Confrontation
  character analysis and, xi,
    xxiii–xxiv
  Reichian character analysis, 28
  self psychology and, xii, 148–154
Consciousness
  fragmentary nature of, xix
  topographic perspective, 18
  unconscious and, 5–6, 83–84
Consensual validation, power of,
  172
Containment, premature
  interpretation, 127–128
Corrective emotional experience

countertransference analysis, 182
as noninterpretive approach, 376
Countertransference
analysis of, 169–194. *See also*
Countertransference analysis
contemporary approaches and,
xxvi
interpretation and, 382
primary processes and, 85
role reversibility,
sadomasochism, 347–348
termination and, 56–57
Countertransference analysis,
169–194. *See also*
Countertransference
case reports, 183–190
as creative construction, 182–183
dialectics and, 169
induced countertransference
concept, 172
interpersonal elements and,
183–184
intersubjectivity and, 169–170
Joe case, 191–194
Kleinian theory, 175–180
object relations theory, 190–191
relativity of the self, 173–174
resistance, of analyst, 171
role and, 174–175, 180–182
selfobject transference, 190
self-syntonicity and, 170–171,
172–173
surface to depth, 173
Cultural relativity
human nature and, 277
impression management and, 198
perversity and, 306
Cure
interpretation and, 376
self and, 113–115
working-through and, 112–113

Deep concept
interpretation and, 82–83
therapeutic alliance, 60–63
Defense(s)
analysis of. *See also* Defense

analysis
case report, 129–135
strategic thought in, 233–273
borderline patient and, 93–94
character armor, 26–27
dream analysis and, 65–67
drive theory and, 64–65
ego-syntonic to ego-dystonic
character style, 94–95
fluid nature of, 64, 65
functional definition of, 81
holistic organization of, 28
homosexuality and, 87–93
interpretation, 28–29, 67–70
positive transference defensive
function of, 17–18
self psychology and, xi–xii,
107–108, 109
transference analysis, 147
working alliance and, 48–49, 64
Defense analysis, 233–273. *See also*
Defense(s)
abreaction, 236–237
antisocial character, 247
case report, 129–135, 242–245,
263–273
character analysis and, 233
character armor, 233–234
character style, 238–240
depressive-masochistic character,
246
drive theory and, 234–235
ego, 260–261
empathy, 252–253
frozen/mobile defenses, 234
hysteric character, 245–246
identity issue and, 251–252
interpretation, of defensive
function, 237–238
multiplicity and, 241–242
narcissistic character, 246
negative transference, 259
paranoid character, 247
personality, 236
resistance, 235–236, 238, 248–249
schizoid character, 246–247
selfobject transference, 259–260

Defense analysis (*Continued*)
  self observation, 261–263
  self-syntonicity and, 247–250,
    253–254
  superego, 260
  transference resistance, 254–256
  unconscious, 240–241, 256–258
Dependence, ego-syntonic to
  ego-dystonic character style
  and, 96–97, 98
Depressive-masochistic character.
  See also Character type and
  style
  borderline-level functioning, 331
  defense analysis, 246
  impression management, 209–210
  pseudoneurotics, role
    reversibility, 370
Descartes, R., 310
Destruction of analyst, identity
  maintenance, 294–295
Developmental factors
  character analysis and,
    xxvii–xxviii
  identity maintenance, 284–285
Dialectics
  changes and, 330
  countertransference analysis and,
    169
  empathy and, xviii–xix
  hierarchical models and, 85
  theory and, xxx–xxxi
  transference analysis, 143
Diffusion. *See* Identity diffusion
Disillusionment, identity
  maintenance and, 279–280
Dream analysis
  defenses and, 65–67
  patient compliance and, 13
Drive theory
  defense analysis and, 234–235
  defenses and, 64–65

Ego. *See also* Structural model
  defense analysis, 260–261
  multiplicity of, 106–107

as participant-observer, 80,
    100–101
  principle of multiple function,
    79–80
  sexuality and, 310
  split in, positive transference, 46
  structural model and, 100
  therapeutic alliance
    autonomy and, 49
    Freud on, 47
  topographic construction of, 83
Ego psychology
  analysis of resistance and, 45–46
  character analysis and, 25
  empathy and, 77
  interaction and, 70–71
  microscopic level and, 99–100
  resistance and, 59–60, 78
  therapeutic alliance and, 55
  therapeutic relationship and, 58
Ego-syntonicity. *See also*
    Self-dystonicity;
    Self-syntonicity
  empathy and, 105
  superego and, 106
Ego-syntonic to ego-dystonic
  character style
  defenses, 94–95
  interpretation and, 96–97
  resistance, 28
  superego and, 97
Ehrenberg, D. B., 183–190
Eissler, K. R., 310
Ellis, A., 249
Empathic character analysis
  character analysis compared, xi
  empathy and, xxv
  subjectivity and, xxi–xxii
Empathy
  character analysis and, 400–401
  consciousness, fragmentary
    nature of, xix
  defense analysis, 252–253
  definitions of, xiii–xiv, xix, xxi,
    xxiii, 407–408
  dialectics and, xviii–xix, xxxi
  ego psychology and, 77

empathic character analysis and, xxv
Freudian position on, 5
impression management, 213
interpretation and, 110
negative transference and, 13–14, 123–124
objectification and, xvii–xviii
perception and, xiv
Reichian character analysis, 29–30
repetition-compulsion and, 382–383
self psychology and, xi–xii, xxiii, 141–142
self-syntonicity and, 112
structural model and, 105
subjectivity and, xiv–xv
therapeutic alliance and, 59
working-through and, 112–113
Erikson, E., 277
Error of humanity, therapeutic alliance and, 54–55

Fairbairn, W. R. D., 379, 380, 383
Fast, I., 279
Fenichel, O., xi, 43, 44, 62, 63, 64, 65, 66, 67, 78, 82, 233, 234, 378, 384, 405
Ferenczi, S., 376
Free association
impression management and, 206
Reichian character analysis, 25
resistance and, 6
therapeutic alliance and, 55–56
French, T. M., 182, 376, 384
Freud, A., 67, 77, 78, 378
Freud, S., xvi, 4–24, 24, 25, 26, 29, 30, 43, 46, 47, 49, 51, 59, 64, 70, 77, 79, 84, 86, 106, 108, 153, 198, 199, 205, 206, 209, 217, 235, 238, 240, 276, 280, 292, 305, 306, 309, 315, 376, 377, 378, 379, 381
Friedman, L., 47–48, 52
Frozen/mobile defenses, defense analysis, 234

Frustration, narcissistic alliance and, 53

Gender, identity maintenance, 279
Gill, M. M., 61, 94, 95, 96, 97, 147, 153, 254, 381, 382, 384
Glover, E., 60
Goffman, E., 205
Goldner, V., 279
Gray, P., 68, 69
Greenson, R., 48, 54, 55, 56, 57, 58, 71, 157
Grossman, W., 100
Guntrip, H., 236, 379, 380, 383

Hartmann, H., 49, 80, 99
Hierarchical models, linear models and, 84–86
Holding environment
borderline patient, case report, 337–338
nonverbal communication, as therapeutic element, 379
Holistic organization
of character, 34–35
of defenses, 28
Homosexuality
case report, 129–135
defense analysis, case reports, 242–245
defenses and, 87–93
Horney, K., 236
Human nature, psychoanalysis and, 276–277
Hysterical character. See also
Character type and style
borderline-level functioning, 331
impression management, 208–209, 219
Hysteric character
defense analysis, 245–246
pseudoneurotics, role reversibility, 370

Identity
changes and, 330
defense analysis, 251–252

428   INDEX

Identity (Continued)
  infantile sexuality and, 310
  maintenance of, 121–122
Identity diffusion
  borderline patient, 330–331
  changes and, 330
Identity maintenance, 275–304
  biology and, 284
  case report, 281–283, 295–304
  character type and, 285–287,
    292–293
  destruction of analyst, 294–295
  developmental factors, 284–285
  disillusionment and, 279–280
  gender, 279
  human nature and, 276–277
  negative transference, 291, 293
  paradox in, 287–288
  private sense of self and, 275–276
  resistance analysis, 291–292
  role reversibility and, 335
  self as illusion, 277–278
  self psychology, 283
  soul murder and, 280–281
  therapeutic relationship and,
    288–291
Impression management, 197–231.
  See also Normality concept
  antisocial character, 216
  case report, 220–231
  cultural relativity and, 198
  depressive-masochistic character,
    209–210
  empathy, 213
  free association and, 206
  hysterical character, 208–209
  manifest content, 220
  narcissism, 200–201
  narcissistic character, 213–214
  negative transference, 212–213
  normality concept and, 197–198
  obsessive-compulsive character,
    207–208
  paranoid character, 215–216
  resistance, 219–220
  schizoid character, 214–215
  self presentation, 205, 210–212

Incest, dream analysis, defenses
  and, 65–67
Individual
  human nature and, 277
  normality concept, 200
  psychoanalysis and, xvi
Induced countertransference
  concept, countertransference
  analysis, 172
Infancy, identity maintenance and,
  284
Infantile sexuality
  identity and, 310
  repression and, 306
Instinct. See Drive theory
Interactive excess, character
  analysis, 403
Interpersonal elements
  borderline-level functioning,
    346–347
  countertransference analysis and,
    183–184
Interpersonal theory, criticism
  from, 413
Interpretation, 375–395
  ambience. See also Ambience
  establishment of, 385–386
  generally, 379–381
  balance in, 377–378
  borderline patient, case report,
    335–337
  case report, 386–395
  character analysis and, xviii,
    375–376
  conflict and, 79
  cure and, 376
  defenses and, 28–29, 67–68
  of defensive function, defense
    analysis, 237–238
  dream analysis, defenses and,
    65–67
  ego-syntonic to ego-dystonic
    character style, 28, 96–97
  empathy and, 110
  Freudian position on, 4–5
  interactive excess, 403
  as interpersonal event, 381–382

management of, 384–385
multiple perspective and, 81
negative transference and, 44
noninterpretive approaches,
376–377
premature, 7–8, 127–128, 175
Rat Man case, 15–16
repetition-compulsion/empathy,
382–383
repression and, 63–64
resistance and, 6–7, 12–13, 18–19
role reversibility, 344–345
sequencing of, 82–83, 108–109,
383–384
structural model, defenses and,
67–70
subjectivity and, xvii
summarization and, 3–4
transference analysis, 155–156
transference and, 382
validation of, 13
Intersubjectivity
countertransference analysis and,
169–170
identity maintenance, 283
self-dystonicity and, 128–129
self psychology and, xiii, 143, 144
transference analysis and, 144,
146

Joe case. See Case reports
Josephs, L., xxix, 207, 371

Kanzer, M., 96, 98
Kernberg, O., xii, 93, 329, 330, 334,
335, 339, 344, 345, 348
Klein, M., 86, 154, 157, 175, 409
Kohut, H., xi, xiii, xix, xvi, xxiii,
xxv, 70, 109, 110, 112, 113,
115–120, 121, 122, 123, 124,
136, 141, 144, 148–154, 156,
157, 163, 198, 200, 214, 252,
277, 283, 285, 289, 309, 310,
329, 338, 344, 349, 381, 384, 407
Kris, E., 45

Lachmann, F., xxii
Language, ambience, establishment
of, 385–386
Lavatory transference, 157–162, 319
Layering, topographic model and,
95
Lesser, R., 135
Lewis, H. B., 105
Lichtenberg, J. D., xii, xiv
Lichtenstein, H., 121, 277, 278, 284,
287, 310
Linear models, hierarchical models
and, 84–86
Loewald, H., 52, 84, 105, 249
Loewenstein, R. M., 47, 60, 82, 83

Manifest content, impression
management, 220
Masturbation, perversity and,
306–307
McDougall, J., 202, 311
Mead, G. H., xx, 409
Memory, sequencing and, 86
Mental illness, normality concept
and, 198
Microscopic level
ego psychology and, 99–100
risks of, 98–99
Mirroring, self psychology and,
xix-xx
Mitchell, S. A., xiii, xix, xxi, xxviii,
107, 110, 131, 134, 277, 283
Mother–infant relationship
self psychology and, xix-xx
subjectivity and, xxii
therapeutic alliance and, 48
Mr. Z case (Kohut), 115–120
Multiplicity
conflict and, 110–111
defense analysis and, 241–242
of ego, 106–107
interpretation and, 79, 81
intersubjectivity and, 144
multiple function, principle of,
overdetermination and,
79–80
self psychology and, 136–137

Mutuality, role reversibility,
348–349

Narcissism
normality concept, 200–201
perversity and, 311–312
Narcissistic alliance, therapeutic
alliance and, 52–53
Narcissistic character. *See also*
Character type and style
borderline-level functioning, 331
defense analysis, 246
impression management, 213–214
pseudoneurotics, role
reversibility, 370
Narcissistic defenses
character armor, 26–27
Reichian character analysis, 34–36
self psychology and, 122
Narcissistic injury
character analysis and, 399–400
character armor and, 28
inflicting of, 29
negative transference and, 44
psychoanalysis as, 19
regression and, 404
Narcissistic neurosis, transference
neurosis contrasted, 217
Narrative
character and, xxi
psychoanalysis and, xv
Negative transference. *See also*
Positive transference;
Transference
analysis of, 120–121, 128
character analysis and, 43–44
defense analysis, 259
emergence of, 122–123
empathy and, 13–14, 123–124
identity maintenance, 291, 293
impression management, 212–213
interpretation and, 7, 18–19, 44
multiple transferences, 145
transference analysis, 157
transference neurosis and, 10
Neutrality
conflict and, 89
nonverbal interaction, 377, 378

sadomasochism and, 318
structural model and, 77–78
therapeutic alliance and, 77
transference analysis, 145–146
Nonverbal communication
neutrality and abstinence, 377,
378
Reichian character analysis and,
26
as therapeutic element, 379
Normality concept. *See also*
Impression management
analyst role and, 201–202
character armor and, 217
deconstruction of, 199–200
impression management and,
197–198
normopathic/normotic illness,
202–205
resistance, 219–220
selfobject failure, 202, 218–219
Normotic/normopathic illness,
described, 202–203

Objectification, empathy and,
xvii–xviii
Object relations theory
countertransference analysis,
190–191
criticism from, 411–413
role reversibility, 346
self and, 137, 143
self-dystonicity, 129
transference analysis, 164
Obsessional neurosis, Rat Man
case, 14–15
Obsessive-compulsive character. *See
also* Character type and style
borderline-level functioning, 331
impression management, 207–208
pseudoneurotics, role
reversibility, 369–370
Ornstein, A., 110, 147
Overdetermination, interpretation
and, 79

Paranoid character. *See also*
Character type and style
borderline-level functioning, 331

defense analysis, 247
impression management, 215–216
pseudoneurotics, role
reversibility, 370
Participant-observer, ego as, 80,
100–101
Patient compliance
dream analysis and, 13
impression management, 207–208
therapeutic alliance and, 56–57
Perception
character analysis and, xx
empathy and, xiv
Personality
conflict and, 80
defense analysis, 236
functioning of, polarities in,
198–199
Perversity, 305–327. See also
Sadomasochism
case report, 319–327
character style and, 312–314
masturbation and, 306–307
narcissism and, 311–312
sadomasochism and, 307–310
self-dystonicity and, 305
sexuality and, 305–306
unconscious and, 315–316
Phenomenology, subjectivity and,
xiii
Piaget, J., 144
Positive transference. See also
Negative transference;
Transference
authority and, 19
defensive function of, 17–18
interpretation and, 5
multiple transferences, 145
superego and, 51
therapeutic alliance and, 46, 77
transference resistance and, 17
Preconscious, unconscious and, 84
Presentation of self. See Impression
management; Self
Principle of multiple function,
overdetermination and, 79–80
Private sense of self, identity

maintenance and, 275–276
Pseudoneurotics, role reversibility,
366–374
Psychoanalysis
historical perspective, 3
human nature and, 276–277
individuality and, xvi
interactive excess and, 403–404
as narcissistic injury, 19
as narrative, xv
strategy and, xvi–xvii
unconscious and, 5–6
Psychopathology, severity of,
character analysis and, 329

Racker, H., 171, 172, 175, 176–180,
382
Rapport, Reichian character
analysis, 29
Rat Man case (Freud), 14–18, 51
Reality testing, consensual
validation contrasted, 172
Regression, narcissistic injury and,
404
Reich, W., xi, xx, xxiii, xxv, 18,
25–41, 43, 46, 70, 98, 153, 217,
233, 234, 235, 236, 255, 276,
378, 405
Reichian character analysis, 25–41
case report, 30–34
character resistances, 26–27
ego psychology and, 45–46
Fenichel on, 43–44
free association and, 25
Joe case, perspective on, 36–41
narcissistic defenses, 34–36
resistance and, 25–26
Sterba on, 44–45
Relational character analysis, xxv
Relational issues
character analysis, xx–xxi
self psychology and, xii–xiii
Relativity, historical perspective
and, 3
Relativity of the self,
countertransference analysis,
173–174

Repetition-compulsion, empathy
    and, 382–383
Repression
    function of, 108
    interpretation and, 63–64
    return of the repressed, 153, 315
    sexuality and, 305–306, 316
Resistance
    character analysis and, xi
    countertransference analysis, 171
    defense analysis, 235–236, 238,
        248–249
    ego psychology and, 59–60, 78
    ego-syntonic to ego-dystonic
        character style, 28
    free association and, 6
    here-and-now, 61
    id and, 78
    impression management, 219–220
    interpretation and, xviii, 5, 6–7,
        12–13
    interpretation of, 18–19
    Rat Man case, 14–15
    Reichian character analysis and,
        25–26
    self psychology and, xi-xii
    structural model and, 10–11
    therapeutic alliance and, 47
    therapeutic relationship and,
        58–59
    transference analysis, 147, 148
    transference as, 8–9
    transference neurosis and, 9–10
    trauma and, 110
    working alliance and, 48–49
    working-through, 10
Resistance analysis, identity
    maintenance, 291–292
Return of the repressed
    perversity and, 315–316
    self-dystonic elements, 153
Role, countertransference analysis
    and, 174–175, 180–182
Role reversibility, 329–347
    borderline character treatment,
        334–335
    borderline-level functioning,

    crisis mentality, case report,
        350–366
    borderline-level functioning and,
        331–334
    change and, 330
    countertransference,
        sadomasochism, 347–348
    holding environment, 337–338
    identity maintenance and, 335
    interpretation, 344–345
    mutuality, 348–349
    object relations, 346
    pseudoneurotics, 366–374
    self psychology, 338–339
    case report, 339–344
Rosenfeld, H., 157–162, 319, 371

Sadomasochism. See also Perversity
    borderline-level functioning,
        332–333
    countertransference, role
        reversibility, 347–348
    identity maintenance and, 335
    perversity and, 307–309
    self and, 312
    self psychology, 338–339
    source of, 309–310
    therapeutic relationship, 316–319
Sampson, H., 162, 240, 242
Sandler, J., 172, 382
Schafer, R., xiii, xv, 120, 121, 122,
    123, 124–127, 136, 405
Schizoid character. See also
    Character type and style
    borderline-level functioning, 331
    defense analysis, 246–247
    impression management, 214–215
    pseudoneurotics, role
        reversibility, 370
Schwartz, D., 135
Self
    character and, xvii
    cure and, 113–115
    identity maintenance, 121–122
    as illusion, identity maintenance,
        277–278
    object relations theory and, 137

presentation of
   character analysis and, 207
   impression management, 205
   self-syntonicity and, 210–212
private sense of, identity
   maintenance and, 275–276
relativity of, countertransference
   analysis, 173–174
unitary self, 110
Self-dystonicity
   intersubjectivity and, 128–129
   and perversity, 305
   return of the repressed, 153
Self-esteem
   self-syntonicity and, 109
   superego and, 106, 107
Selfobject, normalizing, 205
Selfobject failure, normality
   concept, 202, 218–219
Selfobject transference
   countertransference analysis, 190
   defense analysis, 259–260
   transference analysis, 163
Self observation, defense analysis,
   261–263
Self psychology
   confrontation and, 148–154
   criticism from, 406–411
   defenses and, 107–108, 109
   empathy and, xi-xii, xiii-xiv, xxiii,
      141–142
   identity maintenance, 283
   intersubjectivity and, xiii, 143,
      144
   mirroring and, xix-xx
   multiple selves, 110–111
   narcissistic defenses and, 122
   object relations and, 134
   relational issues and, xii-xiii
   role reversibility, case report,
      339–344
   sadomasochism, 338–339
   self-dystonicity, 129
Self-syntonicity. See also
      Ego-syntonicity
   countertransference analysis and,
      170–171, 172–173

defense analysis and, 247–250,
   253–254
defenses and, 108
ego multiplicity and, 107
empathy and, 112
self, presentation of, 210–212
self-esteem and, 109
working-through and, 112–113
Sequencing
   of interpretation, 108–109,
      383–384
   memory and, 86
   topographic perspective and,
      82–83
   transference analysis, 148
Sexuality
   ego and, 310
   Reichian character analysis, case
      report, 30–34
   repression and, 305–306
Sexual orientation, defense
   analysis, case reports, 242–245
Shakespeare, W., 312
Shapiro, D., 155
Shengold, L., 251
Skin ego, topographic model and,
   100
Soul murder
   defense analysis, 251–252
   identity maintenance and,
      280–281
Spence, D. P., xv, 256
Sterba, R., xi, 44, 46, 58
Stern, D., 284
Stolorow, R. D., xiii, 108, 110, 128,
   129, 131, 133, 135, 143, 277,
   339, 408
Stone, L., 379
Strachey, J., 49, 50
Structural model. See also Ego;
      Superego
   Brenner and, 86–89
   defense analysis, 260–261
   ego and, 100
   empathy and, 105
   interpretation, defenses and,
      67–70

Structural model (*Continued*)
  Joe case and, 102–104
  neutrality and, 77–78
  overdetermination and, 79–80
  Reichian character analysis, 26–27
  resistance and, 10–11, 78
  strengths of, 80–81
  surface and deep concepts, 60–63
  therapeutic alliance and, 52
  topographic model and, 78–79,
    101
  utility of, 101
Subjectivity
  empathic character analysis and,
    xxi–xxii
  empathy and, xiv–xv
  interpretation and, xvii
  phenomenology and, xiii
Sullivan, H. S., 80, 205, 277, 381
Summarization, interpretation and,
  3–4
Superego. *See also* Structural model
  defense analysis, 260
  defined, 105–106
  ego-syntonicity and, 105
  ego-syntonic to ego-dystonic
    character style and, 97
  resistance and, 78
  therapeutic alliance and, 49–51
Surface concept
  interpretation and, 82–83
  therapeutic alliance, 60–63

Termination
  countertransference and, 56–57
  narcissistic injury, inflicting of, 29
Theory
  case reports and, xv
  dialectics and, xxx–xxxi
Therapeutic alliance. *See also*
  Working alliance
  critique of, 47–48
  derivation of, 48
  ego psychology and, 55
  empathy and, 59
  error of humanity and, 54–55
  free association and, 55–56
  Freud on, 47

Joe case, perspective on, 71–75
  narcissistic alliance and, 52–53
  necessary but not sufficient
    conditions, 51–52
  neutrality and, 77
  paradox in, 52
  patient compliance and, 56–57
  positive transference and, 46
  resistance and, 47
  structural model and, 52
  superego and, 49–51
  surface and deep concepts, 60–63
  as transference, 53–54
Therapeutic relationship
  ego psychology and, 58
  identity maintenance and,
    288–291
  resistance and, 58–59
  sadomasochism, 316–319
  working alliance and, 403–404
Timing. *See* Sequencing
Topographic model. *See also*
    Structural model
  Brenner and, 88–89
  human nature and, 276
  layering and, 95
  sequencing and, 82–83
  skin ego and, 100
  structural model and, 78–79
Transference. *See also* Negative
    transference; Positive
    transference
  analysis of, 143–168. *See also*
    Transference analysis
  authority and, 17
  interpretation and, 378, 382
  primary processes and, 85
  pseudoneurotics, 366–374
  as resistance, 8–9
  as therapeutic alliance, 53–54
  therapeutic relationship and, 58
Transference analysis, 143–168
  dialectics, 143
  interpretation, 155–156
  intersubjectivity and, 144, 146
  Joe case, 164–168
  lavatory transference, 157–162,
    319

multiple transferences, 144–145
negative transference, 157
neutrality, 145–146
object relations theory, 164
resistance, 147, 148
selfobject transferences, 163
self psychology, confrontation
    and, 148–154
sequencing, 148
surface to depth in, 146–147
Transference neurosis
narcissistic neurosis contrasted,
    217
resistance and, 9–10
Transference resistance
defense analysis, 254–256
positive transference and, 17
Trauma, resistance and, 110. See
    also Narcissistic injury
Trop, J., 129, 131, 135

Unconscious
conscious and, 5–6, 83–84
defense analysis, 240–241,
    256–258
perversity and, 315–316
preconscious and, 84
repression and, 108

sadomasochism, 309–310
superego and, 106
therapeutic alliance and, 48
topographic perspective, 18
Unobjectionable positive
    transference. See Positive
    transference

Wachtel, P. L., xviii
Waelder, R., 79, 80
Weiss, J., 162, 240, 242
Wild analysis, Kleinian analysts
    and, 86
Winnicott, D. W., 236, 276, 278,
    280, 281, 284, 285, 290, 294,
    337, 346, 379, 380, 383, 384
Wolf, E. S., 114, 157, 218
Working alliance. See also
    Therapeutic alliance
defenses and, 64
resistance and, 48–49
therapeutic relationship and,
    403–404
Working-through
empathy and, 112–113
resistance, 10

Zetzel, E. R., 48